THE ETHICS OF GENETICS IN HUMAN PROCREATION

Charles Seale-Hayne Library
University of Plymouth
(01752) 588 588
LibraryandITenquiries@plymouth.ac.uk

The Ethics of Genetics in Human Procreation

Edited by

HILLE HAKER
University of Tübingen, Germany

DERYCK BEYLEVELD
Sheffield Institute of Biotechnological Law and Ethics, UK

Ashgate

Aldershot • Burlington USA • Singapore • Sydney

Published by
Ashgate Publishing Limited
Gower House
Croft Road
Aldershot
Hampshire GU11 3HR
England

Ashgate Publishing Company
131 Main Street
Burlington
Vermont 05401
USA

Ashgate website: http://www.ashgate.com

British Library Cataloguing in Publication Data
The ethics of genetics in human procreation
     1. Human reproductive technology - Moral and ethical aspects
     2. Genetic engineering - Moral and ethical aspects
     I. Haker, Hille II. Beyleveld, Deryck
     176

Library of Congress Catalog Card Number: 00-131628

ISBN 0 7546 1021 7 ✓

Printed and bound by Athenaeum Press, Ltd.,
Gateshead, Tyne & Wear.

Contents

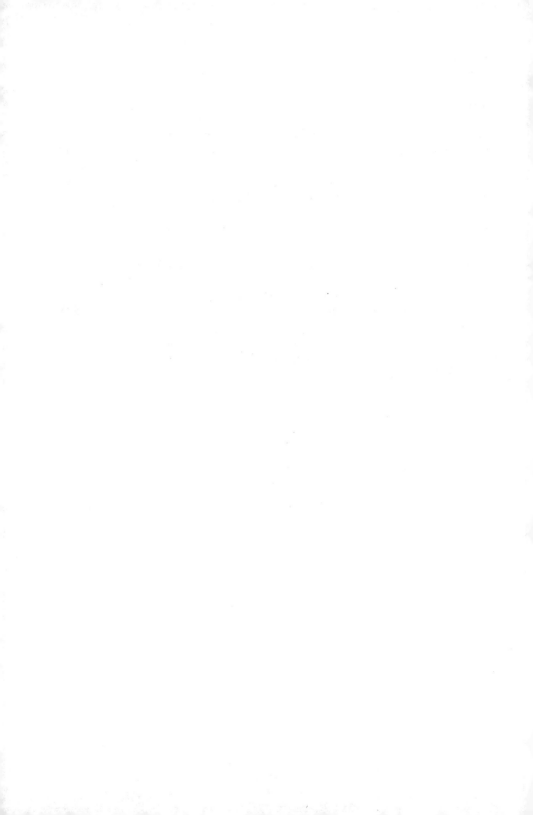

List of Contributors

Jens Badura is a member of the Post-Graduate College Ethics in the Sciences and Humanities, University of Tübingen.

Deryck Beyleveld is Professor of Jurisprudence at the University of Sheffield and Director of the Sheffield Institute of Biotechnological Law and Ethics (SIBLE).

Christian Byk is a judge and Head of the Association Internationale Droit Ethique et Science, Paris.

Ulrich Dettweiler is research assistant at the Kennedy Institute of Ethics, Georgetown University, Washington D.C.

Kris Dierickx is a postdoctoral fellow of the National Fund for Scientific Research (NFWO) at the Centre for Biomedical Ethics and Law of the Catholic University of Leuven, Belgium.

Marcus Düwell is Academic Co-ordinator of the Center for Ethics in the Sciences and Humanities at the University of Tübingen.

Eve-Marie Engels holds the Chair of Ethics in the Life Sciences in the Department of Biology, University of Tübingen.

Sigrid Graumann is a senior researcher at the Department of Ethics and Social Sciences, University of Tübingen and has been Scientific Co-ordinator of the *European Network for Biomedical Ethics* together with Hille Haker.

Hille Haker is a senior researcher at the Department of Ethics and Social Sciences, University of Tübingen and has been Scientific Co-ordinator of the *European Network for Biomedical Ethics* together with Sigrid Graumann.

Christoph Holzem is a former member of the Center for Ethics in the Sciences and Humanities, University of Tübingen.

Micheline Husson is a research assistant at the Institut d'Histoire et Philosophie de Sciences et des Techniques at the University of Paris 1 Sorbonne.

Nikolaus Knoepffler is a member of the Institute 'Technik-Theologie-Naturwissenschaften' at the University of Munich.

Regine Kollek is a professor and heads the research group 'Technology Assessment of Modern Biotechnology in Medicine' at the University of Hamburg.

Walter Lesch is Professor of Philosophical and Theological Ethics at the Catholic University of Louvain in Louvain-la-Neuve.

Gisela Lotter is research assistant at the Chair of Ethics in the Life Sciences in the Department of Biology, University of Tübingen.

Barbara Maier is a gynaecologist at the 'Salzburger Frauenklinik' and teaches medical ethics at Vienna University.

Sheila A. M. McLean is International Bar Association Professor of Law and Ethics in Medicine at Glasgow University and Director of the Institute of Law and Ethics in Medicine at Glasgow University.

Dietmar Mieth is Professor of Social Ethics and Speaker of the Center for Ethics in the Sciences and Humanities, University of Tübingen. He is Co-ordinator of the *European Network for Biomedical Ethics.*

Roberto Mordacci teaches ethics at the University of San Raffaele, Milan.

Anders Nordgren is a research scholar at the Department of Public Health and Caring Sciences (Biomedical Ethics) at Uppsala University.

Onora O'Neill is Principal of Newnham College, University of Cambridge, and Chair of the UK Human Genetics Advisory Commission.

Shaun Pattinson is a PhD student in the Faculty of Law at the University of Sheffield.

Jürgen Simon is Head of the 'Forschungszentrum für Biotechnologie und Recht bei der Europäischen Akademie für Umwelt und Wirtschaft e.V.' in Lüneburg.

Annika Thiem is a member of the Center for Ethics in the Sciences and Humanities, University of Tübingen.

Paul J. M. van Tongeren is Professor of Philosophical Ethics at the Catholic University of Nijmegen and a member of the Centre of Ethics of the Catholic University of Nijmegen (CEKUN).

Jean-Pierre Wils is Professor of Moral Theology at the Catholic University of Nijmegen and Scientific Director of the Centre of Ethics of the Catholic University of Nijmegen (CEKUN).

Hub Zwart is Senior Research Associate at the Centre of Ethics of the Catholic University of Nijmegen (CEKUN).

Preface

This volume contains the papers given in the Third Symposium of the *European Network for Biomedical Ethics* in Sheffield from January 7–9, 1999 on 'Ethics in Human Procreation, Genetic Diagnosis and Therapy', which was organised by the Center for Ethics in the Sciences and Humanities (ZEW) in co-operation with the Sheffield Institute of Biotechnological Law and Ethics (SIBLE).

The papers in this volume deal with a number of overarching issues concerning the ethics of genetics in human procreation.

In Part One, the issue of whether there is a moral right to procreate is considered by Sheila McLean (who argues that this right is only negative not positive), while Onora O'Neill addresses the extent to which parents have duties to their children in relation to the quality of their parenting (and argues that any such duties are only imperfect: a good enough parent does not have to be a perfect one).

In Part Two, Deryck Beyleveld tackles the issue of the intrinsic moral status of the human embryo and/or fetus from the standpoint of theories such as those of Kant, and in particular Gewirth, which might appear to grant intrinsic moral status only to agents (which the unborn, on evidence, are not). He argues that, because we cannot know with certainty which creatures are agents, but are categorically required by Kantian and Gewirthian theories to grant intrinsic moral status to agents, such theories must grant intrinsic moral status to the unborn in proportion to the *evidence* that they might *possibly* be agents.

In a different way, Jean-Pierre Wils' paper in Part Three also addresses the moral status of the human embryo and fetus. However, it does so from a different standpoint, which is the phenomenology (not to be confused with the psychology) of the process by which we recognise the unborn as a subject with moral status, and how various technological developments have affected this process of recognition.

In Part Four, Regine Kollek considers the general social implications of human reproduction being mediated by scientific technology, particularly in relation to the autonomy of women. She argues, centrally, that while the new technologies may appear to extend a woman's choices and give her better control of her biology, this may be an illusion. There is good reason to believe that, under current social living conditions, the new technologies impose new moral obligations on women, which may be more difficult for them to deal with than infertility or disease.

In Part Five, Marcus Düwell considers what constitutes moral reasoning in applied ethics. His most basic thesis is that applied ethics cannot be separated from the justificatory ethics (moral epistemology), because moral relativism makes it impossible to even describe moral conflicts.

In Part Six, Deryck Beyleveld and Shaun Pattinson present a comparative study of legal regulation of assisted procreation, genetic diagnosis and gene therapy in the EU States. They also consider the extent to which different approaches and regulations can be explained by different philosophical ideas about the moral status of the human embryo and fetus.

Finally, in Part Seven, the co-ordinators of the *European Network for Biomedical Ethics* provide an overview of the *Network* and indicate how the issues it raised might be followed up in the future.

Each of the papers in the first six Parts were commented upon by one or more respondents during the Symposium, and these comments were followed by general discussion. Summaries of the discussions of the papers in Parts Two to Six are given in the Annexe.

Acknowledgements

Many scholars from all over Europe contributed to the Symposium at which the papers that make up this volume were delivered, and the *Network* (co-ordinated by Dietmar Mieth) under the auspices of which the Symposium was organised was funded by the European Commission during 1996–1999. We are grateful to all who put their energy, time and money into this project.

We are especially grateful to the European Commission, particularly to Mme. Christiane Bardoux, who was always helpful and sympathetic, and to Mr. Michael von Doering of the University of Tübingen.

At the Sheffield end, we thank Beverley Jepson for helping to organise the social programme. We also very much appreciated the help of students on the MA in Biotechnological Law and Ethics at Sheffield (Fergus Malone, Prakash Modi, Karl Scheeres, Mark Taylor, and David Wengraf), in preparing the conference materials and dealing with problems that arose during the meeting. Above all, we thank Susan Wallace, who made all the travel arrangements, and Shaun Pattinson, who not only ensured that the conference ran smoothly by his efficient organisation of the helpers, but helped with the final editing of the manuscript.

At the Tübingen end, we are grateful to members of ZEW, without whose assistance the event would not have been possible (Jens Badura, Dirk Brantl, Ulrich Dettweiler, Christoph Holzem, Gisela Lotter, Christof Mandry and Uta Ziegler). We are indebted to Glenn Patten for his translations and language advice, and to Dr. Maureen Junker-Kenny for dealing with some unresolved difficulties with language. We thank Dr. Marcus Düwell for his constant support and work in the background, Dr. Sigrid Graumann for her assistance with the co-ordination of the whole *Network*, and Prof. Dr. Dietmar Mieth, not only for his hard work in planning the conference, but also for his co-ordination of all aspects of the *Network* at every stage. Above all, we are grateful to Annika Thiem, who did much of the initial editorial work, and whose help throughout the final period of the *Network's* existence was invaluable.

Deryck Beyleveld and Hille Haker

Ethics in human procreation: An analysis of some dilemmas

Dietmar Mieth

1 Introduction

Why do I, as we come to the end of a very successful network on questions concerning the ethics of human procreation and embryo research in which we have made progress in transparency and achieved better understanding of this field of applied ethics, insist on drawing to attention some dilemmas that need to be addressed in the future? I think that behind our analytical and normative thinking there are some background considerations that must be understood and become more visible than is the case in a more or less biomedical approach. I try to expose some problems concerning the limits of this approach with the intention of encouraging a follow up of philosophical and theological differentiation.

2 The scientific dilemma

On the one hand, science wants to serve knowledge itself. On the other hand, science tries to be socially useful and has a covenant with society. Modern (biological) science needs intervention in nature and instruments for this intervention. The technicalisation of science is not only a result but also a prerequisite of the practice of modern science. Therefore, freedom of knowledge has its limits; firstly, in the social acceptance of its instruments, even with respect to the theoretical aims of knowledge; and, secondly, in the acceptance of practical applications. The scientific dilemma between the insistence on freedom of knowledge, on the one hand, and the necessity of social control, on the other, is perhaps not the central question. In promoting the technicalisation of human procreation, there are always individual needs and social advantages that scientists give as reasons for this technicalisation, including health purposes, but not limited to them. This means that, in the case of biomedicine and the special case of human procreation, science is never only science. The promotion of science often has political implications, giving rise to moral options, and individual as

1

well as social preferences. The dilemma is this: science is not neutral and does not stand above given interests. But all scientists are seen as experts, even if they are only experts for their own paradigm of research and its application. They are not experts for contexts, assessments, ethics, education, and so on. But, in our societies, which have a irreversible contract with science, technology, economics, and their development, the scientific expert is often accepted as an expert for all kinds of knowledge, and this may become a temptation for scientific lobbies. You can easily imagine that a group of scientists could claim to be able to pronounce on a societal development, but you cannot imagine that a group of sociologists would propose a scientific method. Scientists are at the same time members of the scientific community and are high ranking experts just as much as they are citizens. Therefore, it is absolutely necessary to bring societal and ethical dialogue into the scientific community, and not only scientific lobbyism into society.

3   The societal dilemma: increasing individual options, pluralism, tolerance, and the lack of restrictive consensus

Modern, and even more so, postmodern societies are based on individual rights and on their protection by institutions. The liberal state corresponds to a pluralistic society that includes very different options. However, the choices that are made are often not authentic ones but follow social trends and conformity. The conformity present in the ideal of 'authenticity' is one example, the paradox that the more an atomistic concept of individualism is promoted, the more the conformity in concepts of individualisation emerges. People want to be authentic and original, but they choose the same clothes, travel and behaviour, etc., as the expression of this authenticity. Pluralism in society is—this may be a paradox—its own greatest enemy. The same paradox exists for another icon of the liberal state and pluralistic societies, i.e., tolerance. Postmodern tolerance even has problems excluding intolerance from tolerance. Because solidarity is founded on a pluralistic concept, a societal solidarity integrating many differences seems only to be possible in times of great suffering and under the pressure of negative facts (witness Chernobyl). But, in most cases, the distinction between good and evil depends on experiences and on individual or societal options that differ very much depending on the kinds of persons and groups involved. Therefore, a solidarity that goes beyond simple pluralism can only be reached by transparency of interests and argumentation, and by a common understanding through narration and memory in which convictions are formed and need to be promoted or preserved.

4 'Human life' as a controversial social construct

In the same simplifying manner in which C. P. Snow spoke of the two cultures of science and humanities, we can also speak in a heuristic sense of two mentalities in questions of biomedicine. *The biomedical mentality*, involved in the link between experimentation and clinical application, is a mentality *of hope for promotion and acceleration*. Limits are seen as self-evident—for example, that it is forbidden to create human monsters on purpose—or as limited to the present social context, or they are considered to be purely individual limitations set by virtue of specific options, for example in the case of religious groups. In that experts consider themselves responsible for the promotion of interests of health or other great aims in a constantly developing society, they often regard political opposition that opts for the exclusion of restrictions as a mixture of ignorance, conservatism, and fundamentalism. On the other hand, 'bioethics', created by scientific experts and by their philosophical 'servants', is considered to be a kind of a conspiracy against the needs and values of the people. This attitude is often articulated in, for example, Germany.

But it is not necessary to refer to the German debate. As an example of the hermeneutics of suspicion, I will refer to a lecture of Ivan Illich, given in Chicago 1989 to the Evangelical Lutheran Church in America. Ivan Illich (1992) started with the following thesis.

> *'Human Life' is a recent social construct*, something which we now take so much for granted that we dare not seriously question it. I propose that the Church exorcise references to the new substantive life from its own discourse.

For Illich, the new notion of 'life' that is so essential for modern ecological, medical and ethical discourses in the Western tradition is 'the result of a perversion of the Christian message'. In this former understanding, 'life' *(bios, zoe, vita)* means something moved by an internal teleology of the 'soul' (vegetative, sensual or intellectual). Under contemporary conditions, however, the notion of 'life' does not belong to the world of such sacred and contemplative feelings. It is a word that belongs to the field of modern management, to the language of planning so-called 'human resources'. Following Cartesian dualism, 'life' is an objectification and a field of experimental intervention and of manipulation with the intention of improvement. The context of this epistemic presupposition of an unquestioned belief in progress makes a new fetish of 'better life'. Against this background, the current struggle between the two contradictory options 'pro-life' and 'pro-choice' is also cleared up. 'Pro-life' means *'pro vita'*, whereas 'pro-choice' means the best preference for using the 'biological material' for a better quality of the self-determined 'life' of individuals. This understanding of the 'life' of individuals is still connotated with the traditional view of *'vita'*, but it is restricted to an anthropocentric view. What this discourse neglects is the connotation of non-objectivation that had primacy in the 'gospel of life', stated in the gospel as 'I am life' from Moses to Jesus. The modern view has edged out this personalistic view and considers life as a 'value', a good which must be preserved, but which can also be surpassed by social options.

Illich makes five observations about the history of life that we should not forget.

First, life, as a substantive notion, makes its appearance around 1801.

Instead of the religious and philosophical tradition of *psyche, bios* and *zoe,* the term 'biology' means 'a science of life' (Jean-Baptiste Lamarck). 'Life' is from now on a construct of organic phenomena like reproduction, genetic development and so on.

Second, the loss of contingency, the death of nature and the appearance of life are but distinct aspects of the same consciousness.

The loss of contingency here is the loss of dependent and actual connection with the breath of creation. The mechanistic model replaces the creative-processual model.

Third, the ideology of possessive individualism has shaped the way life could be talked about as a property.

It can easily be demonstrated in the debate about patenting life that life is being discussed in its 'elements' not as a 'discovery' but as a result of human 'invention', even if it is identical to its natural state. On the other hand, the instrumentalisation of human life, which we will demonstrate in the options for cloning, is clearly a result of this 'possessive individualism'.

Fourth, the fetishised nature of life appears with special poignancy in ecological discourse.

'To think' of life as a system of correlations between living forms and their habitat is a reduction of imagination and delivers life to all kinds of empirical and also virtual objectivation.

4

Fifth, the pop science fetish of life tends to void the legal notion of person.

The *distinction* between 'human life' and 'human person' created the notion of a 'human non-person', which is not a member of the so-called 'moral community'. 'The new discipline of bioethics', so Illich concludes, 'mediates between pop science and law by creating the semblance of a moral discourse that roots personhood in the qualitative evaluation of the fetish, life.'

I refer to these critical observations of Illich as an important perspective on so-called 'bioethical' questions, because we seldom are aware that, before beginning an ethical discourse, we have to 'exorcise' a language and a language politics that does not allow a truly ethical approach but rather only the semblance of it. 'Bioethics' is an invention of the scientific language of 'biology' and its derivations. This paradigm dominates ethics, legal and social responsibility. This can be demonstrated by an example: the European 'ELSA' group, which is responsible for the research projects of the European Community concerning 'ethical, legal and social aspects' of biotechnology, had 14 members in 1997. Of these, 13 were biologists and only one was a philosopher. It is clear that there is also an interdisciplinary approach to ethics and that interdisciplinarity makes sense in the ethics of sciences and new technologies. Nevertheless, the perception is not mistaken that the paradigm of the life fetish as a fetish of a scientific paradigm is strongly present in this kind of discourse.

Maybe some of Illich's assumptions are a caricature of the more pluralistic world of biology and medicine. However, this experimental approach to the basis of political power and the paradigm of scientific promotion may be helpful for reflecting on motives and presuppositions that are also present if we only speak, for example, about the necessity to help someone who experiences lack of fertility or ambiguous expectations for the health of a future child as suffering.

I think it is a fact that there is a biomedical lobby that also constitutes the background for biomedical and bioethical committees. I will not deny the fact that there are other kinds of lobbies and politically relevant pressure, too. *But the biomedical lobby is defining the language before the ethical and political debate begins.*

5 The politics of language

An example of the politics of language in 'bioethics' is a distinction made regarding human cloning. This will be important for the future of *in vitro* options for experimentation on embryos, concerning which the ethical debate will have nearly the same references as for other *in vitro* options, like PGD.

We have to differentiate between cloning techniques with the intent of *in vivo* development, that is of copying and raising humans, and cloning techniques that are limited to the *in vitro* phase, to the potential embryos before implantation. By transforming embryos into cell-cultures, particular purposes are pursued, for example in connection with therapies to prevent immune-rejection in the case of transplantation, and also in connection with the development of early forms of human organs.

At this point, we are basically talking about science fiction. But as each day passes it becomes less science fiction and more and more scientific reality. However, we are dealing with interesting situations in which a society, with the help of ethical reflection, can explicate its position before the technique as such exists. With respect to the cloning debate, various advisory groups were commissioned to present experts' opinions in order to reach ethical standards: the Clinton Commission in the USA, the already mentioned Advisory Group to the European Commission (GAEIB), and the advisory group to the German Minister of Science, in which the presidents of various research organisations participated. With regard to the cloning of human beings, a distinction was introduced in the EU advisory groups and the US Commission between so-called *'reproductive'* and *'non-reproductive'* cloning. I have already mentioned that we have to differentiate between the *in vivo* and the *in vitro* situation. Our language is not capable of grasping all new phenomena immediately. Any distinction may be misunderstood, and this might be the case with the differentiation between 'reproductive' and 'non-reproductive' cloning. 'Reproductive' means that the cloned embryo is implanted and that a human adult person develops from it. *In vitro* cloning does not yet determine whether an early embryo, which has been manipulated accordingly, will or will not be implanted. And if it is not implanted but rather used for experiments with particular long-term therapeutic goals, then this is called 'non-reproductive' cloning.

The Advisory Group of the EU came to the conclusion that 'reproductive' cloning must be prohibited. The Clinton Commission, using the same terminology, was more liberal only insofar as it demanded a moratorium 'at present.' The formula 'at the present time and the present social context' was not included in the 'conclusion' of the European Advisory Group. In my opinion, this limitation to the *present* time carries with it the assumption that the prohibition of reproductive cloning will—or at least may—be revised in the future. However, it is self-evident that every rule that we formulate under present circumstances *can* be revised in the future. Thus, whoever wants to express this specifically has ulterior motives that should be made explicit. Therefore, it can be said that in fact the Clinton

Commission declared itself in favour of a 'moratorium', whereas the European Advisory Group in favour of a strict ban, but only in the so-called 'reproductive' area. In the 'non-reproductive' area, that is, *in vitro* cultivation of cloned embryos in cell cultures, the EU Advisory Group stated that in those countries that allow experimentation on embryos (such as, e.g., Belgium or Great Britain), *in vitro* cloning should not be forbidden on condition that one is dealing with high-priority therapeutic purposes, on condition that a licensing body, that is, an ethics commission, is consulted, and finally, on condition that the manipulated embryos will not be implanted and become independent human beings. This is also the result of the British Report of the Human Embryology Authority (HFEA) and the Human Genetics Advisory Commission (HGAC) in December 1998.

Even so, I did not sign the declaration of the EU Advisory Group, because I am of the opinion that the distinction between 'reproductive' and 'non-reproductive' cloning was not decided on a *factual basis*, but was rather intended to establish a differentiation in the treatment of 'embryos' and 'humans.' In a 1994 document, I found a statement by the ministerial council of the European Council concerning tissue-banks defining how 'reproductive' and 'non-reproductive' are to be understood in this area. There, egg cells, sperm cells and embryos were considered to be 'reproductive.' Their use as tissue was to be prohibited exactly because they are 'reproductive,' that is because from them human beings could develop. In 1997, the expression 'reproductive' thus was intentionally narrowed to *implanted* embryos by the advisory group in the interest of practicability. This policy, however, was not without precedent: the difference between 'reproductive' and 'non-reproductive' had previously been introduced by an American advisory group on *in vitro* fertilisation. This I call the 'politics of language'.

Non-reproductive cloning today is often called 'therapeutic cloning', and, in my opinion, this is also politics of language. The concept of therapy or the concept of human health plays a very central role in the politics of language. Therefore, I would like to illustrate this with an example from the Human Rights Convention on Biomedicine of the European Council. Article 18(2) of the convention states that the production 'of embryos for research purposes' is forbidden. Article 12 implicitly deals with research on embryos, although it is concerned explicitly with the possibility of sex selection. It states that this selection is possible only if it serves health purposes. As an example of health purposes, sex selection in order to prevent hereditary disease is mentioned. The text does not clarify which method it is speaking about: abortion after prenatal diagnosis, embryo selection before implantation, or possibly also sex selection by centrifuging semen. At the same time, Article 12 states that these health purposes also include 'research for health purposes.' Of course, one wonders at this point what is meant by the prohibition of embryo production for research purposes in Article 18(2)? Are research purposes for health purposes, which elsewhere are always allowed, excluded. If this were the case, then the research purposes of Article 18(2) would mean little, because one could declare any research purpose in this area to have a therapeutic purpose.

With this example I want to make clear that by means of such politics of language the Bioethics Convention simply sets certain problems aside without solving them. This is a problem that we could illustrate with further examples. The Bioethics Convention, as well as its supplementary report on cloning, which was signed in January 1998, leaves the definition of what is a 'human being' to the nation states. One can imagine that, in the attempt to reach a valid European consensus, the openness of this question results in any consensus remaining unclear in a specific case. In the Human Rights Convention on Biomedicine it is not laid down what must be considered a 'human being'.

This has particular significance for the cloning of human beings. It concerns the supplementary report (January 1998), which had been so highly praised in the European press. In this supplementary report, it is stated that it is forbidden to create a human being with the intention of making him or her identical to an already living or deceased person. Someone reading this without bias assumes that this means that any human cloning is forbidden. Yet things are not so simple. The misleading political language is intensified even more by the fact that, in the second paragraph, it is stated that this prohibition is so strict that there are no exceptions. However, when consulting the official explanation things look different.

In this explanation, it is stated that one has to distinguish between three levels of cloning. First, the cloning of cells in general, which is not morally problematic. (I am also of this opinion. Cloning is not morally problematic when dealing with a living being without an independent destiny.) Second, *in vitro* cloning, where 'embryo cells' are carefully looked at. (However, behind 'embryo cells' in the totipotential state, embryos are hidden.) Third, the cloning of 'human beings'. This means that the cloning of 'human beings' is being distinguished from the cloning of embryo cells, and then it is expressly stated that this supplementary report applies only to the cloning of 'human beings'. Thus, I come back to my discussion of the politics of language. Although the expression 'non-reproductive cloning' is not used here, it is clear that the technical distinction that is meant by it— reproductive cloning (No!) and 'non-reproductive' cloning *in vitro* (Yes!)—was adopted by the Human Rights Convention for Biomedicine. Now some interpreters of the Human Rights Convention on Biomedicine claim that this is not that serious a problem, since it is stated in the aforementioned Article 18(2) that one may not produce embryos for research purposes, and this excludes the possibility of using germ cells to create embryos. However, as I have already noted, the concept of 'research purposes' is not yet clear. Is research for health purposes really excluded by this? In the future the courts will seek to clarify this since at present it is not clear from the text. Thus, one cannot assume that there is a total prohibition of human cloning in the Human Rights Convention on Biomedicine and its supplementary report. Such a prohibition does not exist at all in the framework of the UNESCO Declaration, since the Declaration only forbids 'reproductive' cloning.

It seems at least to me to be a political dilemma that we often accept in the political debate a pseudo-ethical discourse in which we speak of the ethical task 'to weigh up risks and benefits'. In most of the cases, the question of what a risk is, and what a benefit is, is a question of ethical reflection on criteria. And, therefore, this discourse is pseudo-ethical as long as the questions regarding the criteria and their foundation is not involved.

6 Pluralism, tolerance, mutual respect—not clarified

In the Opinion of the European Group on Ethics (EGE) No. 12, on Ethical Aspects of Embryo Research, of 23 November 1998, we can read about the diversity of ethical views:

> 1.23 The diversity of views regarding the question whether or not research on human embryos in vitro is morally acceptable, depends on differences in ethical approaches, theories and traditions, which are deeply rooted in European culture . . .

> 1.25 The diversity in policies and regulations concerning embryo research in the Member States of the EU reflects fundamentally differing views . . . and it is difficult to see how, at these extremes [cf. embryo as human life or as human being], the differences can be reconciled.

This kind of introduction to an opinion often leads to the result that a substantial restriction will not be acceptable.

This 'mutual respect' is also mentioned in the EGE Opinion:

> 1.27 Pluralism may be seen as a characteristic of the European Union, mirroring the richness of its tradition and asking for mutual respect and tolerance. [cf. 2.5]

In other papers 'the mutual respect' is precisely focussed on 'moral choices'. Therefore, the more liberal positions always have a political advantage. They cannot be overruled because, if they are, the respect for different approaches and moral choices is not granted. This is what in critical ethics is called a 'repressive tolerance'. You can always suppress substantial restrictions but not a substantial liberalisation.

The ethical discourse on pluralism, tolerance and compromise seems to be very underdeveloped. Most of the members of bioethical committees speak of these attitudes, but the terms remain without clarification. If pluralism is not 'laissez-faire', as the EGE said, what is its meaning? If pluralism is not the same as the lowest restrictive level, how can it be precisely defined? If pluralism has a tendency to compromise, what is the distinction to be made between a practical compromise and an ethical judgment? I am speaking from a concrete experience that I had as a member of a European Project on Pluralism (see Englert). The ethical paradox of the result was that if you take pluralism as the *'norma normans'*, you need no more ethics because all argumentation can be stopped by the norm of pluralism. And if there are no limits to pluralism, then the so called position (reclaiming pluralism) is nothing other than a kind of fundamentalism. If we try to have a moral debate with the goal of consensus, we must begin, for example, by questioning our own moral position and by reflecting on the conditions that are necessary, in order not to be dominated by the power of definition, by the politics of language, or by repressive tolerance. We must also understand that a moral conflict is not directed against the respect for persons. If ethicists have to learn something about scientific specialities and the scientific use of language, the same is true for scientists in the public debate with respect to ethics. In both cases there is a danger of too little education of the public opinion for the conditions of a moral discussion.

References

Englert, Y. (ed.), *Study on Pluralism*, 4th Framework Programme. (Available from the European Commission.)
Illich, I. (1992), 'The Institutional Construction of a New Fetish: Human Life', in Illich, I. (ed.) *In the Mirror of the Past*, New York and London.

Part One

PROCREATION AND PARENTHOOD

A moral right to procreation? Assisted procreation and persons at risk of hereditary genetic diseases

Sheila A. M. McLean

The title of this chapter invites deconstruction. Contained in it are many and varied issues of moral and ethical concern. The most important of these concerns the use of the language of rights in relation to procreation. There is little doubt that the capacity to ascribe to an interest or a desire the title of a human right elevates the interest or desire to a level which is not generally given to other interests or desires. Human rights have been the centrepiece of political and personal struggle in the 20th Century and their importance cannot be underestimated. Reproductive rights—primarily to have access to effective contraception—formed the platform for the early women's movement in the 19th Century, to be followed by more wide-ranging claims provoked by the apparent reluctance of some states to protect individuals from non-consensual intervention in their reproductive choices.[1] From the mass sterilisation programmes in the USA and Nazi Germany in the early part of this Century flowed an intense interest in the reproductive liberties of all citizens, which spawned the assertion that reproductive rights do in fact exist, and challenged legal systems to protect them.

1 A right to procreate?

However, only limited conclusions can be drawn from this. Although those seeking to use assisted reproductive techniques might well wish to claim that they have a right to do so, on analysis this claim is significantly flawed. While it may not always be inappropriate to use the language of rights in respect of reproduction, it is necessary to consider just how far that language can be stretched. Examination of the protection offered to reproductive decisions by the law may help in assessing precisely what kind of rights are in fact recognised.

An appropriate starting point for this analysis would be the United States whose policy of sterilising those thought unfit to procreate has been well documented, as has the legal position taken when such laws were challenged. Throughout the early part of this Century, crude and elementary genetic 'knowledge' was used as the basis for a programme of legislative and social reform designed to enhance the US gene pool. This eugenics policy was also adopted by, or found favour in, a number of other countries, such as the UK, France and some Scandinavian countries.[2] The intention was to maximise 'good' genes by encouraging those thought genetically fit to procreate and to reduce the spread of 'bad' genes by preventing those thought unfit from procreating. The latter group included black people, people who were 'feeble minded' and those who were recidivists. In numerous States, the superintendents of homes for the 'feeble minded' were given the authority to arrange for the sterilisation of inmates, sometimes using this as a prerequisite for release into the community, and often without even telling the individual what was happening to them (see Meyers 1971).

Perhaps surprisingly, given the existence of a written Constitution encapsulating a bill of rights, the law and the courts sided with the eugenicists even in the face of reasoned challenge. Indeed, some judges—like Oliver Wendell Holmes—generally remembered as libertarians, were prepared to hold these statutes to be constitutional. Perhaps the most famous example occurred in the case of *Buck v Bell*[3] where Holmes equated policies of compulsory vaccination with the tying of fallopian tubes, and authorised the sterilisation of Carrie Buck declaring that 'Three generations of imbeciles are enough.'[4] However, although these policies were slow to die out in the US, by the 1930s and 40s, just as Nazi Germany was embarking on its mass sterilisation programmes, there appeared evidence of a change of approach in the USA. This change came about substantially from areas of law other than those specifically dealing with non-consensual sterilisation, but had an inevitable impact on it. In cases such as *Griswold v Connecticut*[5] and *Skinner v Oklahoma*,[6] courts were invited to address the private sexual behaviour of citizens and largely concluded that this was beyond the scope of public control. Creating a so-called privacy right from a cluster of constitutional rights, the law led the way in protecting the sexual and reproductive behaviour of US citizens, with the conclusion that sexual and procreative liberty was a right worthy of vindication.

The question, however, remains what kind of right was identified and protected? In effect, the use of privacy as a model served to generate a negative rather than a positive right. Thus, and this was of direct significance to those subject to possible non-consensual sterilisation, it was a right to exercise existing capacities; not the right to procreate as such but the right to do so if one chose. Further declarations of rights in this area, such as the Universal Declaration of Civil and Political Rights[7] and the European Convention on Human Rights[8] have also referred to procreative rights, but with an interesting slant. Each proclaim the right to marry and found a family, thus arguably constraining the use of rights language within the traditional nuclear family. However, these declarations also contain only a negative right. They presume that the capacity to procreate is present and seek to prevent others from interfering with personal liberty in choosing whether or not to procreate. They do not, and were not intended to, provide a general right to reproduce. For the unmarried, reproductive choice is protected by more general tenets of these declarations concerning the inviolability of the human being. Here again, the right is protective of existing capacity rather than proactively attempting to provide reproductive capacity.

2 Rights in assisted procreation?

With or without the involvement of the law, it seems, therefore, that at best those who are unable to conceive naturally may claim a legitimate interest in reproduction but no right to have their infertility circumvented by the application of modern technologies. The State, therefore, has no obligation to provide such services. However, this does not mean that there are no moral rights which might be asserted once the techniques *are* available. Although the infertile may have no positive claim that resources should be made available, they do have rights which they can expect to see vindicated once they are. Most obviously, perhaps, they have a right not to be discriminated against in the distribution of these services. However, even this right is subject to many constraints—so many, perhaps, that it is rendered of nugatory value.

In the UK at least, there is little provision of infertility services by the National Health Service—the result, no doubt, of political and economic decisions about priorities in health care. Thus, some people are already disenfranchised from gaining access to treatment as a result of financial constraints—arguably a form of economic discrimination. Equally, in husbanding resources, doctors act as moral gatekeepers,[9] deciding which of those seeking treatment should receive it. This can lead to disbarment on a number of grounds such as lifestyle,[10] suitability for parenting and age.[11] And, of course, although not yet so widely considered in the public arena, decisions may also be made on the basis of health status. Indeed, given that health status—at least in relation to self-induced illness—has already been used as a rationing tool in respect of, e.g., smokers, it would be surprising were it not also seen to be of possible relevance in assisted reproduction. This has particular implications for genetic conditions as science can now pinpoint the gene linked to many conditions in advance of pregnancy being established, and can predict with reasonable accuracy the risks posed to any potential child. This issue will be returned to shortly, but there is one other—seldom considered—matter which must be dealt with first.

There remains a considerable shortfall between diagnosis and treatment for genetic conditions.[12] For some, this gap seems likely to expand rather than reduce. It has, for example, been said that

> Forced analysis of the human genome will cause the gap between diagnostic capacity and therapeutic failure to widen more than ever, we shall detect diseases with greater and greater precision, we shall learn to predict at the preclinical or prenatal stage without being able to do anything about the cause. (Schmidtke 1992, p. 209)

However, there is reason to hope that in the future therapy may be available for some of the most disabling conditions. Recent advances, for example in the treatment of cystic fibrosis, mean that the life expectancy of sufferers is considerably extended. With treatment, more of those unfortunate enough to have this genetic disorder can expect to survive to adulthood and may elect to parent. The fact that sufferers can now hope to live into adulthood is a tremendous clinical leap forward, but one which—in reproductive terms—may generate some additional ethical debate. Sufferers still have the gene which causes their illness and therefore are at risk of passing it on. In the knowledge of this, might not the gatekeepers of the technology decide that the infertile person with cystic fibrosis should not be offered infertility treatment because of the risk they pose to future children (and perhaps because their life expectancy may be reduced as a result of their condition)? Even given that embryos/fetuses with cystic fibrosis may be screened out pre-birth using the available screening tools, might it not be argued to be a waste of resources to supply assisted reproduction at all, given that these expensive tests would definitely have to be used, as opposed to the 'normal' infertile person where such tests may not be deemed necessary? And what of those with the gene for late onset genetic conditions, such as Huntington's Disease or breast cancer? Are they to be excluded because of the risk to future generations?[13] Although developments in gene therapy may eventually render this problem largely obsolete, we are a long way from that position yet and it must be taken seriously for the moment.

Similar problems of access may arise in respect of those who carry the gene for a particular condition but who do not themselves suffer from it. Again, pre-implantation genetic diagnosis or prenatal screening may prevent the birth of a child suffering from the condition, but at what cost? Is the deliberate destruction of embryos or the termination of pregnancies less or more morally weighty than a decision not to offer treatment to those known to be at risk of passing on a genetic disorder? This may be an even more problematic question, as carrier status is often misunderstood. Skene, for example, notes that 'In a pilot genetic screening project in Greece, carriers of the gene that causes sickle cell disease were stigmatised by their community and considered ineligible for marriage, except to other carriers' (Skene 1991, p. 238). Of course, the outcome of this policy would not be the avoidance of genetic disease but rather its encouragement, as carriers only pose a risk where they procreate with fellow carriers.

This section can be summed up as reaching the conclusion that the infertile have no right to procreate but that they may have other rights in gaining access to assisted reproduction which centre on the right not to be discriminated against. 'Old fashioned' forms of discrimination may soon be supplemented by new ones, determined by genetic make-up in an eerie reminder of the eugenic policies described above. The fact that the science is more sophisticated in the current situation, is no substitute for reasoned debate about the extent to which the interests of the infertile should be served without prejudice about parenting capacity or the welfare of potential children.

3 Avoiding the birth of a genetically damaged child

It is now intended to turn to the other questions which lie at the heart of this discussion. The fact that an individual is at risk of passing on an inherited condition may have four broad outcomes. First, the person may eschew reproduction altogether, deeming the risk to be too great. Arguably, this choice will become a less popular option as the techniques to avoid or terminate affected pregnancies become more sophisticated and more widely available. Second, the person may—using the technique of IVF—request pre-implantation diagnosis. Third, the woman may be screened in the course of an established pregnancy with the possibility of termination should the embryo/fetus be affected. Or fourth, there may be the possibility of gene therapy prenatally or post birth. The first of these decisions is an entirely personal one, and is unlikely to be a matter adjudicated or commented on in the public arena. However, the last three options merit further consideration.

According to some commentators, the use of pre-implantation genetic diagnosis is still relatively uncommon,[14] although it seems plausible that its use will continue to rise as more and more conditions can be detected. Although doubt has been expressed about this technique, for many it poses the ideal solution to potential problems. Rather than waiting until a pregnancy has been established, pre-implantation genetic diagnosis permits people undergoing IVF treatment the option of selecting only 'healthy' embryos in their bid to have children. Thus, embryos which have the gene which predisposes them to a particular condition can be discarded before conception allowing for the implantation of other embryos which are free from the gene. Not only does this provide elementary reassurance to the intending parent(s), it also avoids the need for pregnancy termination. For many, then, this is a morally less troubling situation than is abortion, since no pregnancy has been established and therefore no child has been created. However, as with all programmes designed to select the healthy from the unhealthy there are dilemmas surrounding the extent to which such selection should be undertaken. As was mentioned above, there are those for whom such a choice is still morally troublesome, making judgments as it does on the worth of a particular potential life, and raising questions about the entire enterprise of screening for genetic problems.[15]

Even more controversially, pre-implantation genetic diagnosis permits the screening out of conditions which are late onset—i.e., they will not affect the potential child until he or she is mature. Such conditions, whilst potentially very serious, need not prevent the individual from having a life which—for them—may be full of quality. For this reason alone, there is cause to be concerned about the decisions which can now confront intending parents as to whether or not to base their reproductive choice on what is currently available in therapeutic terms, or to take the gamble that by the time their potential child has reached maturity there will be therapy or even a cure available for the condition. Equally, there arises the problem of what to do with embryos which are carriers of a particular gene—that is, they themselves would never suffer from the condition, but they could pass it on to future generations if they procreate with another carrier. Few, if any of us, would choose to have a child who suffers from a genetic condition, but the impact of carrier status, as has already been seen, is poorly understood and may lead to the destruction of embryos based on the false belief that in some way they are 'unhealthy' or 'defective'.

3.2 Prenatal screening

In recent years there has been what has been described as an 'evangelistic fervour' (Stone and Stewart 1994, p. 45) for screening. For many years, older women have been the target of screening programmes because of the increased likelihood of them having children suffering from chromosomal abnormalities leading to conditions such as Down Syndrome. But our enhanced capacity to detect genetic disorders opens the door for more wide-reaching prenatal diagnosis, with—as the anticipated outcome—the termination of an affected pregnancy. Many of the problems identified with pre-implantation genetic diagnosis also apply here with the additional moral dilemma of abortion. Furthermore, there is cause for concern that the mere availability of screening will pressurise people into accepting it. In other words, what is now permissible may become effectively mandatory, with prospective parents and health care providers seeking to obviate the costs—emotional as well as economic—associated with the birth of a genetically damaged child. As Hubbard notes,

> As 'choices' become available, they all too rapidly become compulsions to 'choose' the socially endorsed alternative. In this realm, it is amazing how quickly so-called options are transformed into obligations that, in fact, deprive us of choice. (1992, p. 210)

3.3 Fetal therapy

Although still relatively uncommon, it is reasonable to assume that fetal therapy will become a treatment of choice in the future.[16] The capacity to modify genetic conditions, to replace the faulty gene, is surely a major medical advance, but again it will not be without problems. Without being critical of every medical breakthrough, it must be noted that when fetal therapy is considered, there is one other party—namely the pregnant woman—involved. In recent years, the question of women's responsibilities to their fetuses has come to the forefront of legal and ethical debate.[17] In a number of high profile cases, women have been forced into having caesarean sections partly in what has been seen as their own interests and partly in the assumed interests of the fetus. Both in the United States and in the UK, the policy of policing pregnancy and coercing women into behaviour which is against their own judgment is becoming more common, and represents a worrying trend.[18]

One case which poignantly highlights the problems of forcing women to act for the benefit of the fetus is the US case of Angela Carder.[19] This young woman with a terminal illness was forced to have a caesarean section against her wishes in an attempt to salvage the fetus. In an act which is hard to contemplate, a hastily convened court decided to override her wishes and forced her to undergo surgery. Neither she nor the fetus survived. After her death the judgment was reversed. Of the initial decision, Annas makes the following point.

> They [the doctors and the judge] treated a live woman as if she were already dead, forced her to undergo an abortion, and then justified their brutal and unprincipled opinion on the basis that she was almost dead and her fetus's interest in life outweighed any interest she might have in her own life and health. (Annas 1988, p. 25)

Of course, many—if not most—women will have no difficulty in acting during a pregnancy with the interests of their potential child firmly in the forefront of their mind. Even the invasion required if fetal therapy is undertaken would be a burden many would willingly assume if it meant that their child would be born healthy. However, for some women this will not be the case, and—if current legal attitudes can be taken as a template of society's views—these women may well find themselves coerced into decisions which they would not themselves have made.[20] The fact that we may disapprove of such women is no reason to institutionalise such an attack on their fundamental right to reject proposed therapy. As Swartz notes,

> Although it may be morally and ethically appropriate in most cases in which 1) a woman's own health would not be adversely affected and 2) the fetus is viable for the woman to make decisions that would enhance the fetus's chance for good health, legislating morality in these cases raises more questions than it answers. (1992, p. 56)

Although English courts (to the writer's knowledge no Scottish court has considered this issue) have also been prepared to authorise compulsory intervention in pregnancy, recently a court in England gave a woman leave to sue for damages following a forced caesarean section.[21] However, this case is unusual in its individual facts, and does not fit the mould described above so its status cannot be presumed to be definitive of how future judgments will be taken.

4 Having a genetically damaged child

If the ways of avoiding the birth of a genetically damaged child are controversial, so too is the decision of prospective parents to continue with an affected pregnancy. As has already been noted, the anticipated outcome of screening—pre-implantation or prenatal—is that the pregnancy will be terminated or never established. However, there are those for whom neither of these options would be appropriate or acceptable. Their choice, therefore, would be to have the child irrespective of its condition. Although people are free to make such choices, they are not without moral concern.

In exercising their right to make such choices people are deliberately bringing into the world a child who may require long term medical care. To an extent, therefore, the state—as provider of much of this care—may have an interest in not facilitating or supporting such decisions. It may seem somewhat far fetched to imagine states interfering in reproductive choice in this way, but it is by no means inconceivable that they would. Equally, others may have a role to play. In one case in the United States, for example, a woman was told by her health management organisation (effectively her insurer who would normally meet the costs of her health care) that, since the fetus she was carrying was discovered to have the gene for cystic fibrosis, they would pay for her to abort the fetus but would not pay for health care associated with a live birth. Only the threat of litigation forced them to back down.[22] Not only is it unlikely that the threat of litigation will always have this result, it is all too easy to see how this could be expanded into policy.

There are many organisations, state and private, which have an interest in reproductive choice. Like it or not, they are capable of building plausible arguments concerning their 'right' or interest to see the 'correct' choices being made. These choices need not reflect the wishes of the individual but might rather be couched in terms of the economic or other interests of the organisation or the wider community. This potential translation of reproductive choice from the private to the public has consequences which are by no means simple. As Kevles notes,

> Given that changes in individual attitudes inevitably affect the scope of institutional action, both public and private, history surely teaches that serious attention is owed the warnings, however shrill they may sometimes be, of the dissenters from the eugenic revival. (1985, p. 299)

There is, however, one further and more subtle pressure which may be brought to bear on women in these circumstances and this is the notion of reproductive responsibility.[23] It may well come to be seen as irresponsible to choose to have a damaged child, partly because of the impact on the child itself and partly, of course because of the resource problems already alluded to. From the realm of the private, reproductive choice may well re-enter the public arena as social and political policy requires the optimal use of scarce medical resources. The very real threat to procreative liberty which this would entail could be disguised by a number of other morally significant benefits which would flow from such a policy, making it difficult to argue in favour of individual choice.

And, of course, there are the so-called obligations of intergenerational justice.[24] From this perspective, people should not be permitted knowingly to pass on harmful genes to their offspring. Expressed as an aspiration, there can be few objections to this view, but expressed as a policy the potential for coercive enforcement becomes very real. Naturally, we would wish to avoid passing on to our children a condition which may cause suffering, but to require this as part of an ethical (or even legal) framework is a step too far. Indeed, even if this concept remains merely one philosophical approach to parenting, it may have an insidious influence on prospective parents, rendering them less free intellectually to reach the conclusion which is best for them and their family.

5 Conclusion

It can be asserted, therefore, that—in the absence of a right to procreate—the infertile or sub-fertile cannot claim that resources should be made available to them as of right. It is also clear that the genetic revolution poses some increased risk of discrimination against those who are in need of infertility services but who have a history of gene defects in their family. Although it has been suggested that the infertile should not be discriminated against once services are made available it is all too easy to imagine a scenario in which those at risk of passing on genetic disorders are refused services, put at the bottom of the queue or required to make hard decisions after screening. Whether or not these are morally acceptable outcomes is moot. To a large extent, our conclusion on this will depend on the ethical perspective from which we address the issue. If a rigid autonomy based argument is used then, arguably, none of these options is acceptable. People should be free to make their own decisions without coercion, and the choice whether or not to have an affected child is one which should be jealously guarded. From a more communitarian perspective however, it could be said that individual choice is not the trumping value in all situations. The general welfare of the community must also be taken into account.

It seems likely that this latter perspective will become more popular as the genetic revolution continues to tie individuals in the community closer together. Recognition of what makes us alike, and the acknowledged deficit between diagnostic and therapeutic capacity, may lead to the popularisation of ethical theories which are largely discounted by the 20th century's emphasis on individual rights. What will be the outcome of this is impossible to predict, but it is a possibility requiring serious scrutiny now, rather than after the completion of the Human Genome Project, when the ethical debate will be at best tangential to the reality of what can be done.

Notes

1. For further discussion, see McLean 1988.
2. Noted supporters, for example, included Winston Churchill and Marie Stopes. The term eugenics was coined by Francis Galton, a cousin of Charles Darwin, and its application resulted in dramatic legal and social constraints on those thought unfit to procreate.
3. 274 US 200 (1927).
4. At p. 207.
5. 381 US 479 (1965).
6. 316 US 636 (1942).
7. (1948) Article 16(1).
8. (1950) Article 12.
9. For example, s. 13(5) of the Human Fertilisation and Embryology Act 1990 effectively hands over the clinics (and therefore doctors) the right to decide who will or will not receive treatment. Minimal guidance is provided by the exhortation to consider the potential need for a father, but beyond that it appears there is no limitation on the criteria which could be applied.
10. *R v Ethical Committee of St. Mary's Hospital (Manchester), ex parte Harriott* (1988) 1 FLR 512.
11. *R v Sheffield Health Authority, ex parte Seale* (1994) 25 BMLR 1.
12. According to Friedmann 1990, 'there remains a serious gap between disease characterisation and treatment' (p. 411).
13. See Kevles 1985, p. 300: 'Private decision-making in the realm of genetic disorder and disease may ultimately lead to public consequences, and thus to demands for public regulation of reproductive behavior. A sizeable number of people may argue that the right to have genetically diseased children, or even to transmit deleterious genes to future generations, must be limited or denied.'
14. See Furedi 1995, p. 3: 'By 1995, fewer than 1150 cases of preimplantation genetic diagnosis had been undertaken.'
15. See Hubbard and Wald 1993, p. 28: 'The mind-set behind genetic testing rests on a societal view of disabilities which should not go unchallenged.'
16. See Kand 1995, p. 12: 'With the possibility of gene therapy on the horizon . . . it is probable that some parents, who in the past would have chosen prenatal diagnosis with a view to selective abortion . . . in the future will

choose neonatal or prenatal diagnosis with a view to gene treatment, should their child be affected by a treatable genetic illness.'

[17] For discussion see, for example, Harrison 1982; Gregg 1993; Ikenotos 1992; Swartz 1992; Annas, G 1986; Johnsen, D 1986; Lew 1990; and McLean 1998.

[18] See *Re AC* 533 A.2d 611 (D. C. 1987) (first decision). See also *Jefferson v Griffin Spaulding County Hospital Authority.* 247 Ga. 86, 274 S. E. 2d 457 (1981). In the UK, see for example, *Norfolk and Norwich Healthcare (NHS) Trust v W* [1996] 2 FLR 613; *Re S (Adult: Refusal of Medical Treatment)* [1988] 2 All ER 193.

[19] See note 18, supra. See also the appeal judgment in *Re AC.* 573 A, 2d 1235.

[20] For further discussion of the issues raised, see Kolder 1987, p. 1192.

[21] *St. George's Healthcare NHS Trust v S; Regina v Collins and Others, ex parte S, Times Law Report,* May 8 1998; see also *Re MB* 38 BMLR 175 (1997).

[22] This case is referred to in Elmer-Dewitt 1994, p. 39.

[23] See Whittaker 1992, p. 296: 'With the availability of genetic tests, bringing an affected child into the world could be construed by some as reproductive irresponsibility.'

[24] See Fletcher, and Wertz 1991, p. 103: 'The completion of the human genome project will provide a basis for acting on a moral obligation for future generations, a claim that has appeared weak in the past. A generation with such knowledge who neglected to use it to minimise the risks in reproduction could hardly be said to respect the requirements of intergenerational justice.'

References

Annas, G. (1986), 'Pregnant Women as Fetal Containers', *Hastings Center Report,* Vol. 16, No. 6, pp. 13–14.

Annas, G. (1988), 'She's Going to Die: The Case of Angela C', *Hastings Center Report,* Vol. 18, No 1, pp. 23–25.

Elmer-Dewitt, P. (1994), 'The Genetic Revolution', *Time,* No. 3, p. 39.

Fletcher, J. C. and Wertz, D. C. (1991), 'An International Code of Ethics in Medical Genetics Before the Human Genome is Mapped', in Bankowski, Z. and Capron, A. (eds), *Genetics, Ethics and Human Values: Human Genome Mapping, Genetic Screening and Therapy* xxiv, CIOMS Round Table Conference.

Friedmann, T. (1990), 'Opinion: The Human Genome Project—Some Implications of Extensive "Reverse Genetic" Medicine', *American Journal of Human Genetics,* Vol. 46, No. 3, pp. 407–414.

Furedi, A. (1995), 'The Progress Guide to Preimplantation Diagnosis', *A Progress Educational Trust Publication.*

Gregg, R. (1993), '"Choice" as a Double-Edged Sword: Information, Guilt and Mother-Blaming in a High-Tech Age', *Women and Health*, Vol. 20, No. 3, pp. 53–73.

Harrison, M. R. (1982), 'Unborn: Historical Perspective of the Fetus as Patient', *The Pharos*, Vol. 19.

Hubbard, R. (1982), 'Legal and Policy Implications of Recent Advances in Prenatal Diagnosis and Therapy', *Women's Rights Law Reporter*, Vol. 7, No 2.

Hubbard, R. and Wald, E. (1993), *Exploding the Gene Myth*, Beacon Press: Boston.

Ikenotos, L. C. (1992), 'Code of Perfect Pregnancy', *Ohio State Law Journal*, Vol. 53, p. 1205.

Johnsen, D. E. (1986), 'The Creation of Fetal Rights: Conflicts with Women's Constitutional Rights to Liberty, Privacy, and Equal Protection', *Yale Law Journal*, Vol. 95, No. 3, pp. 590–625.

Kand, A. S. F. (1995), 'The New Gene Technology and the Difference Between Getting Rid of Illness and Altering People', *European Journal of Sociology*, Vol. 1, No. 1, p. 12.

Kevles, D. (1985), *In the Name of Eugenics: Genetics and Uses of Human Heredity*, Penguin: Harmondsworth.

Lew, J. B. (1990), 'Terminally Ill and Pregnant: State Denial of a Woman's Right to Refuse a Cesarean Section', *Buffalo Law Review*, Vol. 38, p. 619.

McLean, S. A. M. (1988), The Right to Reproduce, in Campbell *et al.* (eds), *Human Rights: From Rhetoric to Reality*, Basil Blackwell: Oxford.

McLean, S. A. M. (1998), 'The Moral and Legal Boundaries of Fetal Intervention: Whose Right/Whose Duty?', *Seminars in Neonatology*, Vol. 3, No. 4, p. 249.

Meyers, D. (1971), *The Human Body and the Law*, Edinburgh University Press: Edinburgh.

Schmidtke, J., (1992), 'Who Owns the Human Genome? Ethical and Legal Aspects', *Journal of Pharmacy and. Pharmacology*, Vol. 44, No. s1, pp. 205–210.

Skene, L. (1991), 'Mapping the Human Genome: Some Thoughts of Those Who Say "There Should Be a Law On It"', *Bioethics*, Vol. 5, No. 3, p. 233.

Stone, D. and Stewart, S. (eds) (1994), 'Towards a Screening Strategy for Scotland', *Scottish Forum for Public Health Medicine*, Glasgow.

Swartz, M. (1992), 'Pregnant Woman *vs* Fetus: A Dilemma for Hospital Ethics Committees', *Cambridge Quarterly of Healthcare Ethics*, p. 51.

Whittaker, L. A. (1992), 'The Implications of the Human Genome Project for Family Practice', *Journal of Family Practice*, Vol. 35, No. 3, pp. 294–301.

Comment on *A moral right to procreation?*

Anders Nordgren

Sheila McLean discusses two separate but related issues in the ethics of procreation. The first issue concerns whether couples have a moral right to procreation. The second issue concerns whether to avoid or give birth to children with genetic disease.

1 A right to procreation?

McLean argues that couples only have a negative moral right to have children, i.e., no one should be allowed to interfere with their procreative efforts. They have no positive moral right to have children. This implies that involuntarily childless couples have no positive right to assisted procreation. Conversely, the State has no obligation to provide such services. On the other hand, McLean argues that once technologies of assisted procreation are available infertile couples have a positive right not to be discriminated against.

McLean's point of view raises two sets of questions. The first set is about the language of rights: is it appropriate to talk about rights in the context of procreation? If so, in what sense and to what extent? The second set of questions is: should public health care make *in vitro* fertilisation (IVF) and other forms of assisted procreation available to involuntarily childless couples? If so, to what extent?

In her paper, McLean starts with the first set of questions. I prefer to start with the second one. This has to do with my view on rights, which in my opinion only have a derivative status, not a primary one as with McLean. The proper starting point in any discussion about assisted procreation in a public health care system is whether public health care, at least to some extent, has an obligation to provide technologies of assisted procreation to involuntarily childless couples, not whether there is a universal moral right to procreation that public health care should protect.

In my opinion, public health care does have such an obligation. The main argument is that infertility clearly is a clinical disorder. It is a matter of real physiological or—sometimes—psychological obstacles to species-normal functioning. Given the uncontroversial presupposition that public health care has an obligation to give adequate treatment to patients with clinical disorders, it follows that infertility belongs to the domain of public health care. Public health care should take the suffering of these patients seriously. This is also a matter of justice. Public health care has an obligation to provide at least some means to ensure that assisted procreation does not merely become a privilege for the rich who can afford to buy such services in private health care.

However, because IVF is very expensive, and because as many as about 10 to 15% of all couples are involuntarily childless—partly due to a new lifestyle: the postponing of parenthood to the late thirties or early forties—it can be argued that public health care, due to limited resources, can only make such treatment available to a limited extent. But it should never be considered a matter of luxury care. The difficult issue is to determine the number of IVFs to be offered. This is a delicate matter of resource allocation and social justice. In most regions of Sweden—my own country—involuntarily childless couples are entitled to 1–3 IVFs with certain restrictions on the age of the woman. This is a good paradigm. Moreover, Swedish health care regulation in general is articulated in terms of obligations of health professionals, not in terms of rights of patients. This seems wise not only in a legal context but also in a moral one, and not only in health care in general but also in assisted procreation.

However, if we want to talk about moral rights in this context, they should be understood within a kind of limited contractarian framework. The positive right to procreation is not a natural, intrinsic right. If McLean means that there is no natural, intrinsic right to procreation, then I agree. Moreover, if McLean means that it is meaningless to talk about a universal right if it is not attainable for all, then I also agree. But we can talk about a right to procreation in a weaker, contractarian sense. When public health care in a specific national context—or more precisely, the health professionals working in that system—assumes the obligation to provide IVF to involuntarily childless couples, then these couples receive a positive right to IVF in a derivative sense. It is a local or limited right—not a global or universal one—restricted to the public health care system at hand.

2 Giving birth to children with genetic disease?

In her discussion of the second issue, McLean gives an overview of different options for an individual at risk of passing on an inherited condition: to eschew procreation altogether, to request pre-implantation genetic diagnosis and selection, to undertake prenatal testing followed by selective abortion, to use gene therapy on the fetus or child, and to give birth to the child. She also presents some of the moral concerns raised by the last four options. She anticipates pressures from the State and insurance companies not to give birth to children with certain genetic diseases, particularly pressures on people requesting infertility services but who have a family history of genetic disease. McLean stresses that our standing on these issues depends on whether we are committed to a view of radical reproductive autonomy or to a 'more communitarian' view according to which individual choice is not the trumping value in all situations.

I have no objections to McLean's anticipations of certain problems raised by the use of genetics in procreation. They seem well-founded. Moreover, McLean starts with the perspective of the individual. However, at the end she shifts to a more societal one. This is an important move. A key question seems to be, although not explicitly articulated: what policy on the use of genetics in procreation should the government adopt?

In this context, McLean makes a distinction between a view of radical reproductive autonomy and a 'more communitarian' view. In my opinion, the last mentioned view is too vaguely described. With regard to governmental policy on reproductive matters, there are actually two rather different 'more communitarian' approaches to be found. They both state that individual choice is not the trumping value in all situations but they do this differently. According to both views, the government has a legitimate interest in procreation. But this interest is expressed in different ways. In the first case, it is a matter of governmental steering of procreation. This view can be described as a kind of voluntary eugenics (in contrast to the mandatory eugenics in certain countries during the first half of the century). An example of a proponent in the modern bioethical debate is Philip Kitcher who in his 'utopian eugenics' argues that the government should encourage prospective parents not to give birth to children with certain severe genetic diseases (Kitcher 1996, p. 203). Other examples are LeRoy Walters and Julie Gage Palmer who want to use germ-line gene therapy, if it becomes available some time in the future, as a voluntary 'public health program' (Walters and Palmer 1997, p. 88).

According to the second 'more communitarian' view, the government should not specifically try to direct procreation but only put certain restrictions on reproductive autonomy. As with the previous view, there are different versions. The restrictions might differ in normative status. They might be legal restrictions or only governmental recommendations. Moreover, the subjects of restriction might differ. They might concern which characteristics one should be allowed to test for prenatally: very severe diseases, severe diseases, less severe diseases, minor afflictions, disease susceptibilities, late onset disorders, or non-disease traits such as sex (in the absence of sex-linked genetic risks), or intelligence (if possible in the future). They might also concern which interventions on the basis of the test results should be carried out: selective abortion, embryo selection, somatic gene therapy on fetuses, germ-line gene therapy, or genetic enhancement. An example is the view expressed in the Convention of Human Rights and Biomedicine issued by the Council of Europe in 1996. In Article 13 there is a rejection of non-disease genetic intervention and also of germ-line gene therapy. In Article 14 there is a statement against sex selection (Council of Europe 1996).

In sum, there are three different kinds of models for governmental policy on genetics and reproduction:

(1) radical reproductive autonomy;
(2) governmental steering of procreation; and
(3) reproductive autonomy with certain restrictions (see Nordgren 1998).

In my opinion, a version of the last mentioned kind of model is to be preferred. The reproductive autonomy of prospective parents is very important. Briefly stated, my main reasons are as follows: procreation is extremely valuable to the individual, reproductive issues are heavily existentially loaded, there is a pluralism and lack of consensus concerning the ethical aspects of procreation, and, finally, the history of eugenics makes not only mandatory but even voluntary governmental steering of procreation an unattractive alternative.

However, I support certain restrictions on reproductive autonomy. Prospective parents should have reproductive autonomy only within the boundaries of disease. Genetic interventions on non-disease traits do not belong to the domain of health care. Health professionals have no obligation to make such interventions. To draw the line between disease and non-disease characteristics seems more reasonable than to draw the line between serious and less serious diseases, or between some non-disease traits and others. Medicine should keep to the domain of medical conditions. In addition, the distinction between disease and non-disease traits seems much less fuzzy and includes less subjective value judgments than the other two distinctions, although it is not completely strict. An analogy is the distinction between night and day. Night differs clearly from day, although there is nightfall and dawn. Moreover, within the domain of disease traits, the unclear border between serious and non-serious diseases is a further reason to leave the choice to the prospective parents themselves. This view implies that selective abortion, embryo selection, and gene therapy on non-disease traits should be discouraged by the government.

Furthermore, the high value of reproductive autonomy implies that pressures from the State or insurance companies not to give birth to children with genetic disease should, generally speaking, be counteracted. But reproductive autonomy has also a positive side. Public health care should, at least to some extent, have the goal of providing certain reproductive and genetic facilities for those who want to make use of them.

References

Council of Europe (1996), *Convention on Human Rights and Biomedicine*, Strasbourg: Directorate of Legal Affairs.

Kitcher, P. (1996), *The Lives to Come: The Genetic Revolution and Human Possibilities*, Allen Lane: London.

Nordgren, A. (1998), 'Reprogenetics Policy: Three Kinds of Models', *Community Genetics*, Vol. 1, pp. 61–70.

Walters, L. and Palmer, J. G. (1997), *The Ethics of Human Gene Therapy*, Oxford University Press: Oxford.

The 'good enough' parent in the age of the new reproductive technologies

Onora O'Neill

1 Introduction

There have always been many ways in which to become a parent or quasi-parent. Adoptive parents, foster parents, wet-nurses and nannies, as well as many members of extended or reconstructed families and households (grand-parents, uncles and aunts, step-parents) have often acquired parental or quasi-parental roles without taking the familiar route via intercourse and conception through gestation and childbirth to assumption of responsibility for rearing a child. Twentieth Century reproductive technologies have provided numerous new routes to becoming a parent—and of not becoming a parent—that were not previously available. The new routes to becoming a parent are not, of course, anything amounting to expectations or probabilities: many are time-consuming, expensive, unpleasant and have low success rates. Nobody expects these technologies to replace the traditional route to parenthood.[1]

In general, those who use new reproductive technologies try hard to replicate as many features of becoming parents in the traditional way as possible. They want to be genetically related to their children, ideally to be the genetic mothers and fathers of their children and for the woman to be the gestational mother. They are prepared to undergo the rigours of hormonal treatment or surgical correction of infertility, or the disappointments of IVF treatment, in the quest for a child that is genetically and gestationally their own. Only when faced with infertility which cannot be overcome by such interventions, or when they fear genetic disease, will they consider donated eggs or sperm; and then they will generally want donors to look reasonably like themselves, so that lack of genetic relationship will not be obvious.[2] Only when it is clear that the woman cannot, or cannot without high risk, be a gestational mother will they consider surro-

33

gacy as a way of having a child who is (at least partly) genetically related to them.

Expense and risk apart, it is clear that would-be parents generally choose to use new reproductive technologies not to *eliminate* genetic and gestational connection, but to *secure* as much of it as they can in the face of the particular sorts of fertility, genetic or health problems that afflict them. If and when they find that they cannot replicate all the standard genetic and biological connections between parents and child, they typically regret this and seek to minimise the incompleteness of replication. Indeed, it would be hard to see the point of using reproductive technologies if would-be parents did not care at all about genetic and gestational links. For example, a couple who relied on donated egg *and* donated sperm *and* surrogate gestation in effect choose to adopt.[3] New reproductive technologies that rely on donated gametes or on surrogacy are not then seen as good ways to become parents: they are chosen only if other ways are unavailable. Nevertheless they are widely welcomed for their potential contribution to the 'procreative autonomy' of the infertile.[4]

2 'Good enough' parents

Meanwhile our conceptions of being a parent have changed and are changing. For example, in developed societies many people expect to become parents to few children, to have them later in their own lives than used to be common and to take economic responsibility for them for a remarkably long period. They also expect to delegate and to be required to delegate their formal schooling and training very largely to others; they rarely expect to work alongside their adult children. They are more anxious to ensure that their children have skills than to bequeath assets to them (even those with considerable assets live too long and bequeath them too late to secure their children's economic well-being). Despite expecting so small a role in their children's schooling and work, parents often hope to establish emotional and normative bonds with their children which will sustain a close relationship across a very long future, although they may not foresee that they are likely to survive to see their children pensioned.

Hence the questions we can raise about parenting and new reproductive technologies are doubly complex. It is not only that ways of *becoming a parent* are becoming more varied, but that ways of *being a parent*, and including the normative and emotional character of parenthood, change for many reasons. Since it is common for changes of process to change outcomes, we may wonder whether some of the changes in ways of becoming a parent could also affect what it is to be a parent.

34

In this paper, I shall consider only a few ways in which being a parent may be affected by changed ways of becoming a parent. I shall try, in particular, to trace some connections between changes in the ways in which it is possible to become a parent and some of the *normative* and (to a lesser extent) the *emotional* aspects of being a parent. Of course, those who use new ways of becoming parents may not *want* this to affect their way of being parents, and in particular may not want it to affect the emotional and normative aspects of being a parent. On the contrary, they may aspire to be parents in just the way that those who do not use new reproductive technologies are parents, or have traditionally been parents, that is to have the same sorts of emotional and normative relations to their children.

In considering how changes in reproductive technology may affect what it is to be a parent, I shall rely on a quite schematic view of the various types of normative demands usually made of parents, particularly in developed societies. The view is deliberately abstract, rather than anthropologically and socially specific, and so compatible with a wide range of locally specific views of the demands and ideals of parenthood. The reason for considering the types of normative and emotional assumptions about parents and children that are typical in developed societies as background is that (for the time being) many new reproductive technologies are likely to be used only in these societies.[5]

However, in considering the normative aspects of parenthood I do not think it is sensible to consider only those normative demands on parents which are corollaries of children's rights. There are no doubt good reasons behind the huge concentration on children's rights in discussions of the normative relations between parents and children during the last forty years.[6] Parenthood in any developed society is structured by very strong normative requirements, many of them backed by state regulation. Many of the obligations which parents (and others) have to children will be requirements to respect and to meet children's rights, often described as *perfect obligations*, meaning that they are obligations which are sufficiently well specified for them to be claimed by or on behalf of those to whom the obligations are owed.[7]

Some of the rights ascribed to children in contemporary social and legal writing, and the perfect obligations and responsibilities which mirror them, fall on parents because they fall on everybody; others are specific to the role of parent (or to other roles that relate to children).

Children (like others) may have various sorts of rights. In the first place there are the *universal negative rights* that are supposed to be claimable against all others, such as rights not to be abused or tortured or enslaved, where violators can be identified even in the absence of institutions. Many of the universal rights ascribed to children are instances of the universal negative rights ascribed to all human beings: these children's rights are human rights for those human beings who are children.[8]

Other important rights ascribed to children in contemporary social and legal writing are not universal negative rights, in that they are claimable from specifiable others, rather than from all others. Strictly speaking such rights are *special rights*, in that they depend on institutional structures to establish who owes whom what, and hence that there is a claimable right. For children, as for others, important special rights can include welfare rights, rights to subsistence, to medical care, or to education. All of these are unlike universal negative rights, in that they are not claimable against all others, but rather require institutions which ensure that some agents holding certain roles (for example: parents) or agencies (for example: states and state agencies such as schools and medical institutions) are responsible for meeting each, hence every child's claim of a certain type.[9]

The allocation of special obligations to parents is based less on formal procedures or undertakings than on the socially entrenched conception of what it is to take on certain roles or relationships or to make undertakings of less formal sorts. By contrast, the allocation of special obligations that achieve certain other rights for children—rights to schooling, rights to medical care—is often anchored in legislation and formal institutional structures.

Parents who do no more than respect or fulfil those *'perfect'* obligations that correspond to their children's universal rights and to those special rights which it is their obligation to fulfil inflict no injustice on their children. However, if this is *all* they do, their parental performance will be pretty minimal. Yet on some views of ethics, this is all that is required, and any other features of good parenting are emotional attitudes and responses rather than normative requirements, and in particular a matter of emotions and attitudes that fall under the general heading of 'care'.[10] No doubt, care for children (both in the happier and in the less happy sense of the term) is central to being a parent: but it is perhaps not best seen simply as a matter of emotion and attitude. Care too may make strong normative demands, even if there are no rights to care.

This point is overlooked by those conceptions of ethical requirements which hold that all normative demands, and hence all obligations, have counterpart rights, and that everything beyond the domain of rights is a matter either of cultural tradition, of emotional response or of chosen or preferred action.[11] Other, and in my view more plausible, accounts of ethics allow for further ethical requirements which are *obligations without counterpart rights*, often spoken of as *wider* or *imperfect obligations*.[12] If there are imperfect as well as perfect parental obligations, parents who do no more than respect their child's universal rights (for example, not to be abused) and those of their children's special rights that are rights against

36

them (for example: to food and shelter, not to be neglected) may not be very far on the road to being good parents, indeed may be failing in important parental obligations.

Like perfect obligations, imperfect obligations can be divided into those that may be held by all (universal imperfect obligations) and those which are part of specific roles or relationships (special imperfect obligations). Parents are commonly taken to have imperfect obligations of both sorts to their children: they owe them not only the care and concern which everybody is held to owe to the relatively weak and helpless, but a range of support and provision whose lack would not constitute neglect, which cannot be claimed as a matter of right, but which is of huge importance to children. Although children cannot plausibly be said to have a *right* to the cheerful dailiness of family life, to some fun and attention, to some affection and understanding, most people would think that parents have a *responsibility*, an *obligation*, to provide a home and atmosphere which provides some (culturally specific) version of all of these for their children, and that parents who do not do so fail in some of their basic obligations to their children.

In short, a parent who aimed only to respect a child's rights would not be a good parent, not even (as it is sometimes put) a *good enough parent* or *minimally decent parent*.[13] However, even parents who go some way to meeting their imperfect as well as their perfect obligations, so are 'good enough' parents, may be no more. In shouldering not only their perfect obligations but these imperfect, daily obligations, parents may well be much less than ideal or heroic parents; they may not even be particularly good parents, despite providing more than their children have a right to receive from them. 'Good enough' parents may be contrasted with super-parents (variously: ideal, heroic, supererogatory) who provide not only what their children are entitled to, and a 'good enough' degree of care and support, but an exemplary range of further devotion, care and sensitivity even in the face of extreme difficulty. Heroic and ideal parents may be rare, but are not mythical: anybody who knows families with seriously ill or disabled children may well witness shining heroism.

Still, there are many ways in which even 'good enough' parents go very far beyond mere respect for their children's rights. In accepting and fulfilling wider, imperfect obligations, 'good enough' parents usually accept not only the daily round of responsive parenting, but a view of their relationship to their children as long term, moreover as one that they will seek to sustain in the face of vicissitudes and difficulties that might destroy most relationships. The child may be ill, the illness may be a colossal burden; the child may be ill-natured; the child may be a problem at school; the child may get into adolescent troubles of every sort; the child may be a failure in later life. Nevertheless, the parent, even the merely 'good enough' parent, tries to persist.

Knowledge that the parent will persist is of great importance to a child's—or an adolescent's—sense of security and belonging: parental obligations, even when only moderately well discharged, are standardly taken to have a degree of unconditionality which is rarely matched in other areas of life. Colleagues become distant; friends grow apart, couples separate and divorce: but the world is full of examples of parent-child relationships which have survived great vicissitudes and the passing of many decades. Hence it is of great importance to understand what features of parental relationship support this degree of unconditionality of commitment. If this approximation to unconditionality is an important feature of parental obligations—and here I shall simply take it that it is—then the increasing range of ways in which parents may choose not merely whether to have children but what sorts of children to have could be of great significance: for chosen relationships are often hedged with explicit or implicit conditions.

3 Status and contract

Special obligations, whether perfect or imperfect, are often acquired obligations. Many arise from voluntary transactions such as contracts or promises or activities that establish standard expectations. However, the special obligations of parents, including those to whose performance their child has a right, are not usually acquired in these formal ways. There is no moment at which parents formally or contractually take on the massive obligations which they are taken to have, no parental contract.[14]

Rather parenthood has traditionally been taken as a status, and the duties of parents have often been spoken of as 'natural' duties: the child comes into the world as the child of an identifiable mother, and (presumptively) of an identifiable father, and thereby also with identifiable brothers or sisters, grand-parents, uncles, aunts and cousins. In many societies this belonging in the narrow circle of family brings with it determinate forms of belonging to wider circles of clan and tribe, of congregation, community, nation and state. Once a child's status as child of this mother and this father are established, their obligations are also fixed, and so too are wider ranges of obligations of those who form the family and social circles of the parents.

However, some new reproductive technologies have the potential to alter the relation between parents and children by introducing an increasing and a differing range of choice into the process of becoming a parent. As this happens, obligations that were traditionally seen as following from status

38

(as the presumptive natural parents of a child) may come to be replaced, or perhaps partly replaced, by obligations which can be traced in part to choices and voluntary transactions.

An increased range of choice in the process of becoming, or not becoming, a parent was already provided by the development of contraceptive and other reproductive technologies in the early and middle part of the century, and was extended by the legalisation of abortion in many jurisdictions in the later part of the century.[15] Absent contraception, couples can choose between sexual abstinence and—presuming they are fertile and healthy—children. With contraceptive technology, and abortion, they acquire a high degree of choice in the timing and number of their children. There is a profound difference between the lives of families where children appear with unregulated abundance and families in which they are clearly limited, planned and spaced. However, these choices do not amount to choices to have a child with specific characteristics: those who become parents by intercourse, conception and gestation, even if they plan and space their children with care, must (for example) accept the outcome of the genetic lottery.

Nor is the picture of parental obligations changed when parents rely on newer reproductive technologies which have no implication for a child's genetic and gestational connection to themselves, nor therefore for its genetic relation to an extended family, or for its membership of wider circles and communities that follow from these. Hormone treatment, fertility surgery and IVF may be traumatic for would-be parents; so too are some forms of childbirth. But from the point of view of the wider family and society these are simply processes by which a child is born.

The picture begins to change when becoming a parent is contingent in part on the results of prenuptial,[16] pre-implantation, or prenatal genetic tests which are used to avoid having a child with specific genetic or chromosomal problems, or other abnormalities. However, it can hardly be said that those who rely on genetic tests for these purposes are choosing what sort of child to have. The only characteristics they are concerned about are ones that they want to avoid, and they manage this by *not* having a child with such characteristics. Any child they do have will therefore still have been born as a result of a genetic lottery, modified only by the exclusion of one or very few possibilities. Depending on the other views and situation of those concerned, the route to achieving this may be avoidance of marriage to certain partners, the avoidance of implantation of certain pre-embryos, or not bringing certain pregnancies to term. Whichever route is used, there is either no child to be the focus of emotional and normative bonds, or a child who has the genetic heritage of and is born to the parents who bring it up. The effect of these new technologies (whatever their moral implications) are not in the main effects on the children born to couples who have used them.[17]

However, another range of new reproductive technologies introduces wider and different sorts of possibility for choosing that a child with certain characteristics shall be born. The use of donor gametes makes it possible for the infertile, for single women and for homosexual couples to have children who are genetically (partly) theirs and (partly or wholly) genetically related to chosen donors; in effect such choices are somewhat rough and ready choices about at least 50% of a child's genetic inheritance. Surrogacy makes it possible for those who cannot bear a child (whether because of health problems, or because they are men without female partners, or because of age) to have a child who is genetically connected to them. A variety of technologies make it possible to determine a child's sex prenatally—and can be used to choose the sex of children brought to term.[18] Techniques for fixing sex at conception may not be far away. Techniques for choosing a fair range of other characteristics with some degree of control are implicit in the possibility of using donor gametes, and are highlighted by the developing practice of offering for sale sperm complete with glowing descriptions, even videos, of its 'donors' ('vendors'?).[19] Techniques for more specific forms of genetic manipulation may not be far away. Human reproductive cloning,[20] which is currently forbidden or likely to be forbidden in those jurisdictions within which it is feasible, might offer the possibility of choosing a fully determinate and foreseen genetic make-up, whether that of a would-be parent or of some admired third party. The creation of chimaeras with multiple genetic parents offers another prospect of choice in the making of children.

These and other reproductive technologies are not likely to displace the tried and tested way of becoming a parent. But they clearly introduce a widening range of choice into some ways of becoming a parent. It will no doubt take a long while, and a number of hesitations before we can come to clear conclusions about their merits. Here I shall take a preliminary and somewhat sceptical look at them only from one point of view, that of the child whose inheritance they may partly constitute.

4 Parental reproductive choice from a child's viewpoint

In general, there are deep differences between those human relationships which are chosen, and those which are given. If a relationship is given, then there is usually no way of shedding it, although its obligations may be neglected. My brother remains my brother through thick and thin: whether we get on and see one another or do not, the relationship remains. More pointedly, my child remains my child whatever the vicissitudes of life, and in many jurisdictions obligations (for example: in inheritance, financial and medical matters), and the rights which correspond to those obligations, may be legally enshrined.

The same is not true of chosen relationships: whether I remain employed by a given organisation depends both on my employer and on me; either of us can bring the relationship to an end; whether I remain friends with my school mate depends on both of us.

Of course, given relationships are not invariably the best relationships; sometimes they are freighted with emotional difficulties. But they are usually taken to have a certain ineluctable permanence. A simple piece of evidence for this is the effort to which some societies and individuals may go to insist that important chosen relationships are (virtually) given relationships. For example, in many societies marriage is treated as a symbolic equivalent to a given relationship, and the relatives of the spouse are equated with 'blood' relatives (brother-in-law, mother-in-law); equally a classic way of indicating that a chosen relationship is deep and indestructible is to speak of it as if it were a given relationship ('we were blood brothers', 'we were like sisters', 'we were like father and son').

It is evident that given relationships matter deeply to people. For example, adopted persons, even when they have had happy childhoods and love their adoptive parents, often want to make contact with their birth parents. Often they speak of the longing to know their birth parents as becoming stronger with the years, and as particularly strong when they have children of their own, whose genetic grandparents are their unknown birth parents. They may also want to know of and to know any (half) brothers and sisters, or any other genetic relatives. Although one often hears of adopted parents who explain to their children that they were *chosen*, this fact clearly does not always expunge the sense of loss, the sense that *from the child's point of view*, it would have been better *not* to have been chosen, but given.

Similar issues may now arise, perhaps in more acute forms, for children born by using some of the newer reproductive technologies which leave a child with multiple and partly unknown heritage. In principle, the ignorance can be overcome. Questions are already being raised about enabling children born as a result of gamete donation to contact their genetic parents. No doubt we shall soon be discussing enabling those who are born by surrogacy to contact their gestational mothers. However, transparency could raise difficult questions for donors and for surrogate mothers: if their contribution to making the child cannot be disowned, aspects of parenthood with its heavy emotional and normative demands may come to lurk in the one-off altruism (or commerce) of egg donation or surrogacy, or even in the one-off insouciance (or commerce) of sperm donation. The very emotional and normative aspects of traditional parenthood which

41

users of donated gametes, surrogacy (or cloning) hope to attain for themselves may be dissipated by the resulting child having or developing a sense of (also) belonging elsewhere.[21]

Do we have an adequate model for these problems in the experiences, happy and unhappy, of foster families and adoptive families?[22] I suggest that there are significant differences. Foster children and adopted children generally understand that their birth parents did not plan to put them in this situation. The unwanted pregnancy, the breakdown of family life or of parental health that precipitated a decision to place for adoption or fostering are none of them likely to have been deliberate; sometimes they were decisions of public bodies, and strenuously resisted by the birth parent(s). Even a child who was rejected by its birth parent(s) was not usually had in order to reject it. Adopted and fostered children have to face facts that they may find harsh, and in searching for their birth parents may find rebuff and disappointment of many sorts. But they do not have to face the fact that their genetic or gestational parents (or, hypothetically, the person(s) from whom they were cloned) *planned from the start not to have any connection, not to take on any of the emotional and normative demands of parenthood.* Nor do they have to face the thought that the parents who have brought them up *planned from the start for this absence of genetic or gestational links to be the case.* Increase in choice for adults—'procreative autonomy' (or 'reproductive autonomy') exercised in these ways—may seem unaccountable to children born of those choices, who may feel that they have been rejected by their genetic and gestational parents (or, hypothetically, by those from whom they were cloned) and that this rejection was not merely aided and abetted but planned by the parents who brought them up.

Nevertheless, in considering how using new reproductive technologies may affect the ways in which people can be parents, standards must not be set too high. After all, those who take the traditional route from conception to gestation to childbirth often turn out to be no more than 'good enough' parents (sometimes not even that), so more cannot reasonably be asked of those who take a different route. Yet it would be foolish not to acknowledge that this different route is not only different but harder, a route that may make it more difficult to be even a 'good enough' parent. The difficulties that can arise when parental obligations are reassigned to foster or adoptive parents may not fully reveal the ways in which the planned reassignment undertaken in using certain new reproductive technologies may be hard. Fostering and adopting are essentially responses to crisis, and so quite different from uses of new reproductive technologies that disrupt standard genetic and gestational links. In fostering and adoption decisions parental duties are reassigned because parental capacities, or willingness to discharge them, have failed or are predicted to fail, often in radical ways.

Children can often look on their adoption as a result of the unforeseen even unforeseeable misfortunes of their birth parents, and their adoptive parents may be seen as rescuing them from intolerable situations. It may be harder for children to see a *plan* to bring them into the world with a confused and ambiguous heritage[23] and without contact with their genetic parents or gestational mother as amounting even to 'good enough' parenting.

In trying to understand the problems of the new technologies, by which some children may have to face the fact that a confused heritage was planned for them, it may also be useful to consider whether chosen relationships tend to become conditional relationships. We are well aware that contractual and other voluntary relationships are conditional: non-performance on either side may be grounds for complaint, for redress and ultimately for ending the relationship. Would widespread use of those new reproductive technologies which embody most parental choice lead us to revise our views of the character of parenthood, and to see it too increasingly as conditional on the child having and displaying certain planned characteristics?

This is presumably the worry that underlies the thought that advances in reproductive technologies may lead people to want 'designer' babies, and to reject a child who does not measure up to the intended 'design'. This fear arises with the use of donated gametes, of genetic manipulation and (hypothetically) of cloning. In some cases parents might be judged to have chosen not merely to have a child, who at least looks vaguely like them, but specifically to have a child with determinate characteristics. From the child's point of view, even if it likes having the characteristics, any thought that it has been chosen to have those characteristics may not be a happy one. If a child is wanted for its intelligence, or its sporting prowess, or its genetic connection to a celebrity, then he or she may feel pushed to live up not only to parental ambitions (like many another child), but to the parental design. A quite distinctive and conditional conception of parental commitment might emerge, in which parental duties are felt (by the child? by the parent?) to be contingent on achieved resemblance and performance. We know all too well from twin studies that even natural clones do not resemble one another in all ways. It is quite certain that getting the gametes of the famous, even cloning the famous, will fail to reproduce the fancied phenotype. As parental relationships are increasingly chosen relationships, there may be a risk of sliding towards a increasingly conditional view of parenthood.

5 Tentative conclusions

It is hard to estimate the degree of disruption a multiple heritage may bring. Will would-be parents who plan to have children of confused or ambiguous heritage be 'good enough' parents if their way of proceeding is acceptable not only to them but to their extended families? Will they be 'good enough' if they greatly desire the birth, although their extended families cannot accept the child as part of the family? Or is an arrangement 'good enough' provided all parties accept the normative demands of parenthood and any wider familial or social obligations? Or would an important corollary and requirement of moving to greater transparency about origins be the acceptance of some parental bonds and obligations by donors of gametes and surrogate mothers?

Such questions suggest that there may be an important difference between those new technologies which assist infertile couples in begetting and bearing a child, and those which are based upon the deliberate creation of a child with multiple heritage. Where parents rely on medical intervention (surgery, hormone treatment, IVF) to achieve a pregnancy it would seem that nothing differs *for the child*, who is still and all the genetic, gestational and social child of one set of parents. Things may however be different when parental contributions are split, or genetic manipulation takes place. Some new reproductive technologies may give a child grounds to feel not only that the parents who bring it up are not fully its parents (as fostered and adopted children may feel), but that this was something that they planned; others may leave a child feeling that it was had for the sake of a particular characteristic. The parents who bring up a child conceived from donor gametes, or gestated by a surrogate mother, let alone a child who was genetically manipulated or cloned, cannot claim that they rescued him or her from an intolerable situation, as foster and adoptive parents often can. They brought into existence a child who may later experience its confused and perhaps ambiguous heritage as distressing, even damaging. These considerations suggest that appeals to 'reproductive autonomy' should not be the only or central concern in regulating reproductive choice.

John Harris has argued that considerations of fairness must also be borne in mind: although reproductive autonomy might be limited for good reasons it should not be more limited for some than for others. If we do not restrict the reproductive autonomy of the readily fertile, we should not restrict the reproductive autonomy of the less fertile.[24] At first thought the appeal to fairness may seem plausible: given our lax attitude to irresponsible reproduction by the fertile we should be just as lax, or relaxed, about possibly irresponsible reproduction by the infertile. Most societies deal prospectively with foreseeable parental irresponsibility only by interventions of limited effect such as education and persuasion, then use state power retrospectively to remove children from parents who actually endanger or damage them. This asymmetric pattern of regulation has high costs for the children of irresponsible parents. But it is presumably pursued and tolerated not because irresponsible child-bearing commands approval or is seen as a protected expression of 'reproductive autonomy', but because (where education and persuasion fail) reproduction by the fertile can be prospectively prevented only by very grave infringements of personal liberty. When the barrier to reproduction is infertility, it may be easier to limit parental responsibility prospectively without comparably grave—or even any—restrictions of personal liberty, as is standard practice in fostering and adoption decisions. If some reproductive techniques burden children with a confused, even an ambiguous, heritage and parents with added difficulties, their regulation and even their prohibition need not be wrong.

Mere appeals to 'reproductive autonomy', or to fairness, cannot then establish that the infertile—or others—have a right to reproduce by whatever means. There are in fact good reasons for great caution about the validity of claims to 'reproductive autonomy', in the use of reproductive technologies which create confused or ambiguous heritage, and for careful study of the actual experience of any children born by these methods.

Notes

[1]	Some speculative writers have imagined that if wholly artificial reproduction became possible it would be the method of choice. See for example, Huxley 1994; and Firestone 1970.

[2]	A striking practice that symbolises the aspiration for genetic connection has been that of mixing donated sperm with the sperm of the infertile man who is to be the social father—as if the mingling might impart fertility, or the infertile sperm impart its characteristics to the donated sperm.

[3]	They would differ from other adopters only insofar as they 'commission' donors and surrogate mother, and in doing so could, for example, choose to have a child with a direct genetic or gestational connection either to relatives (hence indirectly to themselves) or to chosen others.

[4]	For the phrase 'procreative autonomy' see Dworkin 1993, p. 160. For an approach to reproductive issues centred on the concept of 'reproductive autonomy' see Harris 1993.

[5]	Although contraception and abortion are widely used in some less developed countries, the only novel reproductive technology more used in developing than in developed societies is SDT (sex determination and termination). When elites in developing societies use other new technologies, they typically travel to the first world to do so.

6   *The U. N. Declaration of the Rights of the Child*, adopted by the U. N. General Assembly in 1959, is a basic, influential but opaque document: hazy about children's liberties, rhetorically maximalist about the benefits children should receive and evasive about who holds the obligations that are the indispensable counterparts of all and any children's rights. For philosophical discussion of children's rights, see O'Neill and Ruddick 1979; and Archard 1993, which includes a useful bibliography.

7   For some discussion of differences between perfect and imperfect obligations, see O'Neill 1996; and O'Neill 1998, pp. 445–463. For aspects of the historical background, see Schneewind 1990, pp. 42–63.

8   It may seem odd to stress this point, yet a lot of writing on human rights painstakingly insists that humans of specific sorts also have these rights—as though the matter had been in doubt among those who agree that there are human rights. The point is admirably made by Naomi Mitchison in her Amnesty Lecture (1999, pp. 93–100).

9   For a wider development of this analysis of rights and obligations see O'Neill 1996, Chapter 5.

10 Gilligan (1982) initiated extensive discussion of care and many claims that care and related virtues provided a distinctive, possibly an alternative or even superior, approach to ethics to that provided by theories of justice. Inevitably, discussions of children and families has been a central focus for the 'ethics of care', and mothering (or parenting) have sometimes been seen as paradigmatic of an attitude of care which provides a model for action in seemingly unrelated areas.

11 Communitarians and some virtue ethicists are keen on the idea that central moral relationships are *embedded in cultural traditions*; liberals and in particular libertarians on the idea that they are *voluntary* or *chosen*.

12 See the reference in fn. 8 supra.

13 The phrase 'good enough parent' has had a wide if rather imprecise currency both in psychoanalytic and in ethical writing on families. For some psychoanalytic sources see the work of D. W. Winnicott, as well as Bettelheim 1995. The ethical literature focuses on the idea that parents need to do more than respect children's rights, although they are not required to be ideal parents. See Ruddick 1979; and O'Neill 1988. Writers who base all of ethics on the category of rights have difficulty with the idea of a 'good enough' parent and sometimes use the locution 'minimally decent' in lieu of 'good enough'. See, for example, Thomson 1986; where she refers to 'minimal decency' repeatedly and to the 'Minimally Decent Samaritanism of the mother' (ibid., p. 18).

14 There are exceptions, in particular when parental obligations are shed or reassigned: adoptive and foster parents become parents by formal procedures. Some writers have tried to detect a parallel between parental and contractual

46

obligations. For example, Hobbes writes in *Leviathan* of the infant 'submitting' to its mother in the state of nature; see discussion by Carole Pateman (1988).

[15] For a recent if incomplete history of the development of contraception, see Clarke 1998.

[16] For example, prenuptial Tay Sachs testing among orthodox Jewish communities in New York City, and prenuptial Thalassaemia testing in Cyprus.

[17] A rather different worry is that those who choose to avoid having a child with certain characteristics may come to have negative feelings about persons with those characteristics. However, their thinking may go in the converse direction: they may be trying to avoid having children with characteristics about which they *already* have negative feelings.

[18] See fn. 5 supra. This possibility is worth noting here in that choice of a child's sex differs from using genetic tests to avoid a specific disorder because so many traits are sex-linked.

[19] A more neutral term may be 'sperm provider'. See Daniels 1988. Daniels argues that the role of sperm provider has not been adequately acknowledged. For a sense of current practices in the sale of sperm and for further evidence of that sperm providers may seek a 'voice' in the lives of children they beget see also the advertising by sperm banks on the internet.

[20] The phrase is taken from the 1998 joint report of two UK government bodies, the *Human Fertilisation and Embryology Authority* and the *Human Genetics Advisory Commission*, which distinguishes the use of cloning technologies for human reproduction from their use for other purposes such as the creation of tissues.

[21] Could the trend to transparency be ended in favour of a return to secrecy which denied children knowledge about their genetic origins? This seems unlikely, given that medical practice will increasingly enable, even require, people to know parts of their genetic inheritance.

[22] Step families are another case where parental choice fixes relationships for children in ways which they may find difficult. However these choices are a less apt comparison since they are usually made some distance into a child's life and typically have many other complicating features.

[23] A child's heritage may be viewed as confused as soon as the roles of genetic, gestational and genetic parent do not coincide. It is not only confused but ambiguous when its parent(s) are also related to it in other ways: for example, where the gestational or the genetic mother is also an aunt, or the genetic father an uncle, or where one parent is also a twin sibling.

[24] This might be seen as an appeal to reproductive fairness rather than reproductive autonomy; John Harris (1998) argues for both.

References

Archard, D. (1993), *Children: Rights and Childhood*, Routledge: London.

Bettelheim, B. (1995), *A Good Enough Parent: The Guide to Bringing Up Your Child*, Thames and Hudson: London.

Clarke, A. E. (1998), *Disciplining Reproduction: Modernity, American Life Sciences and The Problem of Sex*, University of California Press.

Daniels, K. (1988), 'The Sperm Providers', in Daniels, K. and Haimes, E. (eds), *Donor Insemination: International Social Science Perspectives*, Cambridge University Press: Cambridge.

Dworkin, R. (1993), *Life's Dominion*, Harper Collins: London.

Firestone, S. (1970), *The Dialectics of Sex: The Case for Feminist Revolution*, William Morrow and Co: New York.

Gilligan, C. (1982), *In a Different Voice: Psychological Theory and Women's Dependence*, Harvard University Press: Cambridge, Massachusetts, 2nd edition 1993.

Harris, J. (1998), 'Rights and Reproductive Choice', in Harris, J. and Holm, S. (eds), *The Future of Human Reproduction: Ethics Choice and Regulation*, Clarendon Press: Oxford, pp. 5–37.

Huxley, A. (1994), *Brave New World*, Chatto and Windus: London.

Mitchison, N. (1999), ' "Women Are Like Cold Mutton": Power, Humiliation and a New Definition of Human Rights', in Jeffries, A. (ed.), *Women's Voices, Women's Rights*, Westview Press: Oxford and Boulder, pp. 93–100.

O'Neill, O. (1988), 'Children's Rights and Children's Lives', *Ethics*, Vol. 98, pp. 445–463.

O'Neill, O. (1996), *Towards Justice and Virtue: A Constructive Account of Practical Reasoning*, Cambridge University Press: Cambridge.

Pateman, C. (1988), *The Sexual Contract*, Polity Press: New York.

Ruddick, W. (1979), 'Parents and Life Prospects', in O'Neill, O. and Ruddick, W., (eds), *Having Children: Philosophical and Legal Reflections on Parenthood*, Oxford University Press: New York, pp. 124–137.

Schneewind, J. B. (1990), 'The Misfortunes of Virtue', *Ethics* 101, pp. 42–63.

Thomson, J. J. (1986), 'A Defense of Abortion', reprinted in J. J. Thomson, (ed.), *Rights, Restitution and Risk*, Harvard University Press: Cambridge, Massachusetts, pp. 1–19.

United Nations (1959), *Declaration of the Rights of the Child*, UN General Assembly: New York.

Comment: *When are parents 'good enough'? Some ethical aspects of parenthood in the age of genetics and of new reproductive technologies*

Walter Lesch

The careful descriptions, distinctions and reflections presented by Onora O'Neill have convinced me so much that it would be a rather strange and artificial exercise to construct my contribution according to the strict rules of the genre of a critical and controversial comment. The following considerations try to suggest some additional points in a similar line of argumentation by exploring the manifold implications of the simultaneously rich and vague concept of the 'good enough' parent.

Moral philosophers and theologians often run the risk of speaking about problems that do not directly belong to the academic sphere of public discourse with its clearly defined topics. Why should we publicly discuss ethical aspects of parenthood that are usually considered to be a *private* affair? Whenever public institutions intervene in family issues, this is a sign of great difficulties and conflicts that cannot be resolved within the family system itself. The 'normal' form of dealing with ethical problems of parenthood only concerns the parents and children immediately involved and is not part of a general debate. On the other hand, reflections upon family life have always been an integral part of moral, social and political philosophy. Families are institutions of public interest and objects of political campaigns and decisions. They are traditional forms of life. But in a pluralistic society they are no longer the only possibility for living together as parents and children. This diversification of life styles and ways of becoming a parent may be an additional reason for theoretical confusion and uncertainty where the status of moral reasoning is at stake. Assisted reproduction and genetic tests unavoidably imply interests outside the inner circle of the traditional family setting.

When future parents ask to have access to genetic knowledge, they need the help of specialists who should know what kinds of tests are to be offered and whether there is still something like 'forbidden knowledge'. Such a problem does not only occur in the rare case of pre-implantation diagnosis. The difficulty is already present when we ask whether future parents should be tested before becoming parents. Are their genes 'good enough'? Or will their reproduction be a burden for themselves, for their child, for society? I certainly will not enter into a detailed discussion of the controversial topic of 'eugenics' here. But we cannot completely disregard this concrete biological aspect of the qualification of 'good' parenthood: the material of reproduction.

Of course the stimulating notion of the 'good enough' parent is taken, as far as I see, from a more innocent context. It was the British paediatrician and psychotherapist Donald W. Winnicott who introduced the idea of the 'good enough' mother into the analysis of maturational processes in early childhood. Winnicott knew very well that there are no completely ideal mothers (and fathers), but there are parents who are able to respond intuitively to the elementary needs of their little daughter or son (see Winnicott 1965). They would be 'good enough' if they managed to encourage the baby to keep on discovering the world by means of illusions of omnipotence. Parents who intuitively know the right moment at which to interact with their children in an appropriate way are to be considered as 'good enough' concerning a child's emotional development, even if such parents are not at all heroes in every respect.

I just want to remind us of this old-fashioned concept of the 'good enough' parent because it demonstrates the distance between the requirements of parenthood in the age of psychotherapy and in the age of genetics. The multiplication of the meanings of the simple word 'good' is going on with an alarming speed and reaches a new quality on the biological level of our genetic constitution. Going beyond the original meaning of the notion coined by Winnicott, and in order to put it in a provocative way, we could now ask: when are parents genetically good enough? When are children genetically good enough? And who should decide about the evaluation of these qualities and the consequences of such an evaluation?

I wonder whether moral philosophers can arrive at more than tentative conclusions in this complex field of research. We have not yet fully understood and accepted the 'genealogy of morals'. Are we already prepared to construct a new 'ethics of genealogy' in the concrete sense of human reproduction, filiation and parenthood?

1 Moral implications of parenthood

There are a lot of traditional answers to the dilemmas of family ethics within the framework of comprehensive doctrines such as Catholic moral theology. For more than thirty years now we can find there the key notion of 'responsible parenthood'. But once again it does not help us to cope with the challenges of the new reproductive technologies. The ideal of 'responsible parenthood' was meant to offer a flexible response in attitudes towards contraception. A couple who want to avoid becoming parents or want to have only a few children would act in a responsible way if they made use of so-called natural methods of contraception. In other words, the regulation of reproduction is not categorically condemned. It is even recognised as a necessity in extreme demographic situations of poverty and population explosion.

The profound conviction behind the idea of 'responsible parenthood' is ultimately a certain concept of parental obligations towards the 'gift of life' (see Gruber 1995). Even without a Christian background most myths and metaphors that we use when we speak about parenthood revolve around this central point: the conception and birth of a child are to be kept out of the realm of calculativeness and instrumental reason. A child is a gift (given by whom?) that illustrates the mystery and the sanctity of life. Don't be afraid that I am planning to switch to an esoteric discourse at this point. I only want to draw our attention to the fact that our everyday concept of parenthood is highly ambiguous because (for more than just sentimental reasons) we stick to the mystification of an extraordinary experience of heteronomy: a child's overwhelming otherness (see Van Tongeren 1995). But at the same time we start to realise that this gift no longer is given: it is up to us to express our wishes, to shape the gift, to influence it, to manipulate it. This would be an expression of the parents' nearly absolute autonomy. Even if conception, pregnancy and birth can no longer be exclusively understood as processes that must not be influenced in any way, the quest for new reproductive technologies is still paradoxically motivated by the desire to have this outstanding experience of being a parent. With Onora O'Neill I suppose that the spectacular wish for a 'designer' baby is not the rule, but rather the exception.

Parenthood is still largely accepted as a *status* with all its moral implications ('natural' duties) and is not conceived as the medically assisted and supervised *contract* that guarantees the perfect child (with the possibility of giving it back in the case of an unsatisfactory result). Nevertheless there is a new range of choice because of the introduction of reproductive technologies and genetic tests with which we can influence the outcome of the lottery of genes. All this does not radically change the moral obligations of parents; it changes the ways of *becoming* a parent.

Of course the legal question of how to regulate intergenerational relations gets more and more complex when social parents are not necessarily both biological parents. But this situation is not so new. There are enough examples of such legal regulations before the era of genetics. The moral aspects of the new ways to parenthood seem to be more intricate. I want to try to locate them in the triangle of parents, children and society with medicine as a part of the social structure.

2 Children's rights, parental ideals and social interests

In this (simplified) version of the social system, children have their own status as individuals and bearers of rights (see Théry 1996). They are certainly not anybody's property (see Smith 1983), and should from the beginning be respected in their right to privacy (see Botkin 1995). They are not just part of a family, but persons who have the right to know where they come from and (at a certain age) to decide where they want to go. This kind of individualism is often connected with a small family consisting only of mother, father (or even only one parent) and a child. If there are brothers and/or sisters their special interests have to be taken into consideration as well.

Most parents have the self-ideal of being a good mother and a good father. At least they sincerely wish to be 'good enough', even if they often fail to accomplish their own ideal of having a consistent moral identity (see Back and Beck-Gernsheim 1990). Society's interventions are limited to the cases in which parents are not only not good enough but obviously bad. This would be the case of a clear violation of the child's rights. In order to react to such disasters of abuse, there are compulsory measures that even allow for separating children from their parents. And in order to avoid a child's suffering under the influence of incompetent social parents, there are, for instance, long lists of criteria for adoption that are largely regulated by the experts' interventions and the points of view of specialists in the fields of psychology, education, social work and law.

All these measures are likely to be accepted even when there is a feeling of injustice at the fact that the 'normal' case of parenthood is subjected to fewer requirements than those that adopted parents have to meet. If some of the high standards for adoption were generalised, a lot of people would lose their 'licence' to be a (good) parent. We are now just starting to realise that the new reproductive medicine has an even more important gatekeeping function than the conventional social means of regulating fostering and adopting. Medicine is no longer just a therapy for biological disorder; it is beginning to change our definition of 'good' parenthood, because it seems to be increasingly elaborating the elements of a precise heritage.

52

3 The ideology of enhancement and the logic of avoidance

In the current bioethical debate the dangers of new reproductive technologies in connection with genetics are usually referred to as the ideology of enhancement, which could be described as the unlimited desire to make things better and to eliminate the burden of biological imperfection. Of course we should take care not to denounce enhancement in general, because it is an integral part of human civilisation (see Parens 1997). On the other hand, there is a new dimension introduced by genetics and the need for ethical consideration does exist (see McGee 1997). Nevertheless it seems that the key question is not so much the logic of improving life that could be affected by certain handicaps but the logic of avoiding the birth of children that will be affected by major difficulties. In other words, is there a duty to avoid the birth of children with hereditary genetic diseases? (See Steigleder 1998.) If this observation is true, the progressing methods of prenatal and pre-implantation genetic diagnosis are contributing to a paradoxical shift in our ideas of parental love. This would no longer be characterised in the first place by the duty to take care of a child, but by the obligation not to give birth to a child with a severe disease, because there are so many diagnoses without corresponding therapies (see Lesch 1998). Will parents be able to be 'good enough' for such children? We can easily imagine different degrees of pressure concerning this logic of avoidance and the role medicine will play in setting new priorities and declaring the standards of health.

4 Liberal and communitarian points of view

The new developments lead to a number of challenges to moral argumentation and demonstrate the limits of the current distinction between liberal and communitarian types of theory. Liberals who used to emphasise the individual's rights must now explain whether they mean the parents' or the child's autonomy (including the moral status of the embryo) (cf., Botkin 1995), and how they want to balance them. Communitarians who are traditionally in favour of family values cannot deny the interaction between family life and its social, political and economic framework, which will influence the readiness to respect the rights of children born with severe handicaps. Whose autonomy? Whose rights? Whose obligations? The standard version of the antagonism between rival moral theories does not give a satisfying answer. The same complexity can be observed in feminist approaches that are very sensitive to the effects of increasing procreative liberties (see Ryan 1990). When liberal thought rediscovers the moral importance of the family this must not necessarily be a turn to more conservative positions. It just shows that the evaluation of bioethical problems in the context of reproductive medicine and genetics also depends on our pre-understanding of good or 'good enough' parenthood (see Castelain-Meunier 1998).

5 Guidelines for 'good enough' parents?

Nevertheless it will be difficult to give a list of concrete guidelines for 'good enough parents'. It would already be an important step towards a contextualised parental responsibility to be aware of the wrong ideals to avoid. These are mainly generated by the scientifically unfounded belief in the possibility of shaping a person's design and destiny in a far-reaching way (see McGee 1997). Ethics cannot take the place of counselling or therapy in the clinical context, but it could help us to get a broader view of practical reason and its rational and emotional contradictions. And, as I would like to add with a certain degree of self-criticism, it should be prepared to move from general considerations to the discussion of hard cases that might transform our reserved scepticism into a greater understanding of some future parents' desires and fears. All this indicates that the question raised by Winnicott in a quite different context continues to point to an acute problem of parenthood and the ideal of unconditional love.

References

Beck, U. and Beck-Gernsheim, E. (1990), *Das ganz normale Chaos der Liebe*, Suhrkamp: Frankfurt a. M.

Botkin, J. R. (1995), 'Fetal Privacy and Confidentiality', *Hastings Center Report*, Vol. 25, No. 5, pp. 32–39.

Castelain-Meunier, C. (1998), *Pères, mères, enfants*, Flammarion: Paris.

Gruber, H.-G. (1995), *Familie und christliche Ethik*, Wissenschaftliche Buchgesellschaft: Darmstadt.

Lesch, W. (1998), 'Zur ethischen Problematik von pränataler Diagnostik und Präimplantationsdiagnostik', *Salzburger Theologische Zeitschrift*, Vol. 2, No. 2, pp. 141–155.

McGee, G. (1997), 'Parenting in an Era of Genetics', *Hastings Center Report*, Vol. 27, No. 2, pp. 16–22.

Parens, E. (1997), 'Is Better Always Good? The Enhancement Project', *Hastings Center Report*, Vol. 28, No. 1, special supplement.

Ryan, M. A. (1990), 'The Argument for Unlimited Procreative Liberty: A Feminist Critique', *Hastings Center Report*, Vol. 20, No. 4, pp. 6–12.

Smith, J. F. (1983), 'Parenting and Property', in Treblicott, J. (ed.), *Essays in Feminist Theory*, Rowman and Allanheld: Totowa, NJ, pp. 199–210.

Steigleder, K. (1998), 'Müssen wir, dürfen wir schwere (nicht-therapierbare) genetisch-bedingte Krankheiten vermeiden?', in Düwell, M. and Mieth, D. (eds), *Ethik in der Humangenetik. Die neueren Entwicklungen der genetischen Frühdiagnostik aus ethischer Perspektive*, Francke: Tübingen/Basel, pp. 91–119.

Théry, I. (1996), 'Les droits de l'enfant', in Canto-Sperber, M. (ed.), *Dictionnaire d'éthique et de philosophie morale*, Presses Universitaires de France: Paris, pp. 490–493.

Van Tongeren, P. (1995), 'The Paradox of Our Desire for Children', *Ethical Perspectives*, Vol. 2, No. 2, pp. 55–62.

Winnicott, D. W. (1965), *The Maturational Processes and the Facilitating Environment*, Hogarth Press: London.

Part Two

MORAL PROTECTION OF THE HUMAN EMBRYO AND FETUS

The moral status of the human embryo and fetus

Deryck Beyleveld

The following positions constitute the political map of the debate on the moral status of the human embryo and fetus.

'Pro-Life': The embryo-fetus has full moral status, equal to that of any adult human, from the moment of conception; or

'Pro-Choice': The embryo-fetus has no intrinsic moral status (i.e., no moral status solely by virtue of its own characteristics).[1] Such status is only acquired at birth or even beyond and, when acquired, is acquired to the full extent possible. Until then, any moral status the embryo-fetus has is derived indirectly from the moral status of those with intrinsic moral status; or

'Compromise': The embryo-fetus has, to begin with, a minimal intrinsic moral status, which increases with its development during gestation. Full moral status is, however, achieved only at birth or beyond.[2]

In this paper, I apply the moral theory of Alan Gewirth (1978) to decide which of the 'pro-life', 'pro-choice', or 'compromise' positions should be espoused. In Gewirthian theory, the supreme principle of morality is the 'Principle of Generic Consistency' *(PGC),* which requires all agents and prospective agents[3] to grant generic rights[4] to all agents. Gewirth demonstrates that the *PGC* is categorically binding on agents by showing that agents deny that they are agents if they do not accept the *PGC* and act in accordance with it.[5] *En route* to proving this, Gewirth proves that an agent denies that it is an agent if it does not consider the sufficient reason why it has the generic rights to be that it is an agent. Consequently, agents deny that they are agents if they do not grant the generic rights equally to all agents (regardless of any of the characteristics they or other agents might contingently possess). So, no additional or stronger generic rights can be conferred on agents by their having characteristics not necessarily possessed by all agents.

Unless agents have a compelling reason to consider the embryo-fetus to be an agent from the moment of conception as they have to consider any adult human to be an agent, Gewirthians must reject the 'pro-life' position—which usually rests on the idea that human life (biologically defined) is the sufficient condition for having full moral status. But which of the 'pro-choice' or 'compromise' positions must Gewirthians espouse?

This paper has five parts. In Part One, I outline Gewirth's argument to the *PGC*. In Part Two, I suggest some contingent and indirect ways in which the embryo-fetus might be protected by the *PGC*. In Part Three, I present Gewirth's view (1978, pp. 142–144), which is shared by Klaus Steigleder (1998), that it is dialectically necessary for agents to accord intrinsic (i.e., direct or non-derivative) moral status to the embryo-fetus

(i) *as a partial agent* (which has some of the characteristics needed to be an agent to at least some degree, without having sufficient of these to the degree needed to be an agent) in proportion to the degree to which it approaches being an agent;[6] and

(ii) as a potential agent.

I argue that Gewirth's use of the analytic 'Principle of Proportionality'[7] to demonstrate (i) is unsound, and that (ii) cannot possibly be true. Thus, James F. Hill (1984, p. 190) is probably right that non-agents *as such* can, at most, have derivative moral status.

However, in Part Four, I argue that it does not follow that the *PGC* does not accord *the embryo-fetus* intrinsic moral status in proportion to its ability to display the characteristics of an agent. Because agents cannot know with *absolute* certainty that the embryo-fetus is not an agent, the *PGC, in its application,* requires that the embryo-fetus be regarded as possibly an agent. Furthermore, through precaution, the *PGC* requires this possibility to be taken seriously in proportion to the degree to which the embryo-fetus has characteristics relevant to empirical judgment of its status as an agent. In addition, because evidence that the embryo-fetus is a potential ostensible agent is relevant to such judgment, *under precaution,* such evidence confers a degree of moral status both on its own and when added to considerations of proportionality. Gewirth and Steigleder are right about the intrinsic moral status of the embryo-fetus, but for the wrong reasons.

In Part Five, I argue that a full picture of the moral status of the embryo-fetus requires more than adding the intrinsic moral status conferred by proportionality and potentiality under precaution to that securable by derivative considerations. Proportionality and potentiality under precaution interact with derivative considerations in mutually reinforcing or qualifying ways.

I conclude that, although individual actions affecting the embryo-fetus must be considered on a case by case basis, Gewirthian theory supports a 'compromise' position on the moral status of the embryo-fetus.[8]

1 Gewirth's argument to the *PGC*

Gewirth argues from the claim of an agent to be an agent within the first-person perspective of that agent. It is appropriate for anyone considering the argument to imagine that he or she is that agent ('I'). The argument can be summarised as follows.

By claiming to be an agent, I claim (by definition)[9]

(1)   'I do (or intend to do) X voluntarily for a purpose E that I have chosen'.

Because E is my freely chosen purpose, I must accept

(2)   'E is good',

meaning only that *I* attach sufficient value to E to motivate me to pursue it. If I do not accept (2) then I deny that I am an agent—which is to say that it is *dialectically necessary* for me to accept (2).[10]

(3)   'There are generic features of agency'.

Therefore, I must accept[11]

(4)   'My having the generic features is good *for* my achieving E *whatever E might be*' ≡ 'My having the generic features is categorically instrumentally good'.

Because I value my purposes proactively, this is equivalent to my having to accept

(5)   'I categorically instrumentally ought to pursue my having the generic features'.

Because my having the generic features is necessary for me to pursue my having the generic features, I must hold

(6)   'Other agents categorically ought not to interfere with my having the generic features *against my will,* and ought to aid me to secure the generic features when I cannot do so by my own unaided efforts *if I so wish'*,

which is to say,

(7)   'I have both negative and positive claim rights to have the generic features' ≡ 'I have the generic rights'.

It follows (purely logically) that I must hold, not only (7), but also

(7′)   'I am an agent → I have the generic rights'.[12]

Consequently, it follows (purely logically) that I must hold

61

(8)   'All agents have the generic rights'.

Since I deny that I am an agent by denying (8), every agent denies that it is an agent by denying (8). Thus, (8) is dialectically necessary for every agent.

2 Arguments for derivative status

2.1 Indirect vicarious protection—the embryo-fetus as part of its mother

The embryo-fetus (post-implantation until birth) is part of its mother's body. *As such,* to harm it is to harm its mother. Hence, its mother's permission is required for any procedures involving it.

However, as a part of its mother, the embryo-fetus has special features. It is different from one of its mother's arms or legs, because (at present, at any rate) her arms or legs (unlike the embryo-fetus) cannot be removed without lasting disability to her. If there were direct duties of the mother not to harm herself in Gewirthian theory,[13] then this would not protect the embryo-fetus, as it would her arm. *Merely* as a part of her body, the embryo-fetus is more like a tumour that spontaneously removes itself at some point.

Thus, *merely as a part of its mother,* the degree to which she values and cherishes it (or the opposite), and what she is prepared to do to or for it, will be decisive in what may or may not happen to the fetus. Of course, matters are complicated if the embryo-fetus must be granted intrinsic moral status (see Part Five), and what the mother may do with the embryo-fetus is, in any case, also limited by duties she has to other agents; but, for simplicity, such complications are, here, to be taken as read.

2.2 Indirect vicarious protection—the embryo-fetus as the property of its parents

Whether an agent owns parts of its body, even after they have been removed from it, is one of the most contested issues in bioethics. In my view, Gewirthian theory supports a strong 'property-in-my-body' thesis.[14] *On such a basis,* it might be argued that not only the mother of the embryo-fetus, but also its father, and, indeed, all its ancestral genetic relatives should, in principle, have some control over the embryo-fetus (in proportion to their contribution to its genetic makeup), and that their desires to protect it are capable of protecting it.

However, this is not so. Once a child attains full moral status, it cannot be the property of anyone. So, its genes, which were once the property of its parents must be regarded as having been gifted to it. Consequently, its grandparents and other removed ancestors cannot claim *any* ownership of the embryo-fetus.

Once a fertilised ovum has implanted, it becomes part of its mother's body. At this point, *assuming that the embryo-fetus has no intrinsic moral status,* although its father retains his property right, its mother becomes the custodian of the embryo-fetus because her part-of-my-body claim takes precedence. Hence, any serious claim that the father has to the embryo-fetus can only apply before implantation (thus to embryos produced for *in vitro* fertilisation.)[15] Even then, the mother should have the greater claim, both because her genetic input to the embryo-fetus (through contributing the mitochondrial DNA) is greater and because she incurs greater risks in production of an *in vitro* embryo.

2.3 Indirect vicarious protection—the embryo-fetus as the beneficiary of contractual undertakings

The generic rights are 'will claim-rights' (which is to say that agents may waive the benefits and protections guaranteed by these rights).[16]

This suggests that, e.g., Catholics may (even if a requirement to do so is not dialectically necessary) grant the embryo-fetus protections (equivalent in weight to generic rights, or even exceeding them), by optionally imposing the correlative duties on themselves.

An obvious difficulty with this suggestion arises if attempts are made (e.g., through legislation) to impose these duties on agents who are not willing to accept them, because no societies exist in which there is absolute consensus. It is possible to deal with this by the 'method of consent' involved in 'indirect applications of the *PGC*', by which democratic decisions may be imposed on those who do not agree with them.[17] However, this has limits; for it is impermissible for the *PGC* to grant the embryo-fetus (or any other being) protections that *override* the conflicting generic rights of non-consenting agents, as doing so contradicts that being an agent is sufficient for maximal moral status.

2.4 Indirect vicarious protection—protection of the embryo-fetus as a means to virtue

In Gewirthian theory, the virtues must be regarded as character traits that dispose one to comply with the requirements of the *PGC,* or that inhibit one from violating them.[18]

It is arguable that to show disregard for the well-being of the embryo-fetus is evidence of a cruel character. Even if the embryo-fetus has no intrinsic moral status, it is similar in many outward ways to human agents. From fairly early on, it looks like a 'little person'. Thus, one might expect (though this requires empirical evidence, which might be culturally specific) that insensitivity to the well-being of the embryo-fetus will correlate with relative insensitivity to the generic rights of human agents. Additionally (or alternatively), cultivation of sensitivity to the well-being of the embryo-fetus might be a means to maintain the virtue of being sensitive to the sufferings of human agents.

2.5 Indirect vicarious protection—protection of the embryo-fetus as a means to protect the sensitivities of agents

Most human agents have strong protective feelings towards unborn children. There is an evolutionary explanation for this, as it is quite plausible that protective feelings for the young, including the unborn, confer an evolutionary advantage. Consequently, to show disregard for the well-being of the embryo-fetus is to cause great distress, even psychological damage to those who have natural, and, indeed generally beneficial emotional responses. Most importantly, to cause them this damage is to violate their generic rights. Again, the embryo-fetus is to be granted protection as a means to protect the generic rights of agents.[19]

2.6 Indirect self-connected protection—protection of the embryo-fetus as a means to protect it as a future agent

Even if the embryo-fetus has no intrinsic moral status as a potential agent, it can, in being a potential agent, have moral status as a *future* agent. For example, it is arguable that a pregnant mother should not smoke because this will damage, not merely the embryo-fetus (putatively a potential agent), but the agent that the embryo-fetus will become if it develops normally. In this sort of argument, the embryo-fetus gains protection indirectly from the generic rights of an agent. However, this agent is a very special agent—it is the agent that the embryo-fetus itself will or might become.

Unless the embryo-fetus has intrinsic moral status, this kind of argument is strictly limited to cases where there is an intention by its mother to nurture the embryo-fetus to agent status. It will not, by itself, protect the embryo-fetus from being terminated before it reaches such status. However, where the intention to nurture the embryo-fetus to agent status is part of the intention that characterises the action being assessed, considerations of 'futurality' may be deployed with considerable force.[20]

3 Arguments for intrinsic moral status I

3.1 The embryo-fetus as a partial agent—the Principle of Proportionality

Gewirth states the Principle of Proportionality as follows.

> When some quality Q justifies having certain rights R, and the possession of Q varies in degree in the respect that is relevant to Q's justifying the having of R, the degree to which R is had is proportional to or varies with the degree to which Q is had. Thus, if x units of Q justify that one have x units of R, then y units of Q justify that one have y units of R. (Gewirth 1978, p. 121)

According to Gewirth, this principle is necessarily true. Given that it is dialectically necessary for agents to take being an agent as sufficient justification for having the generic rights (in full), that it is dialectically necessary for agents to grant the generic rights in part to partial agents in proportion to how close they are to being agents is to be demonstrated by substituting 'being an agent' for Q and 'the generic rights' for R in this principle.

As I have argued elsewhere, however, this principle (as stated) is not necessarily true.[21] While *it is* necessarily true that, when having Q justifies having R, and the possession of Q varies in degree in the respect that is relevant to having Q's justifying the having of R, the degree to which R is had is *a function* of the degree to which Q is had, it cannot be inferred (without further conditions being imposed) that having R is *such a* function of having Q that, if having x units of Q justify that one have x units of R, then having y units of Q justify that one have y units of R for *all* values of x and y.

It is also better to make explicit the conditions that must be satisfied for possession of Q to vary in degree in the respect that is relevant to having Q justify having R. Thus, with it being understood that R can be any property at all, the Principle of Proportionality should be stated as

> When having some quality Q justifies having some property R, and the extent of having Q *sufficient* to justify having R in full is *not necessary* to justify having R to any extent at all, the degree to which R is had is a function of the degree to which Q is had.

By his Argument from the Sufficiency of Agency,[22] Gewirth has shown that being an agent (defined as having purposes that one acts for) is necessary and sufficient for having the generic rights *in full*. While having purposes that one acts for is an *invariant* relational property, to have this

65

relational property it is necessary to have particular capacities and properties (generic capacities of agency). While agents have all the generic capacities of agency to the degree needed to have this relational property, partial agents have the generic capacities of agency to a lesser extent. Gewirth claims that the Principle of Proportionality shows that the degree to which partial agents have the generic rights depends upon the degree to which they have the generic capacities of agency.

This may sound plausible, but it is false. This is because having the generic capacities of agency to the degree needed to be an agent is not only necessary (and sufficient) to have the generic rights in full (so that agents with the generic capacities of agency to degrees greater than that needed to be an agent cannot, thereby, acquire the generic rights to a greater extent), *it is necessary to have any generic rights at all.* This is because, as derived, the generic rights are will claim-rights; i.e., those who have them can always, by their free choice, waive the benefits that exercise of the generic rights entitles them to—provided only that they do not, thereby, neglect or violate their duties to other agents. This is not a function of an arbitrary espousal of the will theory of rights. It derives from the fact that, in the argument to the *PGC,* agents are required to claim the generic rights for themselves, not because they are required to value the generic features of agency for their own sakes, but as instrumental to their pursuit or achievement of their purposes whatever these might be. But, in order to be able to freely waive the benefits of a right, one must have the capacities needed to be an agent. Thus, partial agents cannot have any generic rights.

This objection cannot be evaded by acknowledging that partial agents cannot have any generic rights *strictly speaking,* and claiming, instead, that the Principle of Proportionality nonetheless shows that partial agents have 'quasi-generic rights' (unwaivable protections correlative to duties of agents not to harm partial agents, or to assist them in need) in proportion to their approach to being agents. The Principle of Proportionality can only license inferences about the *quantity* of predication of a quality, it cannot (by itself) license inferences that *alter the quality* of what is predicated. To claim that the Principle of Proportionality licenses inferring that, because *agent*s have the generic rights in full, partial agents have quasi-generic rights to some extent, is to commit 'the fallacy of disparateness'.[23] To have a quasi-generic right is not to have a generic right to some extent. It is to have a different quality of protection from that granted by a generic right.

Thus, if it remains possible that it might be dialectically necessary for the embryo-fetus, *as a partial agent,* to be granted quasi-generic rights, this cannot be because the Principle of Proportionality, operating on the premise that agents are to be granted the generic rights, requires partial agents to be accorded quasi-generic rights.

3.2 The embryo-fetus as a potential agent

According to Klaus Steigleder

> human beings who are not yet agents must possess moral significance for agents for the sufficient reason that they possess the potentiality to become agents. The agent has to attribute to herself dignity by virtue of being an agent. Therefore agency necessarily represents for her an evaluatively and normatively outstanding quality. For it confers on her and every other agent a morally outstanding and unsurpassable status. Now, if a being has the potentiality to become an agent and the agent is aware of this capacity, then the agent must see a morally relevant connection between such a being and herself and her dignity. . . .
>
> . . . It is not possible that agency can possess unsurpassing significance for the agent and in the other case [potentiality for agency] no significance at all. For the agent to judge otherwise would be inconsistent. (1998, pp. 241–242)[24]

But *why must* an agent see a morally relevant connection between a potential agent and itself? *Why* is an agent *necessarily* being inconsistent if it claims that it has full moral status but a potential agent has none? Steigleder does not tell us.

Now, we must remember that Steigleder is claiming that agents must (on pain of denying that they are agents) grant that potential agents, intrinsically, have at least *some* moral status (i.e., that they have at least some intrinsic moral status *for the sufficient reason that they are potential agents*).

Agents possess two kinds of properties: those they necessarily have by virtue of being agents, and those they possess only contingently.

Being an agent is sufficient for full moral status, and possession of characteristics that are necessary for agency is necessary for full moral status. Thus, properties that agents necessarily possess are undoubtedly morally relevant in being necessary for full moral status. However, we have seen that it cannot be inferred *directly* from this that such characteristics are sufficient for some intrinsic moral status.

On the other hand, if a characteristic is only contingently possessed by an agent, then it cannot be morally relevant as being either necessary or sufficient for *full* moral status. Nor can it be morally relevant as being either necessary or sufficient for *some* intrinsic moral status. It is *logically impossible* that an agent could deny that it is an agent by refusing to accept that possession of a property that agents do not necessarily possess is sufficient for some intrinsic moral status.

Now, agents are not mere potential agents (non-agents that are possessors of the potential to become agents). They may once have been mere potential agents, but if so, they no longer are. Being a mere potential agent is not a necessary property possessed by agents. It is not even a contingent property possessed by agents. In fact, it is a property that cannot possibly be possessed by agents. If one is an agent then one is not a mere potential agent and if one is a mere potential agent then one is not an agent. *Ergo,* it cannot possibly be true that it is dialectically necessary for agents to grant that being a mere potential agent, *as such,* is sufficient for the possession of at least some intrinsic moral status.

Therefore, whatever connections might exist between being an agent and being a mere potential agent, even if some of these connections are *in some sense or senses* necessary connections,[25] and even if this can consequently be said to impart moral relevance *of some sort* on being a mere potential agent, it categorically cannot follow from this that *being* a mere potential agent, *as such,* is sufficient to confer at least some intrinsic moral status.

4 The argument for intrinsic moral status II: the embryo-fetus as a possible agent—proportionality and potentiality under precaution[26]

The position we have reached is that, while it is dialectically necessary for agents to grant full moral status to agents, it cannot be dialectically necessary for agents to grant any intrinsic moral status to potential agents *as such,* and (at the very least) it has not been shown that it is dialectically necessary for agents to grant intrinsic moral status to partial agents *as such.*

Agents, potential agents, and partial agents are, however, purely abstract categories. To apply a theory with such an ontology, it is necessary to judge which of the real world objects that we (agents) encounter are agents, potential agents, or partial agents.

How do I (any agent) know whether or not any being I encounter is an agent? Agents (by definition) actively pursue their valued purposes and, as such, have the generic capacities of agency to a particular degree. Thus, the defining characteristic of an agent is, in essential part, a mental state, and its associated capacities are mental abilities.

Since I have direct access to my mental state, I know that I am an agent directly. The problem is that I have no direct access to the mind of any being other than myself. When I infer that another being is an agent, I do so on the basis of observing that the being displays in full the characteristics and behaviour expected of an agent. However, if a being is, on such a basis, ostensibly an agent, it remains possible that it is nothing but a programmed automaton with no mind. No amount of empirical observation can prove otherwise. The relevance of empirical evidence cited for a being's status as an agent depends irreducibly on unfalsifiable and unverifiable metaphysical assumptions.

Does it follow that I can deny that there are any agents other than myself without denying that I am an agent? I think not!

Although I must concede that it can never be known *with certainty* that an other (X), who is ostensibly an agent, is in fact an agent, the presumption 'X is an agent' and the presumption 'X is not an agent' are *not* on a par *morally*. If I mistakenly presume X to be an agent, I might have to restrict my exercise of the generic rights, but I do not deny myself (or any other agent) the status of a possessor of the generic rights. But, if I mistakenly presume X not to be an agent, then I do precisely that—I deny an agent the status of a holder of the generic rights.

Since the dialectical necessity of the *PGC* renders the *PGC* absolutely categorically binding, there can be no justification for violating the *PGC*. Thus, to risk the possibility of violating the *PGC, when this can be avoided,* is to violate the *PGC*.

Where X displays the characteristics and behaviour expected of an agent and is hence, an 'ostensible agent', it will (by the very nature of the case) be possible to treat X as an agent, and to avoid the risk *altogether* of mistakenly denying that X is an agent, by presuming X to be an agent and acting accordingly.

It follows that it is dialectically necessary to accept:

> Where X is an ostensible agent, the metaphysical possibility that X might not be an agent, is to be wholly discounted, and X's display of the characteristics and behaviour expected of an agent is to be taken as sufficient evidence that X is an agent.

Implicit in this argument, which amounts to a moral argument for other minds, is the following Precautionary Principle:

> If there is no way of knowing whether or not X has property P, then, insofar as it is possible to do so, X must be assumed *to have* property P if the consequences (as measured by the *PGC*) of erring in presuming that X *does not have* P are worse than those of erring in presuming that X *has* P (and X must be assumed *to not have* P if the consequences of erring in presuming that X *has* P are worse than those of assuming that X *does not have* P).[27]

Suppose, instead, that X (as far as I am able to ascertain) only exhibits characteristics and behaviour sufficient for me to infer that X is a partial agent. Although X is apparently only a partial agent, I cannot infer that X *is not* an agent. Just as I cannot *know with certainty* that X *is* an agent when X is an ostensible agent, so I cannot *know with certainty* that X *is not* an agent when X is apparently only a partial agent!

So, even though X is apparently only a partial agent, the possibility remains that if I suppose that X is not an agent, and act accordingly, X is an agent, and I will have deprived X of the protection of the *PGC* to which X is entitled. Thus, the *PGC* imposes a duty on me to do whatever I can to avoid this consequence—*provided, as always,* that my doing so does not violate more important provisions of the *PGC* (see further below).

However, where X is apparently only a partial agent, it is not possible to avoid this consequence *altogether.* I can, indeed, refrain from harming (and can assist) X in ways that would safeguard the benefits that X would receive *if* X had the generic rights and chose to exercise them. I can, indeed, recognise duties not to harm (and to assist) X in various ways. However, it must not be forgotten that if X is, in fact, an agent then the *PGC* requires X (thereby) to be accorded the generic rights, the benefits of which X may waive. But, by not displaying in full the characteristics and behaviour expected of an agent, X fails to demonstrate (even under precautionary reasoning) that X has the capacities by virtue of which it is able to waive the benefits of what it is entitled to. Thus, the duties of protection that I must recognise that I have towards X, where X is apparently only a partial agent, are unavoidably paternalistic, which is at odds with what X is strictly entitled to *qua* being an agent (should that be the case).[28]

All other things being equal, conflicts between the duties I owe under precautionary reasoning to two beings (X and Z) that are both apparently only partial agents are to be handled by a criterion of avoidance of more probable harm, according to which:

> If my doing y to Z is more likely to cause harm h to Z than my doing y to X (and I cannot avoid doing y to one of Z or X) then I ought to do y to X rather than to Z.

Where y = failing to observe a particular duty of protection, and h = mistakenly denying a being the status of an agent, we can infer by this criterion that

> If my failing to observe a particular duty of protection to Z is more likely to mistakenly deny Z the status of an agent than is my failing to observe this duty of protection to X (and I cannot avoid failing to

observe this duty to one of Z or X) then I ought to fail to observe my
duty to X rather than to Z.

Since I am more likely to mistakenly deny that a being is an agent the
more probable it is that it is an agent, it follows that *(all other things being
equal)* my duties of protection to those who are more probably agents take
precedence over my duties of protection to those who are less probably
agents.

The moral status of a being may be measured by the weight to be given
to the duties of protection owed to it by an agent. In such terms, it follows
that the moral status of beings who are more probably agents is greater
than that of beings who are less probably agents. In other words, the moral
status of beings is *proportional* to the probability that they are agents.

Given that X's full display of the characteristics and behaviour expected
of an agent must (under precautionary reasoning) be viewed as sufficient
evidence that X is an agent, it follows that display of such characteristics
and behaviour to a lesser degree must be viewed as less than sufficient
evidence (but evidence nonetheless) that X is an agent.

Thus, we establish the following conclusion:

> Apparent partial agents (which category includes the embryo-fetus)
> are owed duties of protection by agents in proportion to the degree to
> which they approach being ostensible agents—not *qua* their being
> partial agents—but *qua* their possibly being agents.[29]

However, *all things considered,* the *PGC* does not require agents to do
everything they possibly can to cater for the possibility that the embryo-
fetus is an agent. Such actions could have *PGC*-relevant costs for other
beings with moral status. In theory, conflicts between the duties owed to
the embryo-fetus and duties owed to other beings are to be adjudicated by
use of a needs calculus that weighs the risk of *PGC*-relevant harm to the
embryo-fetus of action to protect the *PGC*-relevant needs of conflicting
parties[30] (taking into account the *PGC*-relevant 'utility'[31] of such action to
the conflicting parties) against the risk of *PGC*-relevant harm to the
conflicting parties of action to protect the *PGC*-relevant needs of the
embryo-fetus (taking into account the *PGC*-relevant utility of such action
to the embryo-fetus).

The risk of *PGC*-relevant harm to the embryo-fetus is a function of

(i)   the probability that the embryo-fetus is an agent;
(ii) the severity of *PGC*-relevant harm to the embryo-fetus (assumed to be
      an agent) of action to protect the *PGC*-relevant needs of the conflicting
      parties (suppose, only its mother); and

(iii) the probability of such action causing this *PGC*-relevant harm to the embryo-fetus.

The risk of *PGC*-relevant **harm** to the mother is a function of

(a) the probability that the mother is an agent;
(b) the severity of *PGC*-relevant harm to the mother (assumed to be an agent) of action to meet the *PGC* relevant needs of the embryo-fetus; and
(c) the probability of such action causing this *PGC*-relevant harm to the mother.

The *PGC*-relevant utility to a party of action to protect its *PGC*-relevant needs is a function of

I   the magnitude of *PGC*-relevant need of that party for this action;
II   the probability that this action will meet this need;
III   the severity of *PGC*-relevant-harm of this action to that party; and
IV   the probability that this action will cause this harm to that party.

Furthermore, since different actions may be taken to try to protect the *PGC*-relevant needs of the embryo-fetus and its mother, the needs calculus must be applied to the various alternatives available to decide on the right course of action in conflicts.

Suppose that we are considering the permissibility of abortion to save the life of the mother (who is an ostensible agent). To simplify matters, suppose (which is certainly an unreal scenario) that failure to abort will, with virtual certainty, lead to the death of the mother but will, with virtual certainty, save the embryo-fetus. Suppose, too, that abortion will, with virtual certainty save the life of the mother and not cause her *or any other relevant beings* any significant harms.

Under such simplifying assumptions, we need, in effect, only consider (i) against (a), and it is clear that we must abort the embryo-fetus (unless its mother chooses otherwise—in which case we must still consider the harm that the death of the mother might cause to other relevant beings), for the probability that the mother is an agent $=1$, and whatever we think about the embryo-fetus, the probability that it is an agent is <1 (and very much so at any stage of its development).

However, it should be obvious that using the needs calculus is straight-forward only when we have a one-variable conflict. Its application becomes much more difficult if the conflicting parties differ in the values to be attached to two or more of the relevant variables. This is because a one variable conflict requires only a relative ordering of the relevant prob-abilities or the magnitudes of *PGC*-relevant need/harm, whereas a multi-variable conflict requires the significance of a particular probability to be weighed against a particular magnitude of harm/need or a different sort of probability. For this to be done objectively, it is necessary to put absolute commensurable values on the kinds of harm, need, and all the relevant probabilities involved.[32]

Whether or not this can be done, is beyond the scope of this paper. If it cannot be done, then multi-variable conflicts will only be relatively unproblematic in extreme cases. Beyond that, it will be necessary to defer resolutions of conflicts to the *PGC* derived 'method of consent',[33] to good faith decisions of authorised persons attempting to apply the above calculus.

What then of potentiality under precaution?

Under precautionary reasoning, the embryo-fetus is to be viewed as a possible agent that does not exhibit in full (as far as we can tell) the characteristics and behaviour expected of an agent. So viewed, if the embryo-fetus happens to be an agent, then its failure to display itself as an ostensible agent is not because it is not an agent; it is because something is preventing it from displaying the qualifying characteristics or behaviour (or from displaying them in ways that we can interpret properly).[34]

So, if the embryo-fetus is an agent, despite apparently being only a partial agent, then the proper story to tell is not that, as it approaches being an ostensible agent, its potential *to be* an agent is being realised, but that, as it approaches being an ostensible agent, its potential to express itself as an agent is being realised. Suppose, then, that the embryo-fetus is an agent. From this it follows that the embryo-fetus does have the generic rights in full. As such, it must be accorded additive rights to expand its capacities for purpose-pursuit. Because its development of the ability to display in full the characteristics and behaviour expected of an agent will be necessary for it to be able to extend its generic capacities for purpose-pursuit, it must be accorded the right to develop its potential to display in full the characteristics and behaviour to be expected of an agent.

Of course, because the embryo-fetus is apparently only a partial agent, we cannot treat it as having such a right. But we can protect it *qua* the presumption that it is an agent, by accepting a duty to allow its potential to display the characteristics and behaviour of an ostensible agent to develop (and to assist this development, when necessary). Furthermore, this duty will be subject to proportionality reasoning, because the more the embryo-fetus displays the characteristics and behaviour expected of an agent (to the point of being an ostensible agent) the more seriously we must take the possibility that it is an agent.

However, we cannot conclude from this that we have a duty to protect the life of a *potential agent as such* (and other conditions of its being able to develop into an agent) in proportion to the degree to which it approaches being an agent. The potential that is the basis of our duty to protect the embryo-fetus' development is not the potential of the embryo-fetus *to be an agent,* but the possible potential of what is possibly an agent unable to display in full the characteristics and behaviour expected of an agent to develop the ability to do so.

Nevertheless, *because evidence that an embryo-fetus (X) is a potential ostensible[35] agent is evidence relevant to the probability that X is an agent,* precautionary reasoning also supports the following claims.

(1) Evidence that X is a potential agent, *by itself,* requires agents to grant X moral status (in proportion to the strength of this evidence); and
(2) Evidence that X is a potential agent adds to the moral status secured for X by the degree to which X exhibits the characteristics and behaviour expected of an agent. Thus, if Y is apparently only a partial agent with y moral status (by virtue of the extent to which Y displays the characteristics and behaviour expected of an agent) *but not apparently a potential agent,* and X is apparently a partial agent with y moral status *and also apparently a potential agent,* then agents must take more seriously the possibility that X is an agent than that Y is an agent, by virtue of which their duties of protection to X are greater than their similar duties to Y. (And, of course, the degree to which evidence of potential to become an agent adds to X's moral status will be proportional to the strength of this evidence.)

The weakest evidence that one can have that X is a potential agent is that X is a member of a species S (some of) whose members develop into ostensible agents under specified conditions.[36] To this can be added knowledge of correlations between possession of X's specific characteristics and development into ostensible agents by members of S. All factors of this kind being equal, the further X develops in the direction of becoming an ostensible agent, the more confident one can be that X will develop the whole way. Thus, considerations of evidence for potential and considerations of evidence of degree of approach to being an agent are not wholly independent.

Because the evidence that those who do not apply the *PGC* under precaution will use to identify a being as an agent is identical to that which renders it an ostensible agent, and the degree of evidence on the basis of which they will place a partial agent at a particular distance from being an agent will place it at a co-ordinate distance from being an ostensible agent, etc., the results obtained by applying proportionality and potentiality under precaution should not, in principle at least, be different from those that Gewirth or Steigleder argue for.

This, however, does not mean that there is no important difference between the two approaches. The two ways of reasoning about proportionality and potentiality differ radically in their theoretical base. The approaches of Gewirth or Steigleder, in effect, treat proportionality reasoning and considerations of potentiality as deductive extensions of the argument *to* the *PGC*. If they are right, then the *PGC* does not merely state that agents have full moral status. *It* states that partial and potential agents have some degree of intrinsic moral status as well.

In contrast, my approach leaves the *PGC's* ontology unaltered, for considerations of proportionality and potentiality are strictly confined to inductive *application* of the *PGC*. This switch—from attempting to ground the moral status of the embryo-fetus and other 'marginal agents' in onto-logical extensions of the *PGC,* to deriving it in the epistemology of empirical application of the *PGC*—is not trivial. It represents all the difference in the world—that between invalid theses and a valid one.

5 Interactions between intrinsic and derivative considerations

Having established that proportionality and potentiality under precaution both require that the embryo-fetus be accorded a degree of intrinsic moral status, we need to have another look at the sources of indirect protection, for it should be clear that the moral status secured for the embryo-fetus by proportionality and potentiality considerations under precaution affects the derivative sources of status in ways that are sometimes reinforcing and at other times qualifying. For example:

(1) The conclusion that, as a part of her body, the mother may do anything with the embryo-fetus needs qualification. In order to harm the embryo-fetus, she now requires a justification, which must take the form of applying the needs calculus outlined above in her favour. Admittedly, there are difficulties with this, which have already been alluded to. In general terms, it is possible to say only that such conflicts must be dealt with on a case by case basis taking into account all of the considerations that the *PGC* requires to be taken into account—including application of the method of consent, about which some brief comments will be made in connection with (3) below.

(2) If the embryo-fetus is, *ex hypothesi,* an agent, then it may not be owned. Since precautionary reasoning requires agents to take this possibility seriously, the thesis that the embryo-fetus may be regarded as the property of its parents before implantation (and that of its mother after implantation) is no longer acceptable. Were the embryo-fetus known to be an agent, the relationship between parent/s and embryo-fetus would be that of guardianship rather than ownership. However, since this is not known (and the probability that the embryo-fetus is an agent is very small indeed) guardianship imposes over-strong duties on its parents. What is required is that the parents must assume 'precautionary' guardianship—guardianship unless there are coun-

tervailing circumstances. However, this means little more than that a justification using the needs calculus is required for anything harmful to be done to the embryo-fetus.

The most likely harms that might come to the embryo-fetus produced in *in vitro* fertilisation programmes are (a) that it might be used for research, or (b) that it might be discarded as surplus.

Both of these practices can be justified, *if they are necessary,* on the basis of avoidance of the harm that being childless can cause some women. If such procedures are necessary, precautionary reasoning minimally demands that any not to be implanted embryo-fetus be treated with 'dignity'. More tentatively, I suggest that it provides at least *some* basis against the practice of deliberate embryo-splitting (as this *could* be the deliberate splitting, and killing, of an agent), and also for permitting the use of surplus embryo-fetuses by women, other than the genetic mother, who are willing to host them.[37]

(3) Since precautionary reasoning requires the possibility that the embryo-fetus is an agent to be taken seriously, agents must be willing to impose duties on themselves to protect the embryo-fetus in line with the needs calculus. Thus, only when they wish to impose duties on themselves stronger than the needs calculus requires are they waiving the benefits of any of their generic rights. Furthermore, since it is possible that features of this calculus will, for both practical and theoretical reasons, leave room for disagreement on how much weight should be given to, e.g., probability considerations as against severity of harm considerations, there is scope for legitimate disagreement in legal systems as to where lines are to be drawn. One of the remaining tasks for Gewirthian theory is to try to specify as precisely as possible the limits of permissible discretion.

(4) If disregard for the well-being of the embryo-fetus evidences a generally cruel character, then it is plausible to suggest that those who are wholly insensitive to the well-being of the embryo-fetus at a later stage of its development are less likely to care fully for ostensible human agents than those who are only wholly insensitive to the well-being of the embryo-fetus at an earlier stage of its development. In other words, the cruelty or 'brutalisation' effect is likely to be in proportion to the level of development of the embryo-fetus at which an agent's total insensitivity to its well-being ceases. It is important to test this hypothesis, because, if it is confirmed, then quantification of its parameters can assist with setting the limits of permissible discretion in application of the needs calculus. For example, if it were shown (and I hasten to say that I have no reason to believe that this is the case) that those who consider abortion before 21 weeks to be permissible in all cases show no decreased regard for human ostensible agents than those

who are totally opposed to abortion, but those who consider abortion to be permissible after this time do show an increased disregard, then this would be *a* consideration in favour of interpreting the needs calculus so as to prohibit abortion after 21 weeks.

(5) The argument for protection based on the sensitivities of agents does not require attention to be given to the sensitivities of those who are offended by the existence of some *agent* subgroups. The *PGC* grants full moral status to all agents as such, so does not require agents to take into account the prejudices of racists, sexists, and the like. Sensitivities of others need only be taken into account when the actions needed to protect them do not violate what is owed to those protected by the *PGC*. The effect of precautionary reasoning in this connection is to strengthen the derivative protection of the embryo-fetus. Under precaution, those who care for the embryo-fetus are not to be regarded as merely having optional (not irrational, albeit natural) preferences and psychological makeups to be protected. They are to be regarded as having rationally required views and dispositions of character protective of the *PGC* (at least insofar as these are in line with the needs calculus).

(6) Under precautionary reasoning, the intention to nurture the embryo-fetus to agent status, upon which futurality considerations depend, is no longer wholly optional. Precautionary reasoning requires agents to accept duties to allow and assist the embryo-fetus as an apparent potential agent to develop a potential to display itself as an agent (should it be an agent), unless there is a direct conflict with protection owed to those of equal or higher moral status. Unless, there is a *PGC* based justification for not having this intention, the intention is required by the *PGC,* as are the judgments that futurality brings in its wake.

6 Conclusion

In some earlier writings (Beyleveld and Brownsword 1993, pp. 105–106; Beyleveld 1998, pp. 250–251), I suggested that precautionary reasoning could be used to establish moral status for 'uncertain agents' (e.g., dolphins and chimpanzees). At the time, I did not appreciate fully the role that precautionary reasoning has in the epistemology of empirical application of Gewirthian theory as such. However, as I have argued in this paper, such an appreciation entails that precautionary reasoning has application, not merely to beings that approach being ostensible agents closely, but to all living beings.[38] More specifically, whereas I have recently been sceptical (though not wholly dismissive) of the idea that proportionality and potentiality could be shown to be valid grounds for conferring moral status on the embryo-fetus, I now believe that these considerations provide valid grounds for conferring intrinsic moral status on the embryo-fetus.

A great deal of detailed analysis of the implications of applying proportionality and potentiality reasoning under precaution (as well as extensive empirical research) needs to be done before a detailed proposal appropriate to the drawing up of a Gewirthian legislative scheme can be made. What I have done is to provide little more than an outline of principles and considerations to develop in pursuing such a goal.

However, it should be apparent that, in principle, Gewirthian theory does support the 'compromise' position on the moral status of the embryo-fetus.

Notes

[1] Throughout this paper, reference to possession of a moral status is reference to a status that is correlative to moral duties being imposed on those capable of having them.

[2] These are extreme positions. Positions labelled 'pro-life' or 'pro-choice' in public discourse may not be quite as uncompromising as these.

[3] An agent acts, i.e., voluntarily pursues its freely chosen purposes. A prospective agent has the capacity and disposition to act. I use 'agent' to cover both agents and prospective agents.

[4] Generic rights are to the generic features of agency (those capacities an agent needs to be able to act at all or with any general chances of success, *whatever its purposes might be*). Interference with, or deprivation of, a generic feature of agency will interfere (or tend to interfere) with an agent's capacity to act or to act successfully, *regardless of what the action envisaged is*. The generic features of agency are ordered hierarchically into three categories, basic (needed for action as such; e.g., life, mental equilibrium to translate desire into action, and the necessary means to these), non-subtractive (needed to maintain capacities to act; e.g., accurate information), and additive (needed to increase capacities for successful agency in general; e.g., further education) according to the criterion of 'degrees of necessity' or 'needfulness' for action (which also determines which generic rights take precedence in case of conflict with the generic rights of others). (See Gewirth 1978, pp. 62–63; Beyleveld 1991, pp. 88–90.)

[5] My present purpose is not to defend Gewirth's argument but to apply it. See Beyleveld 1991 for an analysis and defence of Gewirth's argument as a whole.

[6] It might be thought that I am misattributing this position to Steigleder; for, while he shares Gewirth's view that beings that are less than agents can have moral status in proportion to their approach to agency, he restricts this claim to 'rudimentary agents', in which category he does not include newborns (see

78

ibid., pp. 243–244), and, by implication, the embryo-fetus. Indeed, he specifically states that 'the potentiality to become an agent is the only characteristic which is directly relevant for the determination of the moral status of human embryos and fetuses' (ibid., p. 244). It should, however, be noted that Steigleder complicates this assertion (if he does not actually contradict it) when he adds that 'the criterion of proximity to agency is applicable to fetuses as well. But here it does not yield definitive and uncontroversial normative results' (ibid., p. 246, fn. 4). All in all, it appears that Steigleder agrees with Gewirth (if only in theory) that proportionality grants moral status to the embryo-fetus (and the newly born); he merely does not consider this to be of any use in specifying duties correlative to this status in these cases.

7   See below.

8   Although my discussion will be conducted strictly within the framework of Gewirthian theory, my arguments (at least in form) are equally applicable to any other moral theory that maintains (i) that morality sets categorically binding requirements on action; and (ii) that agency is the necessary and sufficient condition for full moral status.

9   That Gewirth's method seeks to justify practical precepts to an agent (as defined) is not a function of a *value judgment* that only the views of agents matter. It follows from the fact that practical precepts can only be directed *rationally* at beings having the capacities of agents, and that only for such beings *can the question arise* of what practical precepts may legitimately be followed. To have a practical point of view, one must be an agent.

10   Dialectically necessary procedures contrast with dialectically contingent ones. An argument is *dialectical* if it is propounded relative to some claim made by an interlocutor. Its conclusion is *contingent* where

(i) the claim on which it is based can be coherently rejected by the interlocutor; *or*

(ii) the connection between the premise (claim) and the conclusion is contingent.

Its conclusion is *necessary* where the interlocutor cannot coherently reject the claim *and* the conclusion follows necessarily from the claim.

Dialectical procedures contrast with assertoric ones, where considerations with validity independent of claims made by interlocutors are cited for acceptance of conclusions.

11   By the principle, 'Whoever pursues an end must be prepared to pursue the means necessary to achieve the end'. If I do not accept this principle, I deny that I am an agent (because agents, by definition, do things as perceived means to their chosen ends).

[12] This follows by the 'Argument from the Sufficiency of Agency' (Gewirth 1978, p. 110), which may be presented as follows.

(a) If (7) *does not entail* (7') then I must be able to deny 'I am an agent → I have the generic rights' without denying that I have the generic rights.

(b) To deny 'I am an agent → I have the generic rights' is to assert that my having some property D—a quality not necessarily possessed by all agents—is necessary for me to have the generic rights. To deny 'I am an agent → I have the generic rights' is to assert 'I have the generic rights → I have D'.

(c) The assertion 'I have the generic rights → I have D' logically requires assent to 'I am an agent without D → I do not have the generic rights'. In other words, to be consistent with 'I have the generic rights → I have D', I must consider, *even though I am an agent,* that I do not have the generic rights *if I do not have D.*

(d) However, on the basis of (7), I must, *provided only that I am an agent,* consider that I have the generic rights—which is to say that I must, *by virtue of being an agent,* consider that I have the generic rights, *whether or not I have D.*

(e) 'I must consider, *even though I am an agent,* that I do not have the generic rights *if I do not have D*' contradicts 'I must, *by virtue of being an agent,* consider that I have the generic rights, *whether or not I have D*'.

(f) Since, 'I have the generic rights → I have D' contradicts what (7) entails, 'I have the generic rights → I have D' contradicts (7).

(g) Since, 'I have the generic rights → I have D' is equivalent to denying 'I am an agent → I have the generic rights', to deny 'I am an agent → I have the generic rights', is to deny (7).

(h) Thus, in order not to deny (7), I must affirm 'I am an agent → I have the generic rights'.

(i) Therefore, (7) → (7').

[13] Which there are not. See Beyleveld 1999.

[14] See Beyleveld and Brownsword 1998a and 1998b. We develop this thesis in a book we are currently writing on human dignity in bioethics and biolaw.

[15] Or, if the mother has died and the embryo-fetus can still be rescued.

[16] See further, below.

[17] See Gewirth 1978, pp. 319–322. The method of consent justifies obligations imposed by decisions arrived at by the use of procedures authorised directly by the *PGC* to resolve disputes on matters that the *PGC* cannot resolve (e.g., whether to have a law requiring persons to drive on the left or the right-hand side of the road), or which are so complex as to make agreement between even rational and knowledgeable persons practically impossible. The *PGC's* formal

requirements for the method of consent are discussed extensively in Beyleveld and Brownsword 1986, Chapters 7–9.

18 See Gewirth 1978, pp. 332–333.

19 Once again, this rests on empirical assumptions that need testing.

20 See, e.g., Beyleveld, Quarrell, and Toddington 1998a and 1998b (which is a modified version in German of 1998a).

21 See Beyleveld and Pattinson 1998, where a more detailed critique of Gewirth's application of the Principle of Proportionality is given than there is space for in this paper.

22 See fn. 12 supra.

23 Which Gewirth, himself, formulated. This fallacy is committed where fields or subject-matters are compared on disparate levels or in disparate respects. (See Gewirth 1960, p. 313.)

24 According to Gewirth (1978, p. 142), although the embryo-fetus lacks the generic abilities necessary to be an agent in anything but 'a remotely potential form', it nevertheless possesses the generic rights in a minimal way. Gewirth does not elaborate further.

25 It could be said that being a potential agent is a necessary condition for being an agent. It most probably is, but even so it is not a necessary condition for being an agent in the same way as having some of the generic abilities of agency is. It is a necessary condition for becoming an agent in the future, whereas the generic abilities of agency are necessary conditions of being an agent as such.

26 The argument in this Part is derived from Beyleveld and Pattinson 1998, which develops the argument in more detail.

27 Because of its link to the *PGC,* this principle is dialectically necessary. The reasoning behind *dicta* such as 'Innocent unless proven guilty!' or 'Give the benefit of the doubt' can be subsumed under it. Precautionary reasoning, as such, need not take the *PGC* as the yardstick by which to evaluate the consequences of error.

28 I have argued that Gewirth, by inferring that partial agents have quasi-generic rights, commits the fallacy of disparateness. Although I claim that apparent partial agents are to be granted just such quasi-generic rights, I do not commit the same fallacy.

Whereas Gewirth claims that the Principle of Proportionality licenses inferring quasi-generic rights of partial agents from generic rights of agents, I claim that precautionary reasoning licenses an inference to quasi-generic rights of apparent partial agents (which proportionality reasoning merely qualifies quantitatively). Gewirth requires the Principle of Proportionality, which can only license inferences concerning the degree to which a property is possessed, to license the attribution to partial agents of quasi-generic rights on the premise of a different quality (generic rights) being possessed by different quality beings (agents). In my reasoning, on the other hand, possession of a different quality (quasi-generic rights) is being attributed to agents (the agents that apparent partial agents might be) on the ground that this attribution is required to protect their generic rights (given that if the apparent partial agents are agents, they are agents in a position where they contingently cannot exercise their generic rights). No fallacy is committed here, because both quasi-generic rights and generic rights are attributable to agents.

[29] The behaviour that living beings are capable of exhibiting can be classified in a number of ways. The following sort of classification is particularly relevant to our concerns.

I Patterned organismic behaviour (displayed by all living organisms).
II Behaviour that evidences itself as purposive (as being motivated by feeling or desire).
III Behaviour that evidences itself as intelligent (as being susceptible to learning by experience).
IV Behaviour that evidences itself as rational (value-guided, and characteristic of an agent).

Associated with such behavioural capacities are various biological developments, most important of which relate to the development of a nervous system and brain. Both the degree to which a being displays Categories I, II, and III (short of IV), and the extent to which it possesses structural biological features that correlate with the behavioural capacities are relevant to classifying how close a being is to being an ostensible agent.

[30] The most relevant conflict is always between the embryo-fetus and the possible agent at greatest risk of conflicting harm.

[31] The use of this term, and (more widely) the consequential thinking involved in applying the needs calculus provides no warrant for classifying Gewirthian theory as utilitarian. The values involved in calculating this 'utility' are deontological, in being dialectically necessary (not teleological—meaning, derived by consequential thinking about optional preferences and values). If Gewirthian theory can be classified as a consequentialism, then it is nonetheless a deontological consequentialism. (See Gewirth 1978, p. 216.)

[32] The basic problem is that the Principle of Proportionality provides only a relative ordering: it does not tell us *how much more* probable particular evidence renders it that a being is an agent. Similarly, the criterion of needfulness for action (see fn. 4 supra) does not quantify just how much more necessary for action one generic feature is than another. We also face the classic conundrum as to how, e.g., to compare probabilities of harm with severities of harm. Is a catastrophic harm of minimal probability on a par with a minimal harm that is nearly certain?

[33] See fn. 17 supra.

[34] Thus, one way of explaining why we are required to take more seriously the possibility that a fetus is an agent the closer it approaches to being an ostensible agent, is that the more it displays the necessary characteristics of an ostensible agent the less elaborate and fanciful are the metaphysical stories we have to tell to explain why, despite being an agent, it is unable to display the expected behaviour.

A fairly obvious objection to the argument I have presented is that if the embryo-fetus is an agent then why do I not remember my time in the womb? Why do I only have memories and a sense of self-identity beginning sometime after my second year? A possible answer is that the process of birth causes amnesia. After all, some persons claim to remember birth traumas and even earlier lives under hypnosis. The issue is not whether these stories and others like them are true or even plausible. They only have to be possibly true.

[35] For convenience I will drop the 'ostensible'. Evidence that X is a potential ostensible agent is, under precaution, to be taken as sufficient evidence that X is at least a potential agent, just as the evidence that constitutes X being an ostensible agent is to be taken as sufficient evidence that X is an agent.

[36] Complications, which I will not address here, are created by the fact that these conditions can be specified differently. Thus, the concept of potentiality, like that of a cause (vs. background conditions), is to a degree normative in being dependent on what is taken to be 'normal'.

[37] Even, *perhaps,* for permission to use surplus embryos in this way to be made a requirement of becoming a recipient of an *in vitro* fertilisation programme.

[38] Evelyn B. Pluhar (1995, pp. 252–253) (referring to the fetus) also appreciates that a being should be given the benefit of the doubt about its agency status even when the evidence that it is an agent is not complete. Pluhar, however, like myself earlier, does not elaborate this into a full-scale basis for proportionality reasoning. Furthermore, she presents her thesis within the framework of the mistaken assumption that Gewirth's argument to the *PGC* can operate with the notion that an agent is a being that pursues desired purposes without having the capacities for voluntary or reasoned preferences (on the basis of which the fetus is a near ostensible agent). (Her assumption is mistaken. Without the capacity for voluntary or reasoned choice, a being is not required to *value* its desired purposes, and the argument cannot take even its first step.)

References

Beyleveld, D. (1991), *The Dialectical Necessity of Morality: An Analysis and Defense of Alan Gewirth's Argument to the Principle of Generic Consistency*, University of Chicago Press: Chicago.

Beyleveld, D. (1998), 'The Moral and Legal Status of the Human Embryo', in Hildt, E. and Mieth, D. (eds), *In Vitro Fertilisation in the 1990s: Towards a Medical, Social and Ethical Evaluation,* Ashgate: Aldershot, pp. 247–260.

Beyleveld, D. (1999), 'Gewirth and Kant on Justifying the Supreme Principle of Morality', in Boylan, M. (ed.), *Gewirth: Critical Essays on Action, Rationality, and Community,* Rowman & Littlefield: New York and London, pp. 97–117.

Beyleveld, D. and Brownsword, R. (1986), *Law as a Moral Judgment,* Sweet & Maxwell: London. (Reprinted 1994 by Sheffield Academic Press: Sheffield.)

Beyleveld, D. and Brownsword, R. (1993), *Mice, Morality and Patents: The Oncomouse Application and Article 53(a) of the European Patent Convention,* Common Law Institute of Intellectual Property: London.

Beyleveld, D. and Brownsword, R. (1998a), 'Articles 21 and 22 of the Convention on Human Rights & Biomedicine: Property and Consent, Commerce and Dignity', in Kemp, P. (ed.), *Research Projects on Basic Ethical Principles of Bioethics and Biolaw,* Centre for Ethics and Law: Copenhagen, pp. 33–67.

Beyleveld, D. and Brownsword, R. (1998b), 'Human Rights, Human Dignity and Human Genes', in Brownsword, R., Cornish, W. and Llewelyn, M. (eds), *Human Genetics and the Law: Regulating a Revolution,* special issue of the *Modern Law Review,* Vol. 61, No. 5, pp. 661–680, which is available also as a separate volume published by Hart: Oxford, 1998 (at pp. 69–88).

Beyleveld, D. and Pattinson, S. (1998), 'Proportionality Under Precaution: Justifying Duties to Apparent Non-agents', unpublished paper. (Available from the authors.)

Beyleveld, D., Quarrell, O. and Toddington, S. (1998a), 'Generic Consistency in the Reproductive Enterprise: Ethical and Legal Implications of Exclusion Testing for Huntington's Disease', *Medical Law International,* Vol. 3, Nos. 2 & 3, pp. 135–158.

Beyleveld, D., Quarrell, O. and Toddington, S. (1998b), 'Konstitutive Konsistenz im Bemühen um Nachkommenschaft: Die Relevanz der Absicht, daß potentielle Handlungsfähige handlungsfähig werden, für die moralische Beurteilung von Tests zum Ausschluß der Huntingtonschen Krankheit', in Düwell, M., and Mieth, D. (eds), *Ethik in der Humangenetik: Die neueren Entwicklungen der genetischen Frühdiagnostik aus ethischer Perspektive,* Francke: Tübingen und Basel, pp. 120–148.

Gewirth, A. (1960), 'Positive "Ethics" and Normative "Science"', *Philosophical Review,* Vol. 69, pp. 311–330.

Gewirth, A. (1978), *Reason and Morality,* University of Chicago Press: Chicago.

Hill, J. F. (1984), 'Are Marginal Agents "Our Recipients"?' In Regis, E. Jr. (ed.), *Gewirth's Ethical Rationalism: Critical Essays with a Reply by Alan Gewirth,* University of Chicago Press: Chicago, pp. 180–191.

Pluhar, E. B. (1995), *Beyond Prejudice: The Moral Significance of Human and Nonhuman Animals,* Duke University Press: Durham.

Steigleder, K. (1998), 'The Moral Status of Potential Persons', in Hildt, E. and Mieth, D. (eds), *In Vitro Fertilisation in the 1990s: Towards a Medical, Social and Ethical Evaluation,* Ashgate: Aldershot, pp. 239–246.

Comment on *The moral status of the human embryo and fetus*

Nikolaus Knoepffler

In my comment on D. Beyleveld's talk on the moral status of the human embryo and fetus I wish to focus on two points. Firstly I will explain why Beyleveld's rejection of Gewirth's use of the analytical 'Principle of Proportionality' for the embryo-fetus as partial agent and of Steigleder's argument of potentiality of agency of the embryo-fetus is correct, and that his switch from attempting to base the moral status of the embryo-fetus and other 'marginal agents' on ontological extensions of the principle of generic consistency, to motivating it by the *PGC's* epistemology of empirical application represents, to quote his own words, 'all the difference in the world—that between invalid theses and a valid one'. Then I will show why I doubt the 'Principle of Generic Consistency' and that means Beyleveld's starting point.

1 Beyleveld's argument against Gewirth's Principle of Proportionality

Gewirth states the Principle of Proportionality as a pervasive feature of traditional doctrines of distributive justice:

> When some quality Q justifies having certain rights R, and the possession of Q varies in degree in the respect that is relevant to Q's justifying the having of R, the degree to which R is had is proportional to or varies with the degree to which Q is had. Thus, if x units of Q justify that one have x units of R, then y units of Q justify that one have y units of R. (Gewirth 1978, p. 121)

Beyleveld correctly states that it is false to apply this principle to generic rights because you cannot have generic rights partially, but only fully. As he formulates:

> This is because having the generic capacities of agency to the degree needed to be an agent is not only necessary (and sufficient) to have

the generic rights in full . . . '*it is necessary to have any generic rights at all*' (p. 66 in this volume).

Beyleveld correctly states that Gewirth commits the fallacy of disparateness, i.e. the fallacy of the claim that the Principle of Proportionality licenses inferring that, because agents have the generic rights in full, partial agents have quasi-generic rights to some extent. The reason why this is a fallacy comes from the fact that there is a fundamental difference between a quasi-generic right and a generic right to some extent. I will explain Gewirth's failure with an analogy: you cannot say that water becomes partially ice if it gets colder. There is a certain temperature, then there is no water any more, but ice. So you cannot have generic rights partially according to the above principle.

2 Beyleveld's argument against Steigleder's potentiality

According to Klaus Steigleder 'human beings who are not yet agents must possess moral significance for agents for the sufficient reason that they possess the potentiality to become agents' (1998, p. 241).

Beyleveld asks: 'Why is an agent *necessarily* being inconsistent if it claims that it has full moral status but a potential agent has none? Steigleder does not tell us.' (p.67 in this volume). So correctly he states that potential agency is not the same as full agency:

> Therefore, whatever connections might exist between being an agent and being a mere potential agent, even if some of these connections are *in some sense or senses* necessary connections, and even if this can consequently be said to impart moral relevance of *some sort* on being a mere potential agent, it categorically cannot follow from this that *being* a mere potential agent, as *such*, is sufficient to confer at least some intrinsic moral status. (p. 68 in this volume)

I agree with Beyleveld that to confer generic rights on embryo-fetuses is possible if you see them as *possible agents*. So proportionality and potentiality in a different sense can be applied empirically under precaution. Proportionality here means: the more probably something is an agent, the more it should be given full moral status. Potentiality here means the potentiality to express itself as an agent, not to become an agent. Therefore under precautionary reasoning, the embryo-fetus is a possible agent that does not exhibit in full the behaviour expected of an agent. Its failure to display itself as an ostensible agent is not because it is not an agent; it is because something is preventing it from displaying the behaviour.

3 The problem with the Principle of Generic Consistency

Beyleveld accepts Gewirth's argument of the Principle of Generic Consistency. I do not agree with him on this. I will give you the argument in order to show you why I do not agree. The argument runs as follows:

(1) I do (or intend to do) X voluntarily for a purpose E that I have chosen.
(2) E is good.
(3) There are generic features of agency.
(4) My having the generic features is good for my achieving E *whatever E might be* = My having the generic features is categorically instrumentally good.
(5) I categorically instrumentally ought to pursue my having the generic features.
(6) Other agents categorically ought not to interfere with my having the generic features *against my will*, and ought to aid me to secure the generic features when I cannot do so by my own unaided efforts *if I so wish*.
(7) I have both negative and positive claim rights to have the generic features = I have the generic rights.
(7')I am an agent → I have the generic rights.
(8) All agents have the generic rights.

Where is the flaw in the argument? I don't think that there is a problem in (1) to (4). And I even agree with (4) to (5), which commits no naturalistic fallacy, because it only expresses my claim to pursue the generic features. The main problem is in (5) to (6). Why should other agents not interfere with my having the generic features against my will? Why should they aid me to secure the generic features if I so wish? Why should someone who is able to secure his own generic features of agency help others to secure their generic features in case he prefers doing something that is good for him, but not good for others?

(6) is therefore a very strong principle in itself. The world will be a better place if we follow this principle, but this principle cannot be derived from our being agents. It is a moral principle in itself.[1]

Note

[1] See Hare 1984, pp. 52–58. But my thesis that (6) is a very strong principle in itself may be refutable. See Beyleveld 1991, pp. 242–246.

References

Beyleveld, D. (1991), *The Dialectical Necessity of Morality: An Analysis and Defense of Alan Gewirth's Argument to the Principle of Generic Consistency*, University of Chicago Press: Chicago.

Gewirth, A. (1978), *Reason and Morality*, University of Chicago Press: Chicago.

Hare, R. M (1984), 'Do Agents Have to Be Moralists?', in Regis, E. (ed.), *Gewirth's Ethical Rationalism: Critical Essays with a Reply by Alan Gewirth*, University of Chicago Press: Chicago, pp. 52–58.

Steigleder, K. (1998), 'The Moral Status of Potential Persons', in Hildt, E. and Mieth, D. (eds), *In Vitro Fertilisation in the 1990s: Towards a Medical, Social and Ethical Evaluation,* Ashgate: Aldershot, pp. 239–246.

Comment on *The moral status of the human embryo and fetus*

Micheline Husson

In his excellent presentation on 'The Moral Status of the Human Embryo and Fetus' Deryck Beyleveld has discussed problems that are linked to the status of embryo and fetus by referring to the moral theory of Alan Gewirth. From Gewirthian theory he argues in favour of the compromise position and he proposes to apply potentiality and proportionality reasoning under precaution.

My objective is not to contest or to reject the choice of Deryck Beyleveld in its first principle, namely, to apply the moral theory of Alan Gewirth and to reject the 'pro-life' position. I propose to show that with an objective of practical wisdom, there are alternative choices that can open to us ways to exclude none of the positions in the political range of the debate as he has well specified in his paper. It is questionable to presuppose one definite ontology of the human person and one definition of what is constitutive of ethics. In other words, under what conditions can we try to understand the different agents that play a role in the recognition of the moral status of the human embryo and fetus. My concern is that no position should be excluded *a priori* from the rational debate.

I have organised my comments around three topics.

- How is the human embryo and/or fetus apprehended?
- The use of the *PGC* (Principle of Generic Consistency).
- The elimination of the 'pro-life' position.

1 How is the human embryo and fetus apprehended?

In earlier times (before 1970), human embryos and fetuses were remote from sight and remained hidden in the womanly enclosure. One could neither see them, nor appropriate them, nor nurse them separately. Physicians and researchers dealt with pregnant mothers. With biomedical and techno-scientific progress, however, it has become possible to individualise embryos and fetuses. With the development of medical imagery (scan)

91

and of medical techniques (such as amniocentesis, or fetal surgery) the embryo or fetus has eventually become a patient independent of his/her mother. Thus, the question of its status irresistibly emerged (around 1970). We have to note that specific research and therapy on embryos and fetuses required tolerant abortion laws.

Nowadays fetal medicine does exist. For example, one can visualise the embryo in the lesser details from 10 days on. Many diagnoses can be made on fetuses (or even early embryos). Some diagnosed conditions can be treated efficiently. Besides embryos and fetuses emerging as real patients in medical settings, one may not ignore the fact that, as the use of medical technology has become widespread, future parents now more and more put pictures (echographic images) of their fetus in their family album, and some pro-life groups use such images as visual arguments in the abortion debate. The question therefore is inevitable. What is an embryo in itself? What is a fetus?

As noted by Fagot-Largeault and Delaisi de Parseval, according to the Declaration of Human Rights of 1789, 'human rights' begin only at birth. The Universal Declaration of Human Rights adopted in 1948 by the United Nations (UN) states.

> All humans beings were born and remain free and equal in dignity and in rights. They are endowed with reason and conscience and must behave with each other in a spirit of fraternity. (Fargot-Largeault and de Parseval 1989, p. 88)

It suggests that before birth human beings have no specific status or rights.

The French legislation recognises that human beings deserve respect and protection prior to their birth, but it grants them rights only under the condition that they will be born alive. Scientifically, it is difficult to tell exactly when two gametes become one embryo and when this embryo becomes a fetus. The French National Consultative Ethics Committee (CCNE) specified that 'embryonic and fetal life includes all the steps of the zygote from ovum impregnation to the maturation that allow an autonomous life'.[1] I insist on this point, because in his paper, Beyleveld has not underlined it. I agree with him in recognising the difficulty to trace the limit between embryo and fetus with accuracy. Embryonic and fetal life are in a natural continuity. The continuity of individual life makes it a whole that one can hardly dissociate, and the development of fetal medicine has made the human fetus a patient, just as medicine makes a patient of any defective human being. What then differentiates fetuses from other human beings? The CCNE said that they are 'potential persons' rather than 'actual' ones. H. T. Engelhardt says that fetuses are only 'possible' or 'future' persons. The question then arises: should a 'potential' or 'possible' or 'future' person have the same status and rights as any actual person? But on which criteria does one get the status of an actual person: Agency? Consciousness? Citizenship? There is no consensus on that issue. Asking what embryos/fetuses really are allows us to realise how difficult it is to infer their moral status from the status of actual persons or of agents who already exist, because there is both continuity in the development from the first cell to the mature organism, and absence in the early embryo of the criteria by which one may qualify for moral status. I agree with Beyleveld on the indifferent use of the terms 'embryo' and 'fetus', if he thinks that the moral status depends on the degree of maturation of the developing human being. If the process of embryological development is a continuous process, it is impossible to trace a limit from which this one has moral status and that one does not have moral status. In other terms, I think that the moral status of the human embryo/fetus has to be built on the complexity and the uncertainty of what it is exactly.

If the moral status of the human embryo and fetus is difficult to appreciate, we think that it is a reason to try to analyse all existing positions on the subject, including the pro-life position. Beyleveld in his paper rules out the 'pro-life' position without justification (simply referring to Gewirthian theory). He makes the distinction between 'pro-life', 'pro-choice' and 'compromise'. But since the 'pro-life' position does exist, it should be taken into consideration. The 'pro-life' (or vitalist) position (as he acknowledges) consists in saying that the embryo/fetus from its conception has the same moral status as any adult person. Why discard it immediately, rather than looking for its rationale? What I find even more surprising in Beyleveld's argument is that after dismissing pro-life arguments without examining them he takes a prudential stand and recommends acting as if the fetus might be endowed with the qualities of a moral agent, which is a manner of reintegrating in practice what has been eliminated in principle.

2 The use of the *PGC* (Principle of Generic Consistency)

The *PGC* is evidently used to argue that, as the human embryo or fetus is human, it should presumably be treated as a human being. The prudential use made of this evidence amounts to arguing that, should you know nothing else about someone, the mere fact that you identify someone with a fellow creature belonging to the human race implies that you should be careful and 'protect' it. But that does not allow us to resolve concrete moral dilemmas. There is not one uniform way in which human beings should be treated. Respect for an autonomous adult will mean that decisions regarding the conduct of his/her life will be left to his own deliberation and choice, because he is a 'moral agent'. Respect for a young teenager may include directive or even coercive attitudes regarding the conduct of his/her life, on the part of his/her parents, because he has to learn how to become a true 'moral agent'. Respect for a new-born infant will mean care for his well-being, rather non-interference with his 'agency'. Respect for a defective fetus might mean that, given the poor quality of life this human being would have, should he be allowed to be born, he should not be allowed to be born, because he would never be a 'moral agent' anyhow.

Moral dilemmas in medicine often have to do with the degree of 'agency' granted to the patient. Rather than holding a position *a priori,* it is interesting to inquire into the variety of positions held in practice by various groups, about the requirements for 'moral agency'. A. Fagot-Largeault and Delaisi de Parseval have conducted a meticulous analysis of the various positions.

On the one hand, I think that if Beyleveld uses the *PGC* as a principle that recommends to agents the respect of other agents as a necessary condition for morality, I am in agreement with him. In the discussion on the status of human embryos, it is an original approach, because it tells us that the respect for persons whatever they are is an ultimate moral principle, extending beyond the limits of conscious or responsible human life. In other words, to act in agreement with fundamental human rights as if they were our own is a salutary thing as a general principle, because it means that no one (including terminally ill people, including fetuses, including mental patients) should be denied *a priori* his rights to liberty, and to well-being. It is interesting to analyse what follows logically from that. But it does not resolve all conflicts, or all concrete dilemmas. In a democratic society I think that one has to inquire into the ways people resolve their dilemmas, and how they argue when there is a conflict. We have to take into consideration cultural and social arguments of what is morally acceptable in a given context. It is a point of view that Beyleveld does not approach at all in his analysis. I think that knowing how different cultures or different societies consider the question is very important, and that their arguments should have their place in the debate.

3 The elimination of the 'pro-life' position and other considerations

I have difficulty understanding where Beyleveld wants to go when he extends the principle of prudence and declares that if the embryo/fetus is not an agent, this is not because it cannot be like an agent, but because it does not exhibit the qualities allowing us to recognise it as such. Does he then operate with this new principle a reconciliation with the position 'pro-life'? The human embryo or fetus in its initial development is not a full moral agent (it cannot take responsibility for itself). It is at the most a 'potential agent', or a future agent. Then I do not really understand how one can apply without ambiguity the notion of the agent to potential agents, since Gewirth uses this notion to designate human beings who have a will, and who can act responsibly.

There are different ways of conceiving the moral status of the embryo and the fetus. For some, it is not morally acceptable that human embryos or fetuses be used as means towards an end, for example as research tools. There is a moral obligation that they not be used, e.g., for the sampling of embryonic tissues, the constitution of cell banks, or the testing of medicinal substances—all the more as one knows that some research, or genetic engineering, offers other possibilities, such as the use of transgenic animal cells. Does one truly have the need of human embryos to advance research? Is there no alternative or another orientation of research in this case? But to advance research in some areas, is one not constrained to use only cells that are in the beginning of their development and therefore are not yet differentiated? Thereby, one cannot slice. It depends on the situation with which one is confronted at a given time.

Others think that the decision about what to do ought to be left to the mother or to relatives. I, indeed, think that the moral status of the embryo and the fetus depends also on the meaning and value it has for its mother and relatives.[2] It also depends on the circumstances of the conception. It is untenable to consider the embryo to be medical waste. Because, as Engelhardt (1996, p. 255) argues, a desired pregnancy is not appreciated in the same manner as one that is not wanted. Similarly, the status that relatives can grant to an embryo/fetus depends also on the desirability of the former. Therefore, there is a problem of bonds that relatives can have with the embryo/fetus. And, with the progress of research on the embryo, the importance of preserving it also depends on the quality of the embryo/fetus. I think special consideration regarding its moral status is necessary as soon as the embryo and the fetus cease to be considered as cells and are considered as potential agents.

For others again, reconsidering the embryo/fetus with respect to the biomedical mastery that has developed, is indispensable. Indeed, one is now able to maintain alive the 26 weeks premature child. For the sake of progress of biomedical research, does one have the right to use human embryo/fetus cells for all sorts of therapeutic purposes? For the embryo/fetus to become a person it has to have the potentiality to become a person, and such a potential indeed deserves some consideration. But that does not necessarily imply that one should condemn, for example, good research projects to be conducted on embryos/fetuses until 14 days approximately, especially when this research is potentially beneficial to improve the health of patients. The respect that we grant to the embryo or to the fetus can depend on if it is *in vitro* or *in vivo,* if it is viable or not, and on the consideration that agents have for it. This does not mean that we have to renounce the fact that the human embryo/fetus is intimately linked to our human being reality. Under some conditions, research also is linked to our human nature.

Researchers have shown that the fetus (the embryo) actively interacts with the placenta. Embryology has shown that it is a being that, even without having finished its maturation, has all its sense organs developed before birth. Psychiatrists have also shown that 'in the stomach of its mother, the child is already a subject desiring, shows clearly its pleasure or its displeasure'. It is thereby essential, they think, to 'consider the baby as an interlocutor from its prenatal life'. Perhaps with research progress concerning life before birth, it will bring us to reconsider our positions on the status of the human embryo and fetus (and the notion of agency that is ambiguous in the analysis of Beyleveld, will be more clear). This alone will justify the choice of the notion of person or human being when think- ing about the status of the human embryo and fetus.

4 Conclusion

The development of biomedical sciences and the different medical tech- niques gives us a glimpse of new perspectives with which to appreciate the status of the embryo and fetus. But we always have to distrust our different biological sciences and try to avoid actions that would compromise the future of life in general and human life especially. The moral status of the human embryo and the fetus depends on when we situate the beginning of the individual life and how the mother considers it. And, because the adult human being has capacities that the embryo/fetus does not necessarily have, its moral status heavily depends on the adult. I do not think that it is truly necessary to use a supreme morality principle in the analysis of the moral status of the embryo/fetus as Beyleveld has done with the *PGC.* With the evolution of moral and techno-scientific progress, we need not use ready-made principles to answer once for all the fundamental questions of the philosophy or the ethics on the subject. In subjects like the former, it is difficult to say what is the position that should be adopted. We cannot privilege a position more than another, because we think that the funda- mental difference that exists between the embryo/fetus and an adult human being is found only in the degree of maturity. We should try to arrange that there are no longer conflicts of interest between adult agents and agents that are not yet mature. We do not have to forget that the human being is a historical being, whose characteristics are conception, birth, growth, repro- duction, senescence and death. If we do not give a place to the human embryo/fetus, we can too easily deprive more mature humans of their status. We cannot consider in the same manner an embryo *in vivo* and an embryo *in vitro* or, a desired embryo/fetus and one that it is not. We have to respect each others' ideas. If we consider that the embryo/fetus is a 'potential person' or if we use different arguments, as Beyleveld has done, I think A. Fagot-Largeault and G. Delaisi de Parseval are right in stating that 'the sum of texts that have already been published on the embryo—and our different interventions today—on the status of the human embryo/fetus) well inaugurates our capacity to base our choice on a philosophical thought.' I admit eventually the compromise solution. But, basically I am in favour of a pragmatic position. I think that a pragmatic position is philosophically acceptable and that we have to reason from a set of principles that are not always homogeneous.

Notes

[1] See CCNE (1997), avis, rapport.
[2] Some African customs consider the embryo/fetus and placenta have the same status. In Cameroon, for example, like an embryo/fetus, a placenta is also buried (after delivery) because one thinks that it belongs integrally to the child that would be/is born.

References

Article 'Statut du corps humain, de ses éléments et produits', (1996), *Dictionnaire permanent bioéthique et biotechnologies*, Editions législatives: Paris.

Chambon, P. (1993), 'Des organes artificiels vivants', *Revue Sciences et avenir*, No. 553, pp. 14–18.

Engelhardt, H. T. (1996), *The Foundations of Bioethics*, Oxford University Press: New York.

Engelhardt, H. T. (1998), 'Respect de la vie et fondements de la bioéthique', in Noble, D. and Vincent, J. D. (eds), *L'éthique du vivant*, UNESCO: Paris.

Evans, D. (ed.) (1996), *Conceiving the Embryo: Ethics, Law and Practice in Human Embryology*, Martinus Nijhoff Publishers: London and Boston.

Fagot-Largeault, A. (1985), *L'homme bio-éthique: pour une déontologie de la recherche sur le vivant*, Maloine: Paris.

Fagot-Largeault, A. (1990), Article 174 'Le statut de l'embryon humain: analyse des positions du CCNE', *Le Supplément*, pp. 3–13.

Fagot-Largeault, A. (1993), 'Normativité biologique et normativité sociale', in Changeux, J. P. (ed.), *Fondements naturels de l'éthique*, Odile Jacob: Paris, pp. 191–225.

Fagot-Largeault, A. (1995), 'Philosophie, éthique et droit du vivant', *La propriété intellectuelle dans le domaine du vivant*, actes du colloque, Institut de France, Académie des sciences: London, TED, New York and Paris, pp. 9–18.

Fagot-Largeault, A. and Delaisi de Parseval. G. (1989), 'Qu'est-ce qu'un embryon? panorama des positions philosophiques actuelle', *Revue Esprit*, pp. 86–120.

Ferida, P. and Lecourt, D. (1996), *L'embryon humain est-il humain?* Forum Diderot, Puf: Paris.

Gewirth, A. (1978), *Reason and Morality*, University of Chicago Press: Chicago and London.

Huet, S. (1990), 'Bioéthique: faut-il une loi', *Revue sciences et avenir*, No. 526, pp. 74–77.

Kant, I. (1984), *Fondements de la métaphysique des moeurs*, traduction de Delbos, V. Delagrave: Paris.

Lajeunesse, Y. and Sosoe, L. K. (1996), *Bioéthique et culture démocratique*, L'Harmattan: Montréal, Canada, pp. 191–199.

Lery, N. (1998), 'L'embryon à définir: une proposition de synthèse', *Revue Le Supplément*, No. 174.

Mayle, F., Souccar, T., Tourbe, C. and Vincent, J. (1998), 'La vie avant la vie', *Revue Sciences et avenir*, No. 614.

Neirinck, N. (1998), 'L'embryon humain ou la question en apparence sans réponse de la bioéthique', *Les petites fiches*, No. 29.

Nietzsche, F. (1991), *La volonté de puissance. Essai d'une transmutation detoutes les valeurs*, traduction de Albert, H., Librairie générale française: Paris.

Prigogine, I. and Stengers, I. (1986), *La nouvelle alliance: métamorphose de la science*, collection Folio/essai, Gallimard: Paris.

Sève, L. (1994), *Pour une critique de la raison bioéthique*, Odile Jacob: Paris.

Spinoza. (1965), *Ethique*, traduction de Appuhn, C. and G. F. Flammarion, oeuvres III: Paris.

Sureau, C. and Shenfield, F. (eds) (1995), *Aspects éthiques de la reproduction humaine*, actes de congrès, John Libbey Eurotext: Paris, pp. 151–188.

Part Three

AUTONOMY AND RECOGNITION

Autonomy and Recognition

Jean-Pierre Wils

1 Introductory considerations[1]

Since the 1970s, human reproduction has, in every respect, become an increasingly important field for the development and application of genetic diagnostic and therapeutic methods. Fertility technology and procreative methods are opening up this formerly intimate area of human existence. There has also been radical progress in gene technology relating to animals and plants. This, however, has not become public to the same degree. The cloning of animals was the first development to draw attention in spectacular fashion to a technology that recalled science-fiction stories. In contrast, *in vitro* fertilisation, for example, was from the very beginning at the centre of considerable ethical and socio-political controversy. Since then, molecular-genetic studies have enormously increased our knowledge of genetic risks, illnesses and—to a lesser extent—therapeutic possibilities. Prenatal diagnostic methods have become more and more precise. Presymptomatic examinations have begun to confront us with possible and probable illnesses long before they arise.

A moral consensus was then, as today, hardly in sight (see Bayertz 1996). In the meantime, however, IVF has become part of the standard repertoire of prenatal techniques. The far-reaching possibilities of human genetic technology that followed have dramatically increased the room for manoeuvre—or the room for misuse, as some think. Nevertheless, public consciousness of these issues has already decreased considerably. Only spectacular cases still manage to arouse public attention, and then only briefly. Human genetic technology seems, in its complexity and distance from everyday life, to be something that concerns only 'those affected' and 'the experts'. The tendency is, however, for the entire period of prenatal development to become the object of concern for methods that diagnostically, therapeutically and selectively intervene in an area of human life that up until a few years ago was largely immune from such interventions.

Without a doubt, our idea of life has changed radically since the 1970s. Life has been to a large extent demystified. The air of mystery that once surrounded its origins has been penetrated by the analytical light in which

101

promising research on the cell is being carried out. The nature teleology that once formed the framework of European ethics has lost its plausibility, by reason of a general feeling that it is *superfluous and useless.* Transformations into the area of aesthetics are all that have remained. These have taken on an important function in the area of pre-normative ethics; one can, however, no longer speak of *normative directives.*

In the meantime, our consciousness of the complex nature of constructing ethical norms has also grown constantly. Applied ethics, or 'area-specific ethics', do not have the function of subsuming separate controversial problems under general norms, but rather the task of mediating on the level of an *interpretative or hermeneutical synthesis* between the methodological options or, rather, the substantial principles of a *general normative* ethics on the one hand, and complex *empirical* and *area-specific information* on the other. However, general concepts such as 'life' conceal and obscure this task more than they can contribute anything effective to making it comprehensible.

Let this be said without any intention of giving cause for looking back with nostalgia. To whom would such nostalgia be of benefit, given that it all too often degenerates into a cultural critique based on resentment? Nevertheless, the *position* that we adopt with respect to life has changed. This assertion remains at the same time very imprecise. What is 'life'? There are only concrete living beings, whom we *perceive* in a *particular* way, whom we *encounter* with particular *attitudes, and whom we treat in this way or that.* For this reason it is appropriate to avoid the abstract term 'life', not least because abstract terms often provoke equally general and indiscriminate opinions. In particular, they suggest that the fact that life 'exists' yields a 'meaning' that can perform a useful function as a signpost or point of orientation for working on ethical problems. This is however only infrequently the case. Once we can no longer derive the relevant normative information from *an essential structure of things* and are, accordingly, no longer in the position of *recipients* of this information, we have profoundly changed our relationship to the concrete phenomena. The potential for moral conflict contained by particular phenomena is the result of interpretation, which takes place in the context of our (now *problematic*) ethical tradition, our (*disputed*) basic normative assumptions *and* our (*differing*) preferences and interests.[2]

Terms that played almost no role in classical European ethics have been able to take on importance in this context. In the discussion that follows, attention will be directed towards the two categories of 'autonomy' and 'recognition'. In particular, the notion of 'recognition' clarifies the changed attitude to the morally relevant phenomena: *subjects* that stand in *relationship* to one another now *generate, expound, assess and normatise* moral problems *as such.* The term for the defining feature of such subjects is 'autonomy'. This latter is not a prerequisite for recognition; rather, it is *won* in the struggle *for* recognition and *by means of* recognition. Autonomy is the topic of recognition. Inasmuch as we can only meaningfully speak of autonomy given a background of recognition-relationships, I shall direct my attention to the notion of recognition.

2 What are recognition-relationships? A tentative definition

'Recognition' has been one of the central categories of moral philosophy since Hegel. *Recognition-relationships* are ethically significant in at least two ways. First, they establish the *content* of moral communication, which is mutual respect or mutual consideration for personal individuality. 'Respect-communication' (Luhmann 1978) is an essential component of what ethics is all about. 'Respect' is here not something one has for a person in the sense that *qualities* of his or her personality demand respect, but rather in the sense that this is demanded by *his or her personhood*.

But recognition-relationships also contain necessary (although not sufficient) conditions for communication about aspects of the validity of disputed moral issues, such as the interpretation of what we understand by 'regard' or 'respect'. Recognition-relationships can, for their part, be interpreted as the *morally relevant* basic conditions for such communication, in that asymmetries should be minimised *as much as possible*. In summary, this means: *recognition is a transcendental prerequisite and also a central topic of ethical communication*.

These considerations proceed, however, from an assumption that appears to be so self-evident that it hardly needs mentioning. *Recognition presupposes the visibility of the other person.* In the notion of recognition, different semantically and phenomenologically distinguishable 'layers' are conflated: the normative horizon or the content of moral action, the communicative conditions of ethical validity-disputes and, in a sense, as their anthropological foundation, the perception of the other person as a person. To the extent that the *self of the other* reveals itself to me as another self, the addressee of recognition is—phenomenologically—constituted. Here the notion of perception carries different levels of meaning: the literal seeing of a person, the perceiver's selective attention and—very closely related to this—the *interpretative configuration* of that which is perceived. Perception is the result of a complex construction in which neurologically based principles of form, on the one hand, and individual and cultural patterns of interpretation, on the other, play equally important and selective roles.

3 Perception as a factor in selective attention

But what happens when the identity of the other *escapes* our perception? Here I do not mean contingent—in the sense of place- or time-related—perception, but rather that perception in which we can identify the other as a moral counterpart. What happens when we begin to doubt whether we are dealing with *another self* at all? What happens when the personhood of the other is doubtful, in the sense that his or her identity is an object of scepticism and uncertainty, either because of the particular stage of development at which it finds itself, or even *as such?* Does not all recognition rely upon the certainty of the other's *anthropological* status? And is this status not based on a configuration of the other that sets him or her in a relationship of similarity to oneself?

In using the predicate 'anthropological', I do not refer to the mere fact of belonging to the human species, but to the visible person-like quality of the other as an unanalysable condition for reciprocity, which in turn seems to formulate even the possibility of recognition. 'Visible' means here quite literally the 'perceptibility' of the other as the *configuration* of a personal, or at least person-like, counterpart.

In this context, I want to stay with this notion of 'perception' for a moment. As I have already indicated, an elementary prerequisite for the constitution of moral consciousness is often ignored—the *recognition* of one's own self in the self of the other, the *recognition* of one's own subjectivity in that of the moral counterpart. 'Recognition', however, does not require a counterpart who finds him- or herself at the same stage of development (see Steigleder 1992, p. 283). But without *some possibility of recognising, recognition-relationships as such* are meaningless.

Although this situation can be described up to a point psychologically, it goes beyond every psychological theory. Rather, we are dealing here with a transcendental-anthropological constraint. It is pointless to seek the encounter with the other where there is no common ground. Emmanuel Lévinas' statement, 'As much of him as escapes our understanding, is himself' (1983, p. 115), ultimately abolishes the moral presence of the other. If the other does not become accessible to me as another self, then the basis of the constitution of moral recognition-relationships in general—*that persons are referred and oriented towards each other*[3]—is missing. We need not yet answer the question as to what this common ground consists in. But moral recognition-relationships cannot flourish if the counterpart is only present as 'the absence of any identity'.

This, however, is precisely what happens in the prenatal gene diagnostic and gene therapeutic context: the visibility of the other as a recognisable being with personal or person-like qualities disappears. Furthermore, the decoding of the genome, or rather the genetic manipulation that may follow it, leads to the creation of something I want to call *the possibility of interference with the other's subjectivity.* The situation is paradoxical: while on the one hand the individuality of an emerging human being becomes diagnostically and prognostically accessible, his or her face, the recognisable profile of this individuality, vanishes. At the same time, as our knowledge of concrete subjectivity is constantly increasing and the decoding of a specific genome makes the individuality of a human being literally public, we lose the anthropological contours of this individuality.

Looking at kinds of perception in our society, Paul Virilio (1989, p. 24) has spoken of a 'loss of feeling' that has profound consequences for our attitude to the world. Perception takes place under formal conditions that predetermine particular patterns and techniques. We perceive things not with our eyes only but rather within a multi-layered network in which the senses and cultural 'media' combine to form a perspective on reality. Depending on the principles of mediation we use to build up a picture of reality, our relationship to reality changes.

> The forms 'inform us not only about their being, about what they represent materially, but also about their experiences at that moment, in time, . . . about their tangible reality and the effects experienced. (Ibid., p. 9)

Within the context of the modern information and communication society, one can speak of two important effects on perception. First, 'the image has asserted itself against the thing' (Virilio 1996, p. 33); second, 'the thing' is dissected, taken out of its context and a 'shrinkage' (ibid., p. 51) takes place such that it becomes detached from its life environment. Almost all relevant medical innovations—from non-invasive operative techniques through to all the gene diagnostic and gene therapy procedures—take place in a field of *increasing miniaturisation.* Without the intervention of *microscopy,* the object of the operation is not visible. In particular, the decontextualisation and dissection of the object of perception raise its level of abstraction. This 'emancipation of abstraction' (Claessens 1980, p. 380) extinguishes the potential for recognition gained by evolution. We must relate to a *subjectivity* that reveals itself to us in the form of a mathematical representation. Members of our own species reveal them-selves to us in a strange 'demateriality' (Virilio 1996, p. 77), taken out of the normal spatial and temporal horizon of their development.

Virilio has rightly directed our attention—in another context—to the fact that considerable problems of interpretation now arise. Our traditional interpretations lose their integrating effect. The living being in its radical abstraction has rather a disintegrative effect with respect to the 'conserva-tive'[4] potential of our senses. In particular, the way in which the other is in a visual and tangible way present changes radically. Neither skin contact with the other (see Serres 1993), nor the unity of sensory experience in one's own body and the other's sensory experience (this tactile intimacy of two living beings as pregnant women have always known it) remains. *In this way, the sense of the other's reality is undermined.*

Let me emphasise again that the transformation of perception described here is intended only as an observation, although an observation with *direct* ethical relevance. In the course of technical evolution such transformations are inexorable. Nevertheless, they do not leave the *status of our experiences* untouched. Our habits of perception *select* phenomena on the basis of their *technological design* and *manipulate* our experiences *of* the phenomena. To this degree, the *culture-philosophically motivated* question as to 'whether we are soon to lose for good our status as *eye-witnesses* of sensorily perceptible reality in favour of technical substitutes' (Virilio 1996, p. 127)[5] is justified. When a mathematical and chemical formula is substituted for the body, the sensory exterior of the subjectivity of a human being, the body takes on a *phantom status* that banishes it from the world of familiar sensations and *moral attitudes*.[6]

In a certain sense, a *deception of moral sensibility* takes place: moral recognition-relationships, shrunk down to the size of an analysis of cell-substances, appear to evaporate, although we are *really* and *directly* dealing with the specific subjectivity of a (future) human being. This process of the shrinkage of individuality down to microscopic levels obviously causes perception to be *outwitted*.[7] Perception has 'become a trap' (see Welsch 1990, p. 65). Our moral sensibilities can barely keep pace with the stages of abstraction established by the new conditions. The radical and depersonalising distance of a human being, and the abstraction away from all evolutionarily practised patterns of perception over a longer period of time, is too much for any moral sensitivity. After a short phase of intense moral interest, our attention weakens—in the absence of *discernible, that is sensory support from perception.*

4 The conflict about the interpretation of perceptions

These briefly outlined changes are *structural*. They have a *collectivising* effect. To this extent, they are *spontaneous* processes that are to a large extent beyond our ability to influence them. They are the product of technical or rather technological innovations. I would like to clarify this with an example. Since the mid-60s, beginning with the photography of Lennart Nilsson, the *intra-uterine* processes have become visible that, beginning with the nervous journey of the sperm to the egg cell, direct the entire development of a human being in the womb. The zygote becomes photogenic—and all its following developmental steps are now phototechnically documented. Essentially, what happens is initially a revolution of the moral plausibility structures that have been valid up to that point: the moment the interior becomes manifest and the invisible visible, moral consciousness is forced to turn to a field of perception that was previously almost completely inaccessible, and we become witnesses to a technically accessed biological intimacy.

Soon *after* the mid-60s the notion of a 'misplaced concreteness' began to circulate (see Sontag 1986). The zygote is presented as something that, apart from the extent to which it can be 'seen' by means of photographic technology, is strictly imperceptible, but the photography insinuates a concrete other. The body of the woman is opened up and mutates into a 'glass show case' (Duden 1991, p. 44). Ultrasound scanning, now part of the standard repertoire of prenatal diagnosis, brings about a *technologically mediated quasi-communication* at a point in time at which communication could previously not be spoken of. To the degree that the process between conception and birth could now be presented to a seeing public, the interpretation of the processes involved in pregnancy changed accordingly: a train of events, which until well into our century was completely invisible for the vast majority of human beings, and which in addition could hardly be influenced effectively, could now be reconstructed back to the moment of conception.[8]

As soon as pregnancy became visible, a new responsibility arose for the quality of the pregnancy and for that of the growing child. It is easier, initially at least, to argue that a developing child is an 'intra-uterine person' if one can already recognise child-like features at an early stage. New interpretations of the status of children in gestation are made practically mandatory as soon as new features become visible.

Regardless of whether one defends the personhood of the embryo with the new—in a literal sense—evidence, as has often been done, or speaks with Barbara Duden and other feminists of a 'legal fiction in the lower abdomen' (Duden 1991, p. 72), the new visibility gives rise to a conflict of interpretations, which are ultimately concerned with the moral status of the child that has become perceptible.

Regardless of whether one wants to speak of *illusions* or *realities* of perception here, the issue is nevertheless a 'conflict concerning the interpretation of perceptions', which can still be relatively simply related to our 'normal' objects of perception. This changes, however, as soon as this process of accessing new microscopic evidence is itself radicalised. This takes place in the wake of gene diagnosis and gene therapy. Gene frequencies and mathematical proportions now force us to distance ourselves for good from every *prima facie* indication, from everything we can recognise through the mediation of our senses. Our moral sensibility now loses its sensory and orienting point of reference in reality. Perception—and thus moral consciousness as well—seems to be overstrained once and for all. This means that we have to invent new styles, new ways of perception.

Perceptions are full of interpretations. With respect to particular phenomena, moral awareness is constructed in terms of a sensory hermeneutics, i.e., in terms of a constructive interpretation by means of the senses. The senses perceive selectively. Our perceptions contain a 'symbolic pregnancy', which generates 'experiences' out of data (Cassirer 1977, pp. 222ff.).[9] They not only make selections from the inexhaustible over-information of sense-impressions, but also *intervene by interpreting and evaluating* these selections. This happens not only because perception has cortically anchored formal principles at its disposal, which direct the work of selection, but also because this selection is made mandatory by culturally and situationally conditioned *habits of perception.* Our moral awareness does not exist independently of socio-cultural styles of perception, of the habituation of the senses, which consists not least in value-judgments.

The phenomena as such, just as they present themselves to the senses as pure 'data', only reach our consciousness and our moral awareness by way of a complex path of selection and formation. Only by means of the 'background effect' of habits of perception do phenomena gain their own colouring. It is 'the horizon,' writes Maurice Merleau-Ponty in his *Phenomenology of Perception,* 'which guarantees the identity of the object for the searching look' (1966, p. 92). This constitutive function of the interpretative horizon is valid, not only for the laws of perceptional psychology that determine our perceptions, but also for the *culturally sedimentary meaning* of what we perceive. Words, as well as their references in reality and their meanings in our interpretations, are not understood in isolation, cut off from their semantic and value contexts and networks.

> The meaning of a word is not constructed out of a particular number of physical characteristics of an object; it is rather, and primarily, the appearance which this object takes on in human experience …. It is …, so to speak, a part of the behaviour of the world, a particular modification of its style, and the generality of meaning, just like that of an item of vocabulary, is not the generality of a concept, but rather that of the world as type. (Ibid., p. 459)[10]

With reference to this problem of perception, this means that we access the meaning of sensory data first of all in the process of a typical, hermeneutical configuration that pre-empts the power of our subjectivity and the sovereignty of our self-consciousness. Our ability to choose our habits or styles of perception is very limited. We perceive things in 'epistemological fields or profiles' that make the world accessible to us and constitute the phenomena in this world *in their meaning for us*. Therefore, says Merleau-Ponty,

> every seeing ultimately presupposes, somewhere in the depths of consciousness, an overall design or a logic of the world which every empirical perception defines more precisely, but cannot itself create. (1966, p. 461)

There is, as Ernst H. Gombrich (1960) put it, no 'innocent eye' with which we perceive ourselves and the things around us. Our thinking and our behaviour are embedded in 'styles', in concrete hermeneutical ways. Our perception, or, as the Germans say, our 'Wahrnehmung', is at the same time quite literally a 'Für-wahr-nehmen', the taking of something to be true, inasmuch as it is filled with collective assumptions of a theoretical and practical nature concerning reality. These assumptions are 'stylistic structures' (Fleck 1980, p. 40), 'symbolic fields' (Sieferle 1990),[11] in which our perception, thinking, behaviour and judgment take place. This dependence of perception on collective hermeneutical presuppositions, confirmed by the theory of science and since demonstrated in experimental psychology to the point of constructivism, is not only well documented, but also of the greatest relevance for the condition of moral awareness.

The notion that animals can suffer, inasmuch as they are beings sensitive to pain and have elementary feelings at their disposal, largely escaped classical European moral attention. Today, sensitised by behavioural research and zoology, we see animals suffering almost everywhere. Suddenly we *have practically no alternative* to perceiving the situation this way and not that.

The amount of information that the world offers us is potentially unlimited. If we do not want to drown in this flood, we have to be selective. To begin with, we must construct a new world appropriate to finite human beings on the basis of a selection of relevant data. In this way, we stylise and produce a world in which we can live on the basis of selected perception, knowledge, behaviour and judgment. In this collective and cultural *a priori,* a 'world-birth' takes place that we allow to guide our attention (see Goodman 1990).

With respect to the question of a morally correct assessment of facts and situations, this obviously does not mean that questions of validity can be reduced to the identification of collective habits of perception. But the strong relationship that holds between explicit moral opinions on the one hand and the 'dispositional' or 'habitual' carrying out of actions on the other can hardly be underestimated (see Bourdieu 1988, pp. 15ff.). This disposition is the result of fundamental interpretations: we understand the world by subjecting it to a depth-hermeneutics, which initially effects a stylisation of perception: we select relevant data and condense it in our knowledge, our behaviour and our judgments to an elementary picture of the world, to a fundamental interpretation. Our relationship to the world is 'impregnated with interpretation' (Lenk 1993, p. 264). Our perceptions are directed by selective, pictorial configurations of the world in which the individual objects gain their contours and values. *Explicit* reasons for our moral behaviour can then be understood as rational commentaries with which we support, confirm, or possibly criticise and even reject our basic interpretations.

With regard to the problem of recognition, this means that *in recognition-relationships the other is also initially constructed.* There is a sense in which one can say that actual recognition is already based on an *implicit* recognition, in that we have already selected a potential partner. What turns out to be worthy of recognition is already the result of a choice, which is in turn the result of a particular interpretation of reality. The 'struggle' for recognition constructs and establishes not only recognition-relationships, but also the participants in this process.

This all becomes more difficult, though, as soon as one of these participants has become a living abstraction. This is in essence the case with the various techniques of prenatal gene diagnosis and gene therapy, pre-implantation genetic diagnosis and *in vitro* fertilisation. Essentially, what happens now is that, in proportion to the stages of abstraction, the proportion of *imagination* involved in the construction of the other in the recognition-relationship grows. One could even argue that the partner to whom the recognition is due has now him- or herself become *imaginary.* We have to create a relationship to a being that in its microscopic dimensions eludes the sight by which we access the world we live in and which guides our moral awareness. Instead of this 'sight', a forced second order sight comes into play, the sight of a subjectivity that (in the first instance) is not 'there'—*an imagined subjectivity.* But if the recognition-relationship is *imaginary,* is then the moral recognition for its part *illusory?*

At this point it is worth quickly reminding ourselves of Hegel's famous 'struggle for recognition' in his *Phenomenology of Spirit.* After all, there are a number of remarkable parallels to the problems that have so far been discussed.

5 Hegel's 'struggle for recognition'—a brief reprise

'Recognition' is a procedural event in which the subject of the recognition constitutes his or her own respective autonomy in a movement of mutual

110

distancing and identification. Autonomy is the prerequisite of *moral consideration*. But consideration *in the context of recognition-relationships* has a particular appearance, the appearance of a morality that is oriented according to 'rights' and 'responsibilities.'

The initial relationship—that between a Lord and his bondsman—is *asymmetrical*. Hegel describes the genesis of autonomy as a process within which the identifying features of self-consciousness gain, as it were, a kind of social reality. For this reason, we learn something about the 'inside' of self-consciousness as the condition for the possibility of becoming an autonomous subject at all, and also something about those relationships in which autonomy is really constituted and can become the object of recognition and consideration. Recognition-relationships *constitute* subjects worthy of recognition and do not presuppose them. The normative model for this genesis is self-consciousness. This can only be understood, however, on the basis of a dialectic between the self and the other.

The emergence of self-consciousness described here, thus, contains a number of aspects: first, a *phenomenology* of self-consciousness; second, a *social genesis* of self-consciousness; and third, the *constitution of self-conscious relationships* in the sense of moral recognition-relationships. Recognition appears as an ascription that grows out of a complex structure of reciprocal seeing or mutual perception. What is important is that this reciprocity leads one not only to perceive his or her self in the other, but also to *change* this self in the process of the genesis of self-consciousness. If we can describe the result of the 'struggle for recognition' as the establishment of moral autonomy, it then becomes clear that autonomy is not the pre-condition but rather *the result* of recognition. At the beginning of this process, autonomy, viewed as its outcome, is a distant, imaginary result. And the whole process could be described as a procedure in which the *relata*—Lord and bondsman—*imagine* themselves into the position of the other.

The 'self' of consciousness comes into being only when it is confronted with 'otherness', but not only with 'otherness' in general, but specifically with another self, with the self of an other. It is only in the course of this encounter that a consciousness of self as *this* and not *that* self emerges out of a more general self-consciousness. This occurs in the mirror of another self.

> Self-consciousness exists in and for itself when, and by the fact that, it so exists for another; that is, it exists only in being acknowledged. (Hegel 1977, paragraph 178, p. 111)

Hegel describes recognition as a 'motion', as an 'action', the action of the one as 'the action of the other' (ibid., paragraph 181, pp. 111–112).

111

Accordingly, recognition is not merely a relationship one thinks *about*. The recognition meant here arises instead as a transaction that takes place between the *relata*. The dialectic between 'Lord' and 'bondsman' can, as has already been indicated, also be understood as a dialectic between autonomy and becoming aware. Autonomy is not *a given* for recognition, but rather the *product of becoming aware of oneself in the process of being acknowledged and recognised by the other*.

The process described by Hegel has to do with a 'manifold and ambiguous crossing-over',[12] which is expounded in its separate phases, conceived as phases of becoming a self, as becoming *aware* of oneself. When it is emphasised again and again that the procedure is 'ambiguous', this highlights the fact that we are dealing with a mutual seeing as a seeing of ourselves, both literally and metaphorically. In Hegel's own words: 'They *recognize* themselves as *mutually recognizing* one another' (Hegel 1977, paragraph 181, p. 112). The whole procedure would lead to no result if the imagination, in this case the ability to imagine *oneself* in the other, *oneself* present with the other, was not centrally involved. In other words, the self has an imaginary status without being therefore fictitious. It is the result of a crossing-over of viewpoints and, although we are dealing here with an imaginary seeing, the adoption of perspective has to do with the real ability to perceive the other. Following the model of self-consciousness that orients itself according to the phenomenon of sight—and which was rejected by Martin Heidegger (1949, p. 20) as being *ocular*,[13] the genesis of recognition can be understood as a point at which self-consciousness becomes more precise with reference to the sight of the other.[14]

Now, it would be a misunderstanding if one was to conclude from this that all those who do not (or cannot) participate in this dialectic of seeing are for their part overlooked. The struggle for recognition does not mean that *only* those who enter into this struggle have a *right* to recognition. Hegel says explicitly that the 'individual' that does not risk itself in this struggle 'may well be recognized as a *person*' (Hegel 1977, paragraph 187, p. 114). A right to moral respect can also be acquired by such a 'person', but what is missing then is self-respect. A person defined in this way remains in a sense a passive and therefore dependant recipient of respect.

The scope of the dialectic between Lord and bondsman lies in the fact that the self-consciousness of the Lord proves to be dependent on the 'insignificant' consciousness of the bondsman. In *his* struggle for respect, the Lord clings to the 'insignificant' consciousness of the bondsman, while the bondsman orients himself according to the 'essential action' of the Lord, even though the accordance of respect has not yet been *accomplished*. The asymmetry is present in both cases, but only the initially

inferior consciousness of the bondsman still has the chance of a strength-
ened self before it.

> The *truth* of the independent consciousness is accordingly the servile
> consciousness of the bondsman. This, it is true, appears at first
> *outside* of itself and not as the truth of self-consciousness . . .
> servitude in its consummation will really turn into the opposite of
> what it immediately is; as a consciousness forced back into itself, it
> will withdraw into itself and be transformed into a truly independent
> consciousness. (Hegel 1977, paragraph 193, p. 117)

The self-consciousness of the Lord is, in a sense, empty because it has not
experienced the resistance that proceeds from the other, whereas the self-
consciousness of the bondsman initially exists only as consciousness of
dependency. In the process of recognition, by virtue of a continuous
exchange of perspectives—the dangerous exchange of lines of vision—
something is raised to consciousness that was already effective as a facil-
ity—namely, self-consciousness as the *constitutive feature of autonomy.*

> [T]his truth of pure negativity and being-for-itself, for it has experi-
> enced this its own essential nature. For this consciousness has been
> fearful, not of this or that particular thing or just at odd moments, but
> its whole being has been seized with dread; for it has experienced the
> fear of death, the absolute Lord. In that experience it has been quite
> unmannered, has trembled in every fibre of its being, and everything
> solid and stable has been shaken to its foundations. But this pure
> universal movement, the absolute melting-away of everything stable,
> is the simple, essential nature of self-consciousness, absolute nega-
> tivity, *pure being-for-self*, which consequently is *implicit* in this
> consciousness. This moment of pure being-for-itself is also *explicit*
> for the bondsman, for in the lord it exists for him as his *object*. (Ibid.,
> paragraph 194, p. 117)

In this process, a formation of self-consciousness takes place. The genesis
of self-consciousness by means of the dialectically interwoven phases of
successive abrogation of the asymmetric initial positions does not lead to
the disappearance of the counterpart. *The independence of the one proves
to be dependent on the independence of the other.* The one only recognises
himself or herself as independent in the mirror of the independence of the
other. The recognition with which we are concerned here shows that the
dialectical genesis of self-consciousness constitutes the *moral subject of
the first person:* the one constitutes himself or herself as a moral person
only in the process of recognising the independence of the other. Only

when I give the other self-consciousness respect, does the self-respect come into being that makes me a moral person. If, however, the relationship between persons remains asymmetrical, then I encounter the other at best with anxiety, otherwise with condescension.

> Persons always behave towards each other like persons and mutually ascribe to each other the status of subjects and self-consciousness. (Sturma 1997, p. 313)[15]

The dialectic of recognition shows the extent to which self-conscious subjects in the sense of moral persons give rise to each other. 'The moral independence of the first and moral respect for the second and third persons are mutually dependent on each other' (Sturma 1997, p. 315).

6 The dialectic of recognition—a procedure of exclusion?

Nevertheless, there is an important difference between this *general* topography of recognition-relationships and the *special* situation defined by the *fundamental* asymmetry with which we are confronted in genetic and prenatal dealings with 'others'. This is because the elementary conditions for speaking of reciprocity in any sense at all are here missing. Zygotes do not form *relata* in a recognition-relationship. They are at best the object of care and responsible treatment. For this reason, they also do not have the moral dignity that we ascribe to self-aware subjects. This, however, does not mean that they have no moral status. But the conditions for and possibilities of such a status are more complex and controversial than those that arise as a result of recognition-relationships. The reciprocity between moral persons that arises out of the dialectic of recognition can be used as a sort of moral criterion for actions and omissions in this field. In the case of genetic manipulation, however, this option is not open to us.

The dialectic of recognition constitutes subjects with rights, whose autonomy as moral persons is *fought for* and consequently *established* in their 'struggle for recognition' (Honneth 1992). Here, the essential defining characteristics of persons are no longer in the foreground, but rather the norm of final reciprocity between participants and their orientation with respect to universalist moral principles is. According to the successive abrogation of initial asymmetries, or with regard to the ideal of *mutual* recognition in recognition-relationships, autonomy does not dominate the affective assessment that is brought to bear on a *being with needs*. The missing symmetry with regard to vulnerable or needy beings is usually bridged by affective and emotional concern. Recognition-relationships in which moral agents act, however, cannot orient themselves

114

according to affective concern simply because this is unreliable. Sympathy does not reduce uncertainty with regard to the moral status of the addressee.

But even the *social* value placed on the various abilities and characteristics of members of a caring society is not fully applicable here, given that the *conventionality* and *traditionality* of social recognition contradicts the *principle of strict mutuality* on which recognition-relationships are based. Recognition-relationships are concerned rather with the *cognitive respect* that is granted to the other and owed to him or her as a moral person. The *self-respect* gained here is essentially different from the *self-confidence* that arises from emotional attention, and from the *self-worth* that arises from social recognition. This all makes it extraordinarily difficult to determine the place and status of non-autonomous living beings in such relationships. In premodern societies, the moral rights that defend such beings are anchored in affective attitudes and social conventions. But by their 'autonomy orientation' *modern* societies are unable to accept such attitudes and conventions as the foundations of their moral grammar *in principle,* because of the basic emancipatory and egalitarian assumptions that accompany this orientation.

> The conventional morality of such communities builds a normative horizon in which the manifold nature of individual rights and responsibilities remain bound to the variously valued tasks within the social network of co-operation. If, therefore, legal recognition is graded according to the respective value which accrues to the individual in his or her role in the society, this relationship only dissolves in the course of the historical process which subjects legal conditions to the demands of a post-conventional morality. The recognition due to a person in the sense of the law, which in principle must accrue to every subject, is now so divorced from the level of social recognition that two different forms of respect are created. (Honneth 1992, p. 179)[16]

'Legal recognition' and 'social recognition' belong to two different 'systemic' worlds. In the world of legal persons, actions are carried out according to principles 'without concrete respect for persons', that is, postconventionally and according to a universalist perspective. On the other hand, social recognition takes place in a world of concrete individuals together with their contingent social interactions, in which conventions and affective relationships play a dominating role. Whereas the 'first' world—according to its self-understanding—is by nature emancipatory, it can be perceived from the perspective of the 'second' world as *selective* and *eliminating.* This happens when living beings, who in the social world

115

of social relationships belong to the community of moral 'agents' and 'patients' (see Warnock 1971, pp. 151ff.), are *de jure* only partially represented in the world of legal persons. In the former, they are accepted as 'social persons', that is, as persons due to conventional and affective attitudes; in the latter, they do not belong to 'persons strictly' see Engelhardt 1986, pp. 115ff.). Modern law operates on the basis of an *ontology of persons able to act,* not on the basis of a conventional morality with undemonstrated teleological and metaphysical background constructions. The conclusion seems therefore unavoidable

> that out of the vagueness in principle about what constitutes the status of a responsible person, a structural openness of modern law results for gradually extending it and making it more precise. (Honneth 1992, p. 178)

Now Honneth has pointed out that everything depends on 'how the characteristics of a person which give rise to a normative obligation towards him or her can be defined' (Honneth 1992, p. 182). But he reduces this question to the *discourse concerning the application* of universal norms: characteristics that give rise to normative obligations distinguish persons from all living beings to which these norms cannot be applied. Persons are defined by means of characteristics that constitute their ability to think and act. To this extent, the argumentation is circular: the postulation of these characteristics is described as merely an 'empirical recognition' that already presupposes the normativity of these essential characteristics.

In reality, we are by no means dealing with a mere 'empirical recognition'. *Which* characteristics we ascribe to the *primary* addressees of moral responsibility is *crucially, although not exclusively,* dependent on the level of social value we place on their abilities and characteristics in the framework of our individual *preferences* and our *social value judgments. Such preferences and value judgments are socialised in cultural habits of perception.*

The value placed on a human being has to do with a 'gradual assessment of concrete characteristics and abilities' and, as such, presupposes an 'evaluative system of reference points' (Honneth 1992, p. 183). Honneth, however, reduces this secondary, flanking approach, to the task of distinguishing the concrete value put on *individual* persons from the cognitive respect that accrues to persons as legal subjects *in general.* The moral status of human beings who do not in a strict sense belong to the 'moral community' remains precarious in this case as well. But even the status of persons whose characteristics were *up until now* sufficient for participating in it, is by no means guaranteed. For Honneth, there is

116

no characteristic ... which has in itself such clear contours that they can be fixed once and for all; the range of meanings attributable to the proposition that a subject is capable of acting autonomously according to reason can instead only be determined relative to a definition of what is meant by reaching a rational agreement. This is because according to how this legitimating basis procedure is visualised, the characteristics which have to be ascribed to a person if he or she wants to participate on an equal footing must change. *The determination of the abilities which constitutively distinguish the human being is therefore dependent on the subjective prerequisites which make it possible for someone to participate in achieving a rational consensus. The more difficult such a procedure is conceived to be, the more comprehensive the characteristics will have to be which together make up the moral responsibility of a subject.* (1992, p. 185)

Quite apart from the question of what consequences such a position has for the notion of legal accountability, a dangerous reversal of perspectives has taken place here. The demands placed on the rationality of the 'legitimating basic procedure' now decide who can participate on an equal footing in the procedures that lead to recognition. The normative characteristics of personhood depend as 'background assumptions' on what criteria the 'rational procedure' of the legal system applies to the profile of persons. The struggle for recognition is here cognitively narrowed. Only those living beings are *selected* for cognitive recognition and *legitimated* as participants in the procedure that satisfy the growing demands of the criteriology prescribed by the requirements of procedural rationality. This means, however, that in the long run the legal system loses its protective function *as such*. Of course, the *reason for the validity* of ascribing moral rights to particular subjects must be distinguished from the *extent* of the area protected by these rights. It is therefore entirely possible for the circle of addressees of cognitive respect to differ from the circle of those who profit from a legally anchored protective measure (see Düwell 1998, pp. 34ff.). Concepts for gradualisation and scaling can and must mediate here. *But in order for this to succeed, the social value placed on the characteristics of those human beings who only passively participate in protective rights must for its part form an interest that directs understanding and practice in the field of interaction in which the struggle for recognition is being fought.*

What is underestimated in this model of recognition—and this has significant consequences—is the function of *social recognition* in the definition of the circle of addressees or 'patients' in the recognition procedure.[17] Granted, for Honneth this also belongs to the integral scheme of the dimensions of recognition; but its centre lies without a doubt in the area of

117

cognitive respect between ultimately *symmetrically* positioned partners. The struggle for recognition relates to participation in this cognitive discourse of regard. Without the social resource of value ascriptions against the background of evaluative assumptions that view characteristics and abilities as worthy of protection, legal subjects lose in the long run their sense for the complexities of humanity. This model of recognition, with its one-sided cognitive ideal of regard, is therefore open to the danger of becoming a technique instead of an ethic. Niklas Luhman calls such techniques 'a functioning simplification' (Luhmann 1992, p. 21).

But under these conditions, would not the smallest children and demented human beings already fall out of the protected area as this is constituted through recognition-relationships and made concrete in the construction of moral rights? Are they not inhabitants of the 'community of rights'? (See Gewirth 1996.) True, they have neither 'voluntariness or freedom' nor 'purposiveness or intentionality' at their disposal (Gewirth 1996, p. 13). They lack the elementary prerequisites for 'human action'. Are they therefore without rights?

Traditionally, rights are given to persons, but since Locke and Kant, 'persons' and 'human beings' are not simply identified with each other. To the extent that 'persons' are defined as beings capable of action, this 'new' tradition does not differ radically from the 'metaphysical' tradition, but this latter did not direct its attention to the difference between 'persons' and 'human beings' either. For this reason, the criterion of self-consciousness played hardly any role. But as soon as 'self-consciousness' has to discriminate between 'persons' and 'human beings', rights must be *conferred* on 'human beings'. Kant's idea of an 'a-temporal or intelligible person' that enters into a connection with the individual of the species is an attempt to create a relationship between moral rights and the biological characteristics of the human race.

By 'persons', Hegel, too, understands subjects, *to the extent that* they are capable of reflecting on their actions ('reflection of the will into itself') (Hegel 1942, section 105) and of 'expressing their will as a subjective or moral will' (ibid., section 113) in action. The person constitutes the 'ability to have rights'. And entirely in accordance with the result of the dialectic of recognition, the 'commandment of rights' runs as follows: 'Be a person and respect others as persons' (ibid., section 36). In that children, for example, do not participate in this situation of mutual respect, their rights must be given a different foundation: the rights of children are bound to the notion of 'life' (ibid., section 174). This life is specified by means of 'self-feeling' as characteristic of the human soul: the 'feeling soul' or 'simple ideality, subjectivity of feeling' (Hegel 1970, section 403, p. 122). becomes in 'self-feeling' the ability of individuality 'to distinguish itself in itself and to awake to the capacity for judgment in itself

118

according to which it has *particular* feelings and exists as a *subject* with regard to these, its terms of definition' (Hegel 1970, section 40, p. 160). Physical sensitivity to oneself already belongs to the sphere of influence of self-aware personhood that can justify passive rights.

Hegel leaves us in no doubt that we are dealing with a differentiated mode of sensing one's own body, by virtue of which protective rights are already established. Nevertheless, we are not dealing with persons in the sense in which they are mutually produced in recognition-relationships here either. Once a distinction has been drawn between membership of the species and personhood by means of consciousness- and action-criteria, one can only avoid the impending exclusivity—literally 'shutting out'—of personhood by way of a *gradualism*. As it turns out, there is development biological and anthropological evidence that can function as an empirical indication of this gradualism, evidence that already serves Kant and Hegel as a bridge between membership of the species and personhood. So there is no alternative to attempting to distinguish degrees, even when one identifies personhood with membership of the species. With this maximal assumption, however, one would *semantically empty* the notion of person-hood. I agree with Ludwig Siep when he suggests the following two options for such a gradualisation:

> One should either connect personhood with particular active rights . . . . Then, however, a decision will have to be made concerning the ability to have passive rights, or rather the protective rights of non-persons. Or the notion of person stands for individuals of the human species again as 'natura rationalis' . . . . Then a gradation of rights will have to be attempted according to the degrees of development of persons. (Siep 1992, pp. 113ff.)

This kind of gradualism, which seems to me to be unavoidable,[18] saves us at the same time from an over-extension[19] of the notion of recognition. This latter only makes sense in a context of self-reflexive encounter with the other. Here this other must be able to be a sounding board for my own subjectivity. If this is not the case, the meaning of what we call recognition disappears. Adjoining the *narrow* conceptual space of *recognition in a strict sense,* where the autonomy of persons builds the guiding practical interest, is a *broader* conceptual space in which the proximity to the autonomy of persons is produced, amongst other things, by means of an 'evaluative system of reference' with which we evaluate 'specific charac-teristics and abilities' (Honneth 1992) *in a graded fashion.* This evaluative horizon of references, however, is constituted not least by means of habits of perception in which we give living beings a moral contour against the background of our individual preferences, and primarily against the background of cultural value judgments. To the extent that the addressee of these value judgments becomes abstract in his or her anthropological profile, perceptions become necessary that are carried by an emphatic imagination—by the willingness to recognise already in these abstract preliminary stages of personhood the potential bearers of autonomy who only in later recognition procedures will find their way to an ultimate cognitive form.

Notes

1.   This chapter was translated by Glenn Patten.
2.   On the function of interpretation in moral issues, see Lenk 1998.
3.   Jacques Derrida's emphasis on this irreducible 'egoity', against Lévinas' attempt to remove every trace of intentionality from the original encounter with the face of the other, is the point at which his criticism is and remains justified (see Derrida 1976).
4.   See Claessens 1980, p. 317: 'Given the erosive weakening of synthetic reserves and the simultaneously perceptible weakening of synthetic possibilities, the issue of the nineteenth century was already the Angst, i.e., the existentially oppressive feeling of fear in the face of the inability in principle to develop living reality and identity-conserving and identity-giving meaning out of analytical, i.e., dissolved reality.' (Translated by G. Patten.)
5.   Virilio speaks in this context of an 'ethics of perception'.
6.   'It will have been observed that the problem of "bio-ethics" consists in the fragmentation of the conceptual area of the body; on the philosophical level, however, the issue concerns the fragmentation of the duration or, expressed differently, the specific temporality of the body' (Virilio 1994, p. 139).
7.   It is worth considering whether the 'inconsistency in the attitude to embryos and foetuses' described by Eve-Marie Engels is caused by confusions and uncertainties in the perception of such living beings (see Engels 1998, p. 291).
8.   Nevertheless, innumerable techniques for the heightening of male and female fertility have existed for centuries. (See Josephs 1998.)
9.   In his essay on 'the liberating power of symbolic design', Jürgen Habermas has drawn our attention with great precision to the constitutive function of the achievement of symbolic succinctness: 'Acts of symbolising distinguish themselves in the first instance by the fact that they burst genre-specific defined environments by transforming fluctuating sensory impressions into semantic meaning' (Habermas 1977, p. 19). (Translated by G. Patten.)
10.   Translated by G. Patten.
11.   It must suffice here merely to name the works on the theory of science, already classics in their field, which reflect on this issue: Foucault 1973 and 1978; Bachelard 1976; Canguillem 1979; Fichant 1977; and Kuhn 1996.

12 Translated by G. Patten. The Oxford translation is, in this case, not exact: 'The Notion of this its unity in its duplication embraces many and varied meanings' (Hegel 1977, paragraph 178, p. 111).

13 Cf. Plessner 1980; and Beierwaltes 1957.

14 I agree with Dieter Sturma (1992, p. 126) that 'the physical appearance of a person [is] an important feature for re-identifying him or her.' Sturma is also right when he says that this physicality is 'in no sense sufficient for the constitution of the relationship of a person to him- or herself or to others.' But if 'persons always perceive each other in such a way as to assume mutually similar perspectives of consciousness for each other', then the potential for re-identifying someone which includes the person's physical appearance belongs to this change of perspective as a necessary condition. Sturma fails to consider this. It is not true that perspectives of consciousness are only based on an assumption, or rather, that 'they belong to the part of personal existence which cannot be observed.' Granted, there is no presence in the consciousness of the other; but his or her physical appearance—his or her anthropological identification potential—carries the change of perspective. (Translations from Sturma by G. Patten.)

15 Translated by G. Patten.

16 Translated by G. Patten.

17 This, however, does not mean that the obligatory nature of values merely rests on the fact that they are a 'social institution' (Hoerster 1991 p. 21).

18 I share the view that 'potentiality' and 'degree of proximity to the ability to act' are essential and necessary indications for the ascription of moral status to non-autonomous human beings with Klaus Steigleder. (See, most recently, Steigleder 1998.)

19 See, for example, Pröpper 1995. The proposition that because human beings are intended for the freedom of God, even 'in the most extreme, apparently hopeless case' one 'must not close oneself to the possibility of [this freedom's] realisation beyond human possibilities" is a demand which, inasmuch as it goes "beyond human possibilities', cannot be an ethical demand.

References

Bachelard, G. (1976), *Die Bildung des wissenschaftlichen Geistes,* Suhrkamp: Frankfurt a. Main.

Bayertz, K. (1996) (ed.), *Moralischer Konsens. Technische Eingriffe in die menschliche Fortpflanzung als Modellfall*, Suhrkamp: Frankfurt a. Main.

Beierwaltes, W. (1957), *Lux intelligibilis. Untersuchung zur Lichtmetaphorik der Griechen*, Munich.

Bourdieu, P. (1988), *Praktische Vernunft. Zur Theorie des Handelns*, Suhrkamp: Frankfurt a. Main.

Canguillem, G. (1979), *Wissenschaftsgeschichte und Epistemologie. Gesammelte Aufsätze*, edited by W. Lepenies, Suhrkamp: Frankfurt a. Main.

Cassirer, E. (1977), *Philosophie der symbolischen Formen, Vol. 3: Phänomenologie der Erkenntnis*, Wissenschaftliche Buchgesellschaft: Darmstadt.

Claessens, D. (1980), *Das Konkrete und das Abstrakte. Soziologische Skizzen zur Anthropologie*, Suhrkamp: Frankfurt a. Main.

Derrida, J. (1976), 'Violence and Metaphysics', in *Die Schrift und die Differenz*, Frankfurt a. Main, pp. 121–235.

Duden, B. (1991), *Der Frauenleib als öffentlicher Ort*, dtv: Hamburg 1991.

Düwell, M. (1998), 'Ethik der genetischen Frühdiagnostik—eine Problemskizze', in Düwell, M. and Mieth, D. (eds), *Ethik in der Humangenetik. Die neueren Entwicklungen der genetischen Frühdiagnostik aus ethischer Perspektive*, Francke: Tübingen, pp. 26–48.

Engelhardt, H. T. Jr. (1986), *The Foundations of Bioethics*, Oxford University Press: New York and Oxford.

Engels, E.-M. (1998), 'Der moralische Status von Embryonen und Feten—Forschung, Diagnose, Schwangerschaftsabbruch', in Düwell, M. and Mieth, D. (eds), *Ethik in der Humangenetik. Die neueren Entwicklung der genetischen Frühdiagnostik aus ethischer Perspektive*, Francke: Tübingen, pp. 217–301.

Fichant, M. (1977), *Michel Pécheux, Überlegungen zur Wissenschaftsgeschichte*, Suhrkamp: Frankfurt a. Main.

Fleck, L. (1980), *Entstehung und Entwicklung einer wissenschaftlichen Tatsache*, Suhrkamp: Frankfurt a. Main.

Foucault, M. (1973), *Archäologie des Wissens*, Suhrkamp: Frankfurt a. Main.

Foucault, M. (1978), *Die Ordnung der Dinge*, Suhrkamp: Frankfurt a. Main.

Gewirth, A. (1996), *The Community of Rights*, University of Chicago Press: Chicago.

Gombrich, E. H. (1960), *Art and Illusion: A Study in the Psychology of Pictorial Representation*, Phaidon Press: London.

Goodman, N. (1990), *Weisen der Welterzeugung*, Suhrkamp: Franfurt a. Main.

Habermas, J. (1977), *Vom sinnlichen Ausdruck zum symbolischen Ausdruck*, Suhrkamp: Frankfurt a. Main.

Hegel, G. W. F. (1942), *Philosophy of Right*, translated by Knox, T. M. Clarendon Press: Oxford.

Hegel, G. W. F (1970), *Enzyklopädie III*, Werke Bd. 10, Suhrkamp: Frankfurt a. Main.

Hegel, G. W. F. (1977), *Phenomenology of Spirit*, translated by Miller, A. V. Oxford University Press: Oxford.

Heidegger, M. (1949), *Über den Humanismus*, Klostermann: Frankfurt a. Main.

Hoerster, N. (1991), *Abtreibung im säkularen Staat. Argumente gegen den §218*, Suhrkamp: Frankfurt a. Main.

Honneth, A. (1992), *Der Kampf um Anerkennung. Zur moralischen Grammatik sozialer Konflikte*, Suhrkamp: Frankfurt a. Main.

Josephs, A. (1998), *Der Kampf gegen die Unfruchtbarkeit. Zeugungstheorien und therapeutische Maßnahmen von den Anfängen bis zur Mitte des 17. Jahrhunderts*, Wissenschaftliche Verlagsanstalt: Stuttgart 1998.

Kuhn, T. S. (1996), *The Structure of Scientific Revolutions*, Chicago.

Lenk, H. (1993), *Philosophie und Interpretation. Vorlesungen zur Entwicklung konstruktionistischer Interpretationsansätze*, Suhrkamp: Frankfurt a. Main.

Lenk, H. (1998), *Konkrete Humanität. Vorlesungen über Verantwortung und Menschlichkeit*, Suhrkamp: Frankfurt a. Main.

Lévinas, E. (1983), 'Ist die Ontologie fundamental?', in Lévinas, E., *Die Spur des Anderen. Untersuchungen zur Phänomenologie und Sozialphilosophie*. alber: München, pp. 103–119.

Luhmann, N. (1978), 'Soziologie der Moral', in Luhmann, N. and Pfürtner, S. (eds), *Theorietechnik und Moral*, Suhrkamp: Frankfurt am Main, pp. 8–116.

Luhmann, N. (1992), *Beobachtungen der Moderne*, Westdeutscher Verlag: Opladen.

Merleau-Ponty, M. (1966), *Phänomenologie der Wahrnehmung*, de Gruyter: Berlin.

Plessner, H. (1980), *Anthropologie der Sinne*, Gesammelte Schriften Bd. III, Suhrkamp: Frankfurt a. Main.

Pröpper, Th. (1995), 'Autonomie und Solidarität. Begründungsprobleme sozial-ethischer Verpflichtung', in Arens, E. (ed.), *Anerkennung der Anderen*, Freiburg, pp. 95–112.

Serres, M. (1993), *Die fünf Sinne*, Suhrkamp: Frankfurt a. Main.

Sieferle, R. P. (1990), *Die Krise der menschlichen Natur. Zur Geschichte eines Konzepts*, Suhrkamp: Frankfurt a. Main.

Siep, L. (1992), 'Personbegriff und praktische Philosophie bei Locke, Kant und Hegel', in *Praktische Philosophie im Deutschen Idealismus*, Suhrkamp: Frankfurt a. Main, pp. 81–115.

Sontag, S. (1986), *Über Photographie,* Suhrkamp: Frankfurt a. Main.

Steigleder, K. (1992), *Die Begründung des moralischen Sollens. Studien zur Möglichkeit einer normativen Ethik,* attempto: Tübingen.

Steigleder, K. (1998), 'Müssen wir, dürfen wir schwere (nicht-therapierbare) genetisch bedingte Krankheiten vermeiden?', in Düwell, M. and Mieth, D. (eds), *Ethik in der Humangenetik. Die neueren Entwicklung der genetischen Frühdiagnostik aus ethischer Perspektive*, francke: Tübingen, pp. 91–119.

Sturma, D. (1992), 'Person und Zeit', in Forum für Philosophie, Bad Homburg (ed.), *Zeiterfahrung und Personalität*, Suhrkamp: Frankfurt a. Main.

Sturma, D. (1997), *Philosophie der Person. Die Selbstverhältnisse von Subjektivität und Moralität*, Schöningh: Paderborn.

Virilio, P. (1989), *Der negative Horizont. Bewegung/Geschwindigkeit/Beschleunigung*, Hanser: München/Wien 1989.

Virilio, P. (1994), *Die Eroberung des Körpers. Vom Übermenschen zum überreizten Menschen*, Hanser: München/Wien.

Virilio, P. (1996), *Fluchtgeschwindigkeit*, Hanser: München/Wien.

Warnock, G. J. (1971), *The Object of Morality*, London.

Welsch, W. (1990), 'Zur Aktualität ästhetischen Denkens', in Welsch, W., *Ästhetisches Denken*, reclam: Stuttgart, pp. 41–69.

Comment on *Autonomy and Recognition*

Eve-Marie Engels

1 General remarks

Jean-Pierre Wils raises a variety of issues that are not only central to the special subject of our conference but also to applied ethics in general. His overall line of argumentation is to show the close connections between our *moral* attitudes and *moral* inclinations on the one hand and our *everyday* and *scientific views* and *theories* about these subjects on the other hand. In other words, before something or someone can become a subject of moral concern, there has to be a previous process of selection and recognition in which subjects are identified as morally relevant. These processes are dependent on our *historical, social* and *cultural contexts* including *techno-logical* possibilities of interference with human and nonhuman nature. New biological and medical technologies have opened up quite new options of action at the beginning and at the end of human life and new possibilities of interspecies manipulation that challenge our traditional understanding of life and death, of human and nonhuman beings, and of identity. Thus, new subjects come into being that are morally relevant. Technology is one of the most outstanding examples of the *construction* of these new realities. Since applied ethics is a discipline that has emerged in response to these challenges, it cannot consist in a simple application of traditional ethical principles to new cases, but has to include reflection on the *ontological* and *biological status* of its subjects. It therefore has to include *anthropology, natural philosophy* and the *philosophy of science* as well as the *empirical sciences* dealing with subjects that have become morally relevant. Moreover, it has to imply reflection on the tenability of central traditional moral and philosophical concepts. For this reason I tend to avoid the notion of 'applied ethics' and prefer to speak of 'application oriented ethics' (anwendungsbezogene oder -orientierte Ethik). I suppose that this is the reason why Wils talks of 'area-specific ethics'.

The theoretical framework in which Jean-Pierre Wils sets his arguments can be characterised as *constructivist*. Our visual as well as conceptual world views are constructions depending not only on our particular historical, social and cultural contexts with their specific thought styles, but also on our natural, physiological outfit that allows us to perceive only objects of a certain size. To use the language of evolutionary epistemology: our unaided senses only allow us to perceive the world of the middle dimensions, the so-called 'mesocosm'. This physiological structure can have an important impact on our moral attitudes and thus has to be taken into account in bioethics. This, however, does not mean that questions of moral judgment and justification can be reduced to natural or cultural habits of perception. On the contrary, the detection of habits and attitudes that we usually are not aware of can become important for raising our moral sensitivity and for expanding the circle of our ethical reflections. In order to support this approach, I want to point to another example that has been mentioned many times in the history of ethics. It is our tendency or disposition not to behave equally benevolently or altruistically towards everybody. David Hume, for instance, writes in his *Treatise of Human Nature*:

> In general, it may be affirm'd, that there is no such passion in human minds, as the love of mankind, merely as such, independent of personal qualities, of services, or of relation to ourself (1975, p. 481)

> ... A man naturally loves his children better than his nephews, his nephews better than his cousins, his cousins better than strangers, where every thing else is equal. (Ibid., pp. 483–484)

Nevertheless, neither Hume, as he particularly made clear in his *Enquiry Concerning the Principles of Morals,* nor we would claim that this bias towards a gradual benevolence depending on the degree of relatedness and friendship should be the basis for a social ethics in a just society. During the last thirty years there has been much research in social psychology on the mechanisms of promotion and inhibition of helping behaviour. All these studies can be relevant for raising our moral sensitivity.

2 Special issues

I now come to the specific issues that Jean-Pierre Wils raises in his paper and which are centred on the concepts of *recognition* and *autonomy*. By the notion of autonomy Wils characterises subjects, agents or persons whose relationship is defined as one of reciprocal recognition and respect for each other as persons. These relationships of mutual recognition are the very basis of autonomy and of morality. For Wils the notion of recognition implies the perception of someone else as a person, and perception itself is twofold: it means the *literal* seeing of someone else, which presupposes

126

the visibility of the other being *and* it implies a certain *interpretation* of what is seen. The recognition of someone else as a person presupposes that there are common features between the other self and me, that there is some kind of identity. Wils' *central thesis* is that in the context of the new technologies (prenatal and pre-implantation genetic diagnosis, gene therapy, *in vitro* fertilisation) the visible profile of the individual disappears whereas the individuality of an emerging human being is inferred by gene diagnosis. Our moral sensitivity cannot keep pace with this kind of *abstraction* and *invisibility*. Our perception has become a trap. Whereas I think that Wils is right in pointing to the fact that our perception can become a trap and thus reduces our moral sensitivity, I do not think that this holds for the technologies that are discussed here.

I think that the development of *in vitro* fertilisation and the technologies of prenatal diagnosis are a good example for showing that new morally relevant subjects can arise from new technologies. Before the introduction of *in vitro* fertilisation (IVF) the term 'embryo' was used in medical embryology for the embryo after its implantation in the uterus, and the etymological roots of 'embryo' in Greek and Latin also lead us to its definition as 'fruit of the womb'. Before IVF, the embryo's existence was connected to the diagnosis of a pregnancy, and therefore its protection began from this moment on. In today's reproductive medicine, however, the term 'embryo' is already used for the early stages of development from fertilisation on. And the discussions about the appropriate *biological designation* of the fertilised egg *in vitro* (embryo, pro-embryo or pre-embryo, etc.) as well as the discussions about its *moral status* show an increase in moral sensitivity in connection with the invention of a new technology.

There are examples in the history of biology that show that the invention and use of instruments, like the microscope, have *increased* the sense of concreteness and directed the imagination towards a theoretical construction of embryos or 'little animals' as complete miniature organisms either in the sperm or in the egg, that only have to grow. This was the preformation theory in embryology that replaced the theory of epigenesis by the end of the 17th Century and which was again replaced by it at about the end of the 18th Century.

Moreover, by the use of such enlargers and magnifiers even the smallest organisms have come into our field of vision and can become an object of admiration and respect. Organisms that were not visible and thus for many people not existent until now, fascinate the observer because of their complexity considering their smallness.

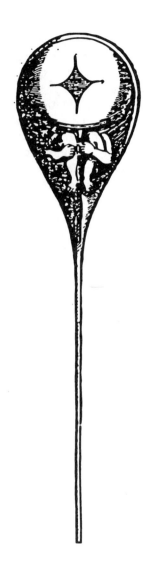

From: Nicolas Hartsoeker: *Essay de Dioptrique*. Paris 1694, page 230

Before gene diagnosis and other reproductive technologies had been developed, the embryo was not more visible than it is now, nor did it possess a higher degree of concreteness and personhood than now. In the context of abortion the question of the embryo's moral status has been raised long before it came up again in the debates about the new technologies.

I agree, however, with Wils in pointing to the ethical problems that arise from taking the concept of a *person* and thus the idea of *reciprocal recog-*

nition as a basis for respecting and treating other beings as deserving our protection. I think that this is a good example for showing how traditional philosophical and ethical concepts are challenged in the new context of bioethical problems. The traditional concepts of recognition and autonomy are too limited if we want to protect all those human and nonhuman living beings to whom these concepts are not applicable.

I would plead for the protection of *all* humans including very early embryos as well as severely handicapped people. But I would have a problem with the idea that *only* humans have to be protected for their own sake. Without being able to argue it in detail in this comment, I think that a form of respect for living beings including zygotes as well as other minute organisms can be cultivated that is not based on the reciprocal recognition of human beings as persons but which instead grows out of the recognition of a form of self-organisation and complexity that was not created by the human being but which is an essential feature of life and therefore also of human life. I would not want to drop the notion of life, because I think that this would have detrimental effects on our understanding of living beings that we want to respect and to protect. 'Life' is a notion under which we can subsume living beings without adopting a teleology of nature in the traditional sense.

Gene diagnosis does not necessarily mean a *loss* of concreteness. One danger may even lie in attributing *too much* concreteness to just one aspect of the growing human being, to his/her genetic outfit. In most cases the phenotypic expression of the genetic constitution of a human being depends on many conditions, and the *idea* of a *genetic determinism* is a more severe threat to autonomy than the new technologies as such. The idea of an omnipotent genetics, often conveyed by the media and by some overzealous scientists may entice the credulous public into believing utopian visions of constructing ideal human beings or nightmares of genetically manipulated marionettes, both of which are the expression of an outdated prescientific image of the human being.

Finally, I would like to make a critical remark on the idea of increasing degrees of protectability depending on the development of the embryo or fetus. The problem with any kind of progressive gradualism is that the lines of demarcation between the stages of development are arbitrary. And this does not only hold for the development of the embryo and fetus but also for evolution as such. The idea of an ascending organic scale in nature, which was a basic assumption in traditional natural philosophy, has become highly controversial in the context of evolutionary theory. Instead of starting with grades of protectability inherent in embryonic development I would propose granting a *prima facie* right to live to the embryo at all its stages of development. This does not exclude decisions against the life of the embryo in conflict situations. But it makes a difference for the protection of the embryo whether we begin with the assumption of grades of protection inherent in its developmental process or if this is our last resort in case of conflicts. And I would want to make a plea for extending this view to our treatment of all living beings.

References

Engels, E.-M. (ed.) (1999), *Biologie und Ethik,* Reclam: Stuttgart.
Hume, D. (1975), *A Treatise of Human Nature: Being an Attempt to Introduce the Experimental Method of Reasoning Into Moral Subjects* (ed.) by Selby-Bigge, L. A., Clarendon Press: Oxford. Reprint of the original, London 1739/40.

Comment: *Autonomous decisions in assisted procreation and genetic diagnosis*

Kris Dierickx

In many discussions concerning assisted procreation, genetic testing and screening, autonomy plays a crucial role. With Kuitert (1989, pp. 56–57), I would like to make a distinction between two forms of autonomy: societal autonomy and anthropological autonomy. The former means that humans, in contrast with animals, for example, are not bound by instincts of determinate behaviour but can make a rational choice between several alternatives, and this can be seen as a typical human condition, a capacity. This is the kind of autonomy that is discussed in the paper of Wils. Before focussing on this concept of autonomy, I would like to underline the importance of the societal form of autonomy by which Kuitert means not being forced by others, and that might be considered as a right. To preserve people from coercion, from the loss of autonomy in this sense, ethics has developed the instrument of informed and free consent. The qualification 'free' in the context of assisted procreation and genetic testing is not always evident. Looking at the example of a genetic screening programme or a pre-implantation genetic screening initiative offered in a fertility centre, the practical realisation of respect for the autonomy of the persons involved is not evident. In general most people agree that one has the right not to participate in such a screening programme. But how free is the participation in an, in itself, unasked offer of genetic diagnosis that takes place on the initiative of others, e.g., the fertility centre, the public health authorities, etc. Several studies show that the explicit offer of a screening technology has a strong imperative character (see Tijmstra 1991). The tendency to binary thinking ('They can say, "your chances are 100 to one", but for me it is "yes or no"') and the anticipation of decision regret ('Later I will have to say: I should have done it at that time') mean that this kind of 'chance offering' technology is not so free of obligations. The same can be said if social consequences are related to non-participation. These consequences can be situated in the broader social domain or within the family. At the first level, cases are known of pregnant couples that are (in)directly forced by their insurance company to undergo a genetic diagnosis (see Billings *et al.* 1992; and Nys 1994). But not using actual medical possibilities in the domains of assisted procreation or genetic diagnosis will not be appreciated and free of any pressure at the level of the family either (see Livingstone 1994). In Belgium, for instance, we have almost 10,000 treatments for medically assisted procreation in 35 fertility centres on somewhat more than 100,000 births. In this context, it is clear that the autonomy of subfertile or infertile couples can be threatened by their own wishes, the existing and frequently explicit expectations of the parents (in law), the partner, and society. The same can be said for pre-implantation genetic screening. If a fertility centre offers couples the opportunity to have the fertilised egg screened for several genetic mutations, the autonomy and freedom of the future parents to say 'no' to such an offer and thus to increase their chance of giving birth to a child with a genetic disease could be strongly limited.

A very explicit curtailment of autonomy is found in carrier screening programmes where the government or the public health authorities impose a programme for genetic diagnosis (see Lappé *et al.* 1972; and Reilly 1977). The increasing possibilities for influencing the genetic qualities of people and their offspring leads, for certain groups, to the obligation to prevent identifiable genetic afflictions. If people with a known increased genetic risk do not use these preventive possibilities, so say the proponents of genetic control by the authorities, then the government has the right, if not to say the obligation, to bring them to 'better thoughts'. They (see Verber 1980; and Fletcher 1988) base their vision on several arguments: significant cost savings; preventing a genetic apocalypse; the reduction of the frequency of 'bad' genes; the harm that will be done to handicapped children by letting them be born; the advantage of collecting much data and information for scientific research. It is clear that there is no place for autonomy in such an enterprise.

Along the lines of Virilio's 'loss of feeling', one could speak in this situation, where large groups are forced to participate in a genetic diagnostic test, of a shrinkage of the participants who are more considered as dematerialised and abstract numbers, taken out of the normal spatial and temporal horizon of their development than as concrete human beings with their own life story and context (see Virilio 1989). The object of perception here is only present in the form of genetic data and a genetic constitution, and individuality loses its anthropological contours so that the other's reality is undermined. And I follow Wils when he states that this transformation of perception has an ethical relevance. The depersonalising distance of human beings as cell-substances influences our moral sensitivity and sensibility.

132

On the other hand, one could ask if moral sensibility's loss of sensory and orienting points of reference in reality has to have the same consequences in our highly technological world of today. Videoconferences bring real persons together virtually and concrete individuals start virtual relationships via the Internet, which sometimes even lead to marriage. Is it possible that this new visibility could lead to a second moral sensibility (in the sense of Ricoeur: deuxième sensibilité morale—deuxième naivité)?

1 Lévinas

For some authors it is clear that the (in)visibility of the other human being is rather relative. In order to illustrate this I want to show what an author like Emmanuel Lévinas (1961) means with the appearance of the other as visage. At first sight it looks simple: a visage is a visage. But looking closer, we are confronted with an obvious misunderstanding. If we hear 'visage', we spontaneously assimilate it with face, physiognomy, and the expression of the face; then the character, social standing and the past and context out of which the other becomes visible and describable. The visage seems to fall together completely with what the other allows us to see by his appearance and behaviour. In various forms of medical and therapeutic assistance, too, we start from a diagnosis, literally, a methodological and technological professionalised observation.

Lévinas, however, means by 'the visage of the other' not his face or appearance, but the peculiar fact that the other—not only in fact, but also in principle—falls in no manner together with his or her appearance, image, photo or evocation. The other is invisible, states Lévinas provocatively. That is why in the vision of Lévinas we cannot speak about a phenomenology of the face, because phenomenology describes what appears. The visage, however, is what in the face or appearance of the other escapes from our look. The other is different, that is, irreducible to his appearance, and therein he reveals himself as visage (see Lévinas 1947). The other is not only more in fact—in the sense that we can always discover more about him—but also in the sense that he can never be reflected or caught in one or another image. He is essentially, and not only in fact or temporarily, a transcending movement. The epiphany of the visage is therefore always confusing, an epiphany by which the other remains enigmatic and forces himself upon us as an irreducible entity, separate and different, a stranger, in short, as the Other. The appearance of the other means *dis-order, extra-ordi-nary* and *e-normous* externality: an irreducible otherness. As the *in-visible*—this means we cannot be reduced to his face and appearance—the other appears by not appearing. This is why the visage is so vulnerable in his appearance (as face). It is tempting

133

to reduce the other to myself; in extreme terms, this is the denial of the other, physically incarnated in the murder (see Lévinas 1974).

But for Lévinas in this temptation to murder lies the ethical meaning of the visage. At the moment that I am drawn to reduce the other to his appearance, I realise, as a being with the same origins, that what I could do is not permitted. This is the core of the ethical basic experience that is given rise to from the visage, namely the interdiction to fix the other in his appearance. It is by the appearance of the visage of the other that I become *re-sponsible,* in the passive sense of the word. A responsibility in spite of myself: a heteronomous responsibility (see Burggraeve 1985).

2 Love and respect

In Wils' article, it is also stated that for Hegel the constitutive feature of autonomy consists in self-consciousness, which is considered as a condition for recognition relationships. For some authors, it is not necessary that the other human being has a self-consciousness in order to be recognised as a person (see O'Donovan 1986; and Schotsmans 1994). They distinguish persons only by love, by the discovery via encounter and by the promise or the association/relation that this human being is irreplaceable. They call it an act of belief. It is possible to refuse this act of belief. Being a person can in this vision never be proven in the full sense of the word. But without this act of belief we have no reason at all to commit ourselves to a personal relationship with those whose personality cannot yet be recognised, for instance because they are unborn children or severely handicapped children. If we finally come to recognise these human beings as persons, we can only do this after having committed ourselves in a personal interaction with them. The concept of person indicates for them no static entity, no tableau, but rather a story. As in the ancient Greek theatre, the *'personae dramatis'* are not merely faces, but characters whose appearance (the person) might be recognised independent of which actor is interpreting it. In analogy, for them a person is an individual appearance that receives continuity by means of a story. They prefer to speak about 'person' instead of mere qualitative categories (such as ratio) characterising the personality. These characteristics and qualities can be verified (by attitude and biological tests, e.g.; testing the brain functions) and lead to the excavation of the concept of person. For the above-mentioned authors, the ultimate foundation of respect is love, not self-consciousness.

3 Responsibility

I would like to finish my comment with some thoughts about the new responsibility that arises for the quality of the pregnancy and for that of the emerging child as soon as the pregnancy becomes visible by prenatal ultrasound scan or genetic diagnostic test. In contemporary clinical medicine concerning assisted procreation and genetic diagnosis there is an increasing focus on individual responsibility. But the concept of responsibility is a complicated one. We would like to make a distinction between two kinds of responsibility (see Ricoeur 1991; and Frankena 1973). In the first sense we use the proposition 'X is responsible for Y' when Y is an act already performed. We hold X responsible for having done Y. In the second sense we use the proposition 'X is responsible for Y' when Y still has to be carried out. We hold responsible for having to do Y in the future. This distinction between the first and the second context points to an important difference between the practical uses of the concept of responsibility. In practice, 'responsibility' apparently has a prospective and a retrospective force.

Prospectively, responsibility is assigned to the individual for his future health. To attribute this kind of responsibility to someone is equivalent to saying that he has an obligation to preserve his health. The retrospective ascription of responsibility implies a particular evaluation of what has happened, and combines causality with culpability. If an individual has a health problem he is held causally responsible because of his unhealthy life-style in the past: this means disapproval and blame.

The possibility of the widening of procreative options by genetic diagnosis and counselling is in practice sometimes linked with the argument that individuals or couples who are not using these possibilities, should be responsible themselves for the harmful or negative (financial and other) consequences. If, for instance, a couple of which both the partners are carriers of a recessive genetic mutation decides not to undergo a prenatal or pre-implantation genetic diagnosis to check if the fetus has the particular genetic disorder, or decides not to abort the pregnancy of a fetus with the disease, in this view, the couple should be considered responsible for the pain and the harm of the child. If so, there is no longer harm that happens to someone, but only harm that has been caused. In fact, in this kind of reasoning, personal responsibility has been moralised. In this way responsibility has been stretched endlessly. One can be held responsible for everything that happens. Nothing can happen of one's own. With ten Have and Loughlin (1994), we could speak here about a moral hypertrophy of responsibility.

References

Billings, P. R. *et al.* (1992), 'Discrimination as a Consequence of Genetic Testing', *American Journal of Human Genetics* Vol. 50, pp. 476–482.

Burggraeve, R. (1985), *From Self-development to Solidarity: An Ethical Reading of Human Desire in its Socio-political Relevance According to Emmanuel Lévinas*, Peeters: Leuven.

Fletcher, J. (1988), *The Ethics of Genetic Control: Ending Reproductive Roulette*, New York.

Frankena, W.K. (1973), *Ethics*, Englewood Cliffs NJ: Prentice Hall.

Kuitert, H. M. (1989), *Mag alles wat kan? Ethiek en medische handelen*, Ten Have: Baarn.

Lappé, M. *et al.* (1972), 'Ethical and Social Problems in Screening for Genetic Disease', *New England Journal of Medicine*, Vol. 282, pp. 1129–1132.

Lévinas, E. (1947), 'Le temps et l'autre', in Wahl, J. *et al.* (eds), *Le choix le monde, l'existence*, Arthaud: Grenoble/Paris, pp. 125–196.

Lévinas, E. (1961), *Totalité et infini. Essai sur l'extériorité*, Nijhoff: The Hague.

Lévinas, E. (1974), *Autrement qu'être ou au-delà de l'essence*, Nijhoff: The Hague.

Livingstone, J. *et al.* (1994), 'Antenatal Screening for Cystic Fibrosis: A Trial of the Couple Model', *British Medical Journal,* Vol. 308, pp. 1459–1462.

Nys, H. (1994), 'Genetics and the Rights of the Patient: Informed Consent and Confidentiality Revisited in Light of Reproductive Freedom', in Westerhäll, L. *et al.* (eds), *Patients' Rights: Informed Consent, Access and Equality*, Stockholm, pp. 137–154.

O'Donovan, O. (1986), *Begotten or Made?*, Clarendon Press: Oxford.

Reilly, P. (1977), *Genetics, Law and Social Policy*, London.

Ricoeur, P. (1991), 'Postface', in Lenoir, F. (ed.), *Le temps de la responsabilité. Entretiens sur l'éthique*, Fayard: Paris, pp. 259–260.

Schotsmans, P. (1994), *De maakbare mens. Vruchtbaarheid in de 21ste eeuw*, Davidsfonds: Leuven.

Ten Have, H. and Loughlin, M. (1994), 'Responsibilities and Rationalities: Should the Patient Be Blamed?', *Health Care Analysis,* Vol. 2, pp. 119–127.

Tijmstra, T. (1991), 'The Imperative Character of Screening Technologies', in Mantigh, A. *et al., Screening in Prenatal Diagnosis*, Academic Press: Groningen, pp. 65–70.

Verber, M. (1980), *Is It Ethical to Make Genetic Screening Compulsory? Reflections on Neonatal and Heterozygote Screening Programs*, University of Rhode Island.

Virilio, P. (1989), *Der negative Horizont. Bewegung—Geschwindigkeit/Beschleunigung*, Hanser: München/Wien.

Part Four

SOCIAL IMPLICATIONS

Technicalisation of human procreation and social living conditions

Regine Kollek

Reflections on reproductive medicine and genetics quite often do not mirror the specificities of the social contexts of which these developments are part. These contexts need to be analysed in order to understand the dynamics by which modern reproductive and genetic technologies are developed, implemented and accepted—not only as material practices, but also as a specific way to conceptualise human inheritance and procreation under the conditions of late modernity.

In this paper, I would therefore like to argue that deeper insights into the social structures and institutions as well as cultural practices relevant to procreation are needed for an adequate understanding and hence social shaping of reproductive and genetic technologies. Second, the new technologies impart the impression that they extend women's choices and give them better control of their biology. In contrast to this, I would like to question this widespread belief and argue that under current social living conditions, artificial reproductive technologies (ART) and the new genetics lead to new moral obligations, which may be even more difficult for women to deal with than infertility or disease. Third, reproductive and genetic technologies are not only medical treatments, but are also loaded with symbolic meanings and interpretations. These meanings have not yet been explored sufficiently. Their analysis should help to understand better the force with which they penetrate clinical practice and become integrated into daily life. Finally, I would like to explore some of the problems created by current bioethical discourse.

1 Conceptual framing of social living conditions at the turn of the second millennium

The ethical problems and social implications associated with the new reproductive and genetic technologies have been described in detail by many authors. An adequate understanding of these developments and their implications, however, is not possible if we consider their consequences for the individual alone. Rather, such an understanding requires a theoretical framework able to conceptualise social structures and developments that are basic for the career of these technologies and their successful implementation in the medical system and society.

Central to my analysis is the concept of individualisation. It has been put forward by Anthony Giddens (1991), and by Ulrich Beck and Elisabeth Beck-Gernsheim (1992, 1994, and 1996). It refers to specific social developments that are especially characteristic for post-World War II, western industrialised and democratic societies. Individualisation means that in such societies individuals tend to leave traditional social structures and relationships that are at the core of traditional systems of power and support. In doing so, traditional orientations, belief systems and guiding norms are lost. This, however, does not mean that the individual now is free to do voluntarily whatever he or she wants, since at the same time he or she experiences new forms of social entrenchment and control (see Beck and Beck-Gernsheim 1996, p. 206). In developed democratic societies, however, this control is not exerted by external authorities; instead dominant rules are internalised and become effective from within, apparently based on free and autonomous decisions. The relevant question therefore is, *which rules guide modern forms of procreation, where do they come from, to which social and cultural context do they relate, and what kind of function do they have?*

Although there is considerable controversy about the concept of individualisation, several phenomena that are included in it have been described independently by other authors. Other phenomena embraced by the concept are not new. In 1840, Alexis de Toqueville (1969, p. 506) already described the disposition of citizens to isolate themselves from others as individualism. Furthermore, the concept is well known in classical sociological thinking. According to this view, modern societies developed by means of the transformation of traditional communities that were based on larger groups and dominated by kinship-models. Such transformed societies are characterised, among other things, by the growing dominance of private ownership, profit motives, industrial production, mobility, large urban centres and bureaucratic professionalism (see Knorr-Cetina 1997).

It is thought by sociologists that these developments undermined what has been perceived from our perspective as the 'embeddedness' of individuals in traditional social structures (see McFarlane 1979). This singularisation left traces in the self-perception of modern individuals and their relations to social structures and institutions. It results in anonymous social relations and 'divided' identities, which are used by individuals to act according to each actual social context or sphere. Some theorists like Berger and his colleagues (1974, p. 196) thought that this 'alienation' was the 'price' individuals and societies have to pay for individualisation. According to Giddens,

> modern life is characterized by profound processes of the reorganization of time and space, coupled to the expansion of disembedding mechanisms—mechanisms which prise social relations free from the hold of specific locales, recombining them across wide time-space distances. The reorganization of time and space, plus the disembedding mechanisms, radicalize and globalize pre-established institutional traits of modernity; and they act to transform the context and nature of day-to-day social life. (1991, p. 2)

An equally important phenomenon of modern societies is that they differentiate into a variety of belief systems. This pluralism undermines the plausibility and meaning-bestowing quality of any of such system. They become useless as providers of orientation and certainty. According to Berger *et al.* (1974, pp. 184–185), we are therefore not only 'homeless' in society, but also in the cosmos.

The rise of capitalism and industrialisation, and the transformation of traditional structures of production resulted in the decay of larger social structures. After World War II, most Western countries experienced an expansion of the social welfare state, which carried the process of individualisation even further, since individuals were not as dependent on family support as before. Traditional roles became less clearly defined and more subject to human agency compared to more traditional roles that were determined by class, gender and race.

On the one hand, these transformations result in an increase of choices and non-linear 'patchwork' biographies that do not resemble biographical patterns of former generations. On the other hand, however, a pluralisation of life styles can be observed. Life styles are also no longer bound to traditional roles, but multiply as societies become more and more heterogeneous by education, permeability of traditional social structures, migration, mobility, and so on. But life styles are not only a result of individual preferences but also an element of self-production and self-composition, which are characteristic of a society in which traditional ways of securing the self by accepting one of the predetermined roles in society are no longer an option. The different elements of life styles do not need to be invented anew all the time. All of them can be used by individuals in order to put together their own specific life styles. Furthermore, individuals are no longer bound to the place where they were born or have grown up. Increasing personal and professional mobility has contributed to the fact that most people change social contexts and the belief systems associated with them more and more often during their life time. The same is true for the roles that they play in these contexts. This 'lifting out' of social relations from local contexts is exactly what was meant by Giddens when he coined the term 'disembedding', which is 'the key to the tremendous acceleration in time-space distantiation which modernity introduces' (1991, p. 18).

This freeing from prescribed biographies, local contexts and life styles must certainly be regarded as an element of emancipation and liberation. It is the dominant conviction in western societies that we—at least in essence—are free to shape our personal lives ourselves, and that we have a high amount of control over them. But this real or perceived increase in freedom and control and the new complexity of biographies and social roles was and is also connected with an increasing degree of individual responsibility and accountability. This applies not only to daily activities but also to conditions that are basic for individual and social life like health and procreation.

The changing status of tradition in contemporary life and the ambiguities associated with it have therefore severe consequences. Individuals are thrown back on their own emotional and cognitive resources to construct a coherent life course, identity and forms of togetherness for themselves (see Beck and Beck-Gernsheim 1994 and 1996; Giddens 1994; and Heelas 1996). The perception that the course of our life is no longer prescribed by tradition has created the idea that we can 'construct' our lives ourselves. All these developments together pose quite a challenge for the individual. Flexible life styles and patchwork-biographies require, among other things, as Karin Knorr-Cetina put it, 'the will to sustain a certain amount of emotional oscillation, ambiguity and social creativity' (1997, p. 4). Many people do not possess the psychological means to deal with the great freedom of choice or the contingency of contemporary life (see Bauman 1996, pp. 92ff.). They look for orientation, which is not provided any longer by traditional roles, life styles or institutions of society. In this situation, private and personal relationships gain more and more importance. Since large families do not exist any longer, and the average number of children per couple today statistically is less than two in Europe, the number of family members belonging to one generation becomes smaller. The one child couple becomes the rule, and the traits and characteristics of this child become more and more important. In contrast to the decreasing importance of such horizontal relationships, the importance of vertical relationships between members of a family belonging to different generations grows as much as the perceived dependency and feeling of mutual responsibility among members of such vertical family lines. These developments are additionally promoted by the increasing life expectancy in western industrialised societies.

Like other social institutions and systems, the medical system was also affected by individualisation. In the context of general liberalisation and democratisation of the 1960s and 1970s, patients' rights and principles like self -determination, autonomy and informed consent became established and a guiding norm for physicians as well as for patients and clients (see Beauchamp and Childress 1994; and Fox 1994). Especially for women, these transformations have had far-reaching consequences. The greater control of fertility and ability to choose when and how often to give birth to children allowed women to plan their lives more rationally and made it easier for them to participate in public and professional activities. Later on, ART brought relief for many women and couples from the often painful experience of infertility. Furthermore, IVF and other inventions in the field of reproductive medicine and genetics have now offered new possibilities that extend our control over the process of reproduction and which—at least in principle—allow women to choose freely not only the time of procreation and number of children, but also the state of health, sex, and—perhaps soon with the progress of the human genome project—behavioural traits and other phenotypes of their offspring, independent of their own genetic endowment and fertility or that of their husband or partner. The new genetic and reproductive technologies are therefore a perfect match for modern, individualised life styles that are characterised by the need as well as the desire to plan and to structure the course of one's own life rationally and in accordance with the requirements of modern living.

2 Controlling fertility and genetics—and reducing uncertainty?

Basic to the application of modern reproductive and genetic technologies is the assumption that women or couples profit from them and that they can help to reduce uncertainty with respect to reproduction. It is not clear, however, on what basis these assumptions are made. Although it is not questioned that assisted reproduction can help to overcome female and male fertility problems, and that genetic tests can unveil a growing number of chromosomal or genetic alterations, it is much more controversial whether these new options are really beneficial for women, and whether they can in fact reduce risk and uncertainty connected to reproduction and the planning of life.

First of all, it is rather uncertain whether one or repeated treatments with ART will finally result in the birth of a child. The low efficiency of IVF is still the most disputed feature of this treatment. Baby take home rates are in general not much higher than 15 to 20% per embryo transfer. Considerable effort was invested to increase IVF efficiency—with limited success. Success rates depend on the social and medical context in which these technologies are used (see White 1998).

A second question is whether the baby conceived by IVF will be healthy. This is not apparent since the baby can be at risk for several reasons. First of all, the number of twins and triplets and the number of children born prematurely is still much higher in women giving birth after IVF than among women not treated by any method of assisted reproduction. Higher grade pregnancies are mainly observed when doctors are allowed to transfer more than 3 *in vitro* fertilised embryos. This is often the case when costs for IVF treatments are not covered by health insurance, which is common in the US but not in European countries. Second, an increasing number of IVFs are performed with the help of intracytoplasmic sperm injection (ICSI), which was introduced during the early 1990s. In Germany, ICSI is applied in more than 50% of all IVFs. The most alarming fact concerning this development is that the method has not been adequately evaluated in controlled clinical trials. Although some groups maintain that there is no increase in malformation after ICSI due to the method itself, it is not entirely clear yet whether or not this method of injecting the male gamete mechanically into the oocyte leads to a higher percentage of children born with malformations than traditional IVF (see Kurinczuk and Bower 1997). Although this technique can help males with fertility problems to father their own child, it may also help to transmit existing genetic dysfunction in cases where infertility is due to genetic or chromosomal alterations, which in turn legitimise prenatal or even preimplantation genetic diagnosis, if couples want to make sure that the fetus is not affected by the father's genetic problem that has led to infertility.

Concern about genetic or chromosomal aberrations or developmental problems after applying methods of assisted reproduction is not new. From the very beginning the prevention of such problems was one of the major objectives of reproductive medicine. The combination of IVF together with the new techniques of chromosomal and genetic disorders offered unprecedented powers to biomedicine: the power to decide who is to bear children and which fetus is permitted to survive. The English sociologist Hilary Rose has pointed out that such a fusion of powers

144

was symbolized in the agreement that Lesly Brown[1] was required to sign as a condition of her being treated with the new experimental techniques, that she would have an abortion if the fetus was abnormal. (Rose 1994, p 177)

This vision of immaculate products of assisted reproduction was and is an integral part of these techniques. The more gene tests become available as the human genome project proceeds, the more the future of children to come is drawn into the present by the diagnostic means developed by expert cultures. The concept of risk becomes fundamental to the way both lay men and women and technical specialists organise the social world. Under the conditions of modernity, the future is continually drawn into the present (see Giddens 1991, p. 3).

Abortion of a wanted pregnancy, however, is a traumatic experience for most women (see, e.g., Donnai *et al.* 1981; Black 1991; White van Mourik *et al.* 1992; and Turner 1994). It can be compared with stillbirth rather than with abortion of an unwanted child within the first three month of pregnancy (see, e.g., Lloyd and Laurence 1985; and von Gontard 1986). Many women and couples develop feelings of guilt after aborting such a desired pregnancy, which sometimes lasts very long (see, e.g., Black 1991 and 1994; and Sandelowski and Jones 1996). Especially the fact that she has actively decided against the child after the diagnosis, is hard to bear for most women. Personal responsibility for the loss of the pregnancy hurts and is experienced as extremely difficult (see von Gontard 1986). Abortion is not only a traumatic experience for women, who have probably gone through different cycles of IVF and waited long to become pregnant, but physicians and geneticists too may feel that their reputation is tarnished by the birth of a child with chromosomal, genetic or developmental abnormalities. But it took little more than a decade after the birth of Louise Brown to develop pre-implantation genetic diagnosis (PGD), which now makes it—at least in principle—possible to avoid abortions after IVF. PGD can be used to examine embryos genetically after IVF and before implantation. The positive aspect of possibly avoiding an induced abortion, however, has to be contrasted with the fact that the treatment may be even more of a strain for women than conventional IVF. Whereas in routine treatment only five or fewer embryos are needed, massive stimulation of ovaries is necessary in the context of PGD in order to obtain a sufficient number of embryos for genetic examination and selection (see Edwards 1998, pp. 9ff.). The high costs of the treatment and possible health problems for the women are often neglected when PGD is propagated as a method to avoid abortions.

Despite medical, psychological and ethical questions and problems associated with PGD, a small but increasing number of women in the US,

Great Britain and some other countries do use these methods, which are regarded as being able to ensure the birth of healthy children and avoid the risk of abortion at the same time. Many people know that this is not entirely true, since numerous developmental problems and genetic alterations will not be detected by these tests, and misdiagnoses occur in about five to ten percent of all cases. Therefore, a verification of PGD results by amniocentesis and prenatal genetic diagnosis is recommended by PGD-specialists.

In Germany, PGD is not practised yet, and it is currently debated whether it is in fact prohibited by the embryo protection law or not. Since interest in PGD research with embryos and embryonic cells grows, there is an increasing pressure—indicated by newspaper headlines complaining that German research has to stop when it starts to become interesting—to revise the law, legalise PGD formally and make embryos or embryonic cells available for research or commercial purposes.

Fundamental to such efforts to change the existing law are arguments that connect PGD and embryo research to health. In the context of modern, highly individualised societies, health has become one of the highest ranking norms. The desire for it seems to be completely natural and self-evident. No reason needs to be given to substantiate this assumption. In contrast to this, health or disease was perceived as fate in pre-industrialised societies, and it could be accepted as something the individual was not able to control. The genetic endowment of children was prone to pure chance: it was the result of 'genetic roulette', as Fletcher (1988) put it. Today, there is growing awareness that the structures and processes of the body involved in health and disease can be controlled by modern medicine, and especially genetics. Hence, health is not perceived any longer as a gift of God, but as result of 'good genes' and 'healthy life styles' and therefore prone to human or medical intervention, respectively. It becomes the result of personal decisions, and at least partially a duty of a responsible citizen. He or she has to ensure that health is maintained by adequate prevention. In this sense, modern efforts to maintain health and to prevent disease are not solely the product of personal wishes or fears. Rather they are part and package of modern life, and refer to new biographical patterns, their options and demands (see Beck-Gernsheim 1993, p. 203).

In this context, it seems to be highly rational to overcome fertility problems by the use of IVF, to participate in prenatal screening programs or to take advantage of PGD, if indicated and available. The use of such services confers the impression of being in control of one's biological destiny. Or, as the English anthropologist Sarah Franklin stated in her study on assisted conception,

146

consumer choice and technological enablement represent new free-doms to construct the future, be it individual, national or global, to precise specifications. (1996, p. 166)

This impression is, at least in the USA, but also for example in Italy, care-fully fostered by advertisements. Those who do not choose, or cannot afford to participate in prenatal screening, may be portrayed as irresponsi-ble or even reckless, placing more than a necessary burden on health insurance and social security systems. This implicitly promotes the notion, as Angus Clarke put it,

> that genetic endowment and chosen lifestyle together determine one's future health, while the importance of material circumstances (espe-cially poverty) in creating ill health will be glossed over. (1997, p. 101)

In addition to this neglect of social factors influencing health and disease, the 'genetification' of health and disease (see Lippman 1991) constitutes a fundamental change in our understanding of human nature.

> From moral beings, whose character and conduct is largely shaped by culture, social environment and individual choice, we are transformed in our perception to essentially biological beings, whose 'fate' according to [the former human genome] project herald James Watson, 'is in our genes'. (Kaye 1992, p. 77)

This construction of a new self-definition seemingly sanctioned by the biological sciences constitutes a highly reductionistic and deterministic 'dehumanization of thought' that is dangerously seductive in this period of 'cultural crisis and moral uncertainty', when many people in Western countries are individually and collectively '[c]onfused about who we are, . . . how we should live,' 'and where we are going' (ibid., p. 80 and p. 84).

Hence, a close connection can be seen between the characteristics and demands of modern societies that are constitutive of individualisation, and the attractiveness of genetics and controlled procreation for many people. The 'possessive individualism' (Rose 1994, p. 171), which is characteristic of modern societies, is one of the driving motives that makes the use of modern reproductive and genetic technologies not only acceptable, but in many cases also desirable to women. It also makes it very difficult to limit or to restrict individual access to these new possibilities by moral argu-ments or legal means. This does not necessarily mean that a high propor-tion of the population would undergo prenatal testing, participate in genetic screenings or procreate by using IVF. But the promise of certainty that is assigned to these methods and their perceived capacity to create 'healthy' families and to ensure the endurance of family bonds, transforms them into a set of procedures that are thought to provide orientation and reduce uncertainty. This is—in many cases—an illusion. Many women know for example that they cannot be certain of the outcome of IVF. But at least they can hope for the certainty of knowing they did everything possible to succeed. But, as Sarah Franklin and others have shown, this is precisely the certainty that IVF takes away. Women get into a 'no-win' position of 'indefinite irresolution' (1996, p. 173). They become technologically dependent, because there will always be a new method to try. In the many cases of failure they are left without consolation.

Furthermore, the desire for healthy children can hardly be realised without ambivalence and conflicts. For example, explicit differences between articulated opinion and uptake of genetic tests are constantly observed (see Shiloh 1996). In a German study, about 50% of individuals at risk responded positively when confronted with the question, whether they wished to perform prenatal or direct genetic testing for Huntington's Disease (see Kreutz 1996). Actual uptake, however, was, and is, not much higher than 5–10%.[2] Similar observations are made with respect to PGD. Although many women support PGD as an important option, the risks for the embryo, the low efficiency of IVF, and moral reservations are reasons why a substantial proportion even of those women at risk for genetic disease would prefer PND to PGD as the method of choice in order to prevent the birth of a child with genetic disease (see Snowdon and Green 1997).

Outside of the interview situation, that is, in real-life contexts, many different arguments and reasons come together: severity of the expected condition, previous knowledge about and experience of it, existing therapies, biography, and the normative frame in which the actual situation is placed (see Parsons and Atkinson 1993). Such discrepancies between principles and personal decisions cannot only be interpreted as behavioural or normative inconsistencies of the people involved. Rather they are—according to Irmgard Nippert (1997)—the result of the very process of decision making under the conditions of moral and biographical uncertainty. The desire to have a healthy child has to be balanced with values that have to be taken into consideration as well. The moral conflict that exists between social expectations and abortion cannot be denied. Observed discrepancies therefore have to be regarded as an indication that in such a situation many conflicting interests and needs are present at the same time (see Shiloh 1986, p. 85).

In this context, the underlying concept of 'needs' itself has to be problematicised. Needs, as far as they go beyond vital necessities, are socially constructed, culture bound and historically contingent. They can be created by technical or medical inventions, or by advertisements. With respect to a 'need' for prenatal diagnosis it has been shown that there are important cultural differences. For example, to know about the sex of the fetus in order to be able to abort female fetuses seem to have become a need for women and a socially well-accepted practice in China or Korea,[3] whereas in Europe or the US it is rejected by most couples and physicians.

Furthermore, in most contemporary cultures, childcare is still the responsibility of women. It is expected that they do everything possible to give birth to a healthy child. If women want to work and to have a career similar to that of their male colleagues, they in most cases feel that they could not adequately care for a handicapped child. Under such conditions, a 'need' for prenatal diagnosis may indeed develop, which soon may be transformed into a 'right'. When a women is older than about 35, she will find it difficult to reject for example ultrasound or the triple test (see Lippman 1991, p. 28). Conforming to such a practice gives her the impression of responsible motherhood.

But needs for medical or genetic assistance in the context of procreation are not only products of social or economic living conditions, but also created by the way such developments are offered and the contexts in which they are applied. From pilot studies of carrier screening for cystic fibrosis it is known that the mode of offering a genetic carrier test is much the most important factor influencing uptake of the test (see Clarke 1997, p. 100). Therefore, uptake of genetic tests seems to be less driven by consumer demands than by market push. This is most likely true for uptake of assisted reproduction services as well. Another important factor is how genetic tests become integrated into the medical system. Routinisation of testing and of screening practices certainly promote their uptake. To refuse a test that seems to be an integral part of clinical routine is quite difficult in a situation where most women think that they depend—and actually do depend—on the good will of their doctor. These and other structural features of the health care system contribute to the widespread implementation and acceptance of prenatal testing.

3 Autonomy: limitations of a principle

In many discussions, critique of ART and genetics is rejected with the argument that it is the woman who decides whether to use or not to use the new possibilities of conception and of preventing children with inherited diseases. Such reference to women's autonomy has become one of the strongest, but at the same time also one of the most controversial arguments in the context of assisted reproduction and prenatal diagnosis.

149

According to many philosophers and ethicists, autonomy is regarded as one of the most important principles in genetic testing or reproductive medicine (see, e.g., Andrews *et al.* 1994; and Beauchamp and Childress 1994). A critical evaluation of widespread perceptions of genetics and the mechanisms by which genetic tests are implemented, however, raises the question of how autonomous women's decisions really are.

Whereas the Kantian notion of autonomy was conceptualised comparatively simply as 'the condition of the morally mature human being, who is led by his conscience alone', Beauchamp and Childress need 20 or more single-spaced book pages in order to elaborate on the complexity of the concept of autonomy. This indicates that the concept itself is being increasingly debated, criticised and questioned, together with the paradigm of 'principlism', which dominates US-American bioethics (see, e.g., Fox 1994; and Gert *et al.* 1997). Furthermore, the principle of autonomy is very flexible, and historically and socially contingent. Seen from a systematic perspective, it becomes clear that more than one conceptualisation of autonomy can be valid at the same time. Anne Waldschmidt (1998), a German sociologist, has recently identified four concepts of autonomy that can be described as pursuing different objectives. These are 1. subordination of the self, 2. instrumentalisation of the self, 3. self-thematisation, and 4. self-design. Furthermore, these concepts differ in their basic questions with respect to the social historic context in which they mainly developed, the objective of recommended action, the main imperative, the concept of freedom, the recipient, the notion of the subject, the promise, the relationship between body and mind, and with respect to their consequences for health care practices and the health care system.

It is generally regarded that violation of autonomy threatens the integrity of the individual and offends the dignity of the person. In some situations, it is quite obvious that autonomy is not sufficiently respected. This is the case when women are not adequately informed about prenatal tests and their consequences. From different studies it is known that this more or less uniformly applies to triple tests and sonography, which are usually offered routinely during pregnancy without adequate counselling. The complexity of the principle, however, makes it very difficult to assess whether or not it is violated in a specific situation. For instance, autonomy can be restricted by social expectations. In a Swedish study performed by Sjögren and Uddenberg (1988), 85% of all women involved said that they agreed to prenatal diagnosis voluntarily, and that they would do it again. 15% of the women felt that they had been forced to perform the test. Furthermore, almost all women found that it was difficult to reject amniocentesis, once it was offered (75% definitively, 22% to a certain extent). Even if there was no direct pressure, women felt somewhat obliged to do the test (see ibid., p. 268). This ambivalence could be an indicator of the fact that a women's autonomy in reproductive decision making is limited. Especially for pregnant women over 35 years, PND or PGD becomes something like part of a moral codex, which prescribes the duty of future parents.

Women's decisions are not only influenced by social expectations and the medical context in which counselling takes place but also by the state of technological development and implementation. In a study performed in Germany, Portugal and England, Marteau and Drake (1995) found that the ubiquitous availability of prenatal diagnosis alters the attribution of responsibility for the birth of handicapped children considerably. Questionnaires were given to four groups: men, women, geneticists and obstetricians (891 questionnaires). In all countries, the most important factor for attribution of responsibility for the birth of a child with Down Syndrome was the history of diagnosis of the mother. Women who knew about the possibility of prenatal diagnosis, but did not use it, were regarded as accountable for the handicap of their child, in contrast to mothers who did not know about the screening beforehand. This shows that the availability of prenatal diagnosis and genetic tests already implies some necessity to use it.

The opinion that individuals or couples at risk for genetic disease should make use of prenatal diagnosis is widespread within the population. I now quote from a study that was performed by Nippert (1998, p. 167) and others: when confronted with the sentence: 'People with a high risk for severe handicaps should not have children, unless they make use of prenatal diagnosis and selective abortion' different groups in Germany reacted as follows: with agreement or strong agreement 64.8% of pregnant women and 61.5% of the employed population, but only 11.2% of geneticists. The sentence was strongly rejected by 14.9% of pregnant women, 25.7% of the employed population, and 77.7% of geneticists. With the progress of the human genome project, more and more genetic tests will come onto the market. In the context of PGD, it is possible to select among a number of *in vitro* fertilised embryos the ones that best suit the expectations of the future parents. The application of PGD therefore results as Shoshana Shiloh (1996) put it—in 'bifurcation' of embryonic development: embryos are divided into a fraction that is allowed to develop to maturity, and into another one that will be discarded. PGD, therefore, much more than PND, approaches embryos like consumer objects that are subjected to choice and quality control (see Lippman 1991, p. 23). When having a child becomes such a far-reaching choice, including not only time of conception but also its genetic features, this will have many more consequences than is visible at first glance.

One of the most important questions in this context is how far women or parents will be held responsible for the birth of a genetically handicapped child. In view of such findings, the conjecture of women's autonomy with respect to genetic testing has to be questioned. Any decision for or against prenatal diagnosis or IVF can only be regarded as free if other alternatives of the same quality are available (see Lippman 1991, p. 32). Therefore, in addition to choosing prenatal diagnosis or IVF, there has to be the possibility of giving birth to a child without checking its health or constitution prenatally, even if this decision seems to contradict dominant rationality. As long as handicapped people suffer from open or hidden discrimination in our societies, however, such a decision can never be regarded as free. In this case, the new opportunities provided by reproductive medicine may develop into a duty to produce healthy children (see Hepp 1994, p. 267), even if no direct legal or economic pressure is applied.

Such attitudes and expectations, accompanied by the new reproductive and genetic technologies, will most probably leave their marks on pregnant women. In accordance with the characteristics of individualised, democratic societies, dominant rules or new guiding principles of social behaviour will not be enforced by institutions or law, but rather become internalised, and their prevalence is secured by public discourse and social control. They form the feeding ground for what has been called 'private eugenics', which is performed deliberately by individuals and which does not need to be pushed by legal means.

Pre-occupation with the principle of autonomy, which is mainly characteristic of the US discussion, but extends to Europe as well,

> petrifies individualistic preferences and bends the whole field of social implications of the new genetic and reproductive technologies away from being a question of the community and the larger society. Furthermore, it removes the field from a conception of social justice that pays special attention to the plight of the poor, the disadvantaged, the victims of social prejudice and discrimination. (Fox 1994, pp. 49–50)

How far women's autonomy will in fact be restricted by such mechanisms and developments is hard to say. On the one hand, women are very well able to decide autonomously in the context of reproduction.[4] On the other hand, the direction of such decisions is influenced considerably by the necessity to adhere to social and cultural norms. It is difficult to examine such influences in more detail, since the social expectations regarding pregnant women are subject to continuous change (see Badinter 1998). New developments within reproductive medicine confront women with new possibilities and choices, and alter social expectations. Therefore, there is a continuous necessity to assess critically social structures with respect to the aspects of pregnancy and motherhood that are advanced, and which are restricted.

4 Symbolic meaning of reproductive and genetic technologies

But what are the cultural norms to which women tend or are forced to adhere? The new reproductive and genetic technologies do not only become effective by their social power alone, but also by symbolic meanings that became associated with these technologies from the very beginning and which are a very powerful part of their marketing. This symbolic meaning is conveyed by different notions, situations and mechanisms. It is, for instance, embedded in a specific representation of women's desire for a child, and of ART specialists that promotes specific patterns of interpretation and action in case of unwanted childlessness.

Although infertility has always been experienced by a certain number of women and couples, it first became a socially recognised phenomenon during the 1980s, after the introduction of IVF. In the context of assisted reproduction discourse, the desire of a woman to have a child became (again) something like a natural force that she can resist only at the risk of psychic problems. Similarly, her capacity to endure distress and pain to realise this biological need is seen as something belonging to her nature. Patrick Steptoe, one of the medical 'fathers' of Louise Brown, was convinced that a 'biological need' to reproduce exists, and that women who resist this will react by developing psychic problems.[5] Similarly, but slightly different, the desire of women to have a family becomes naturalised.

This representation of the desire to have a child or a family has far-reaching consequences. It suggests that being childfree is something against nature, and especially against women's nature. Although having no children by one's own decision has been accepted in many western countries as a result of women's liberation, unwanted childlessness still can become a stigma that needs to be avoided (see Pfeffer 1993). The fact that many women in the first years of application kept silent about their use of assisted reproductive technology confirms this assumption, although this attitude changed after the new technologies became more socially accepted. Furthermore, the ever growing possibilities of assisted reproduction make it more and more difficult for couples seeking medical advice for fertility problems not to use the new offers. Performed not by regular gynaecologists, but by highly specialised experts, IVF confers the impression of a high quality and efficient medical treatment. 'From being something of a pariah group, associated with messy and undignified procedures, infertile women and men were now the potential recipients of glamorous,

153

highly scientised medicine' (Pfeffer and Woolett 1983). In the conjunction of reproduction and technology, two of the most powerful Euro-American-Symbols of future possibility are combined: children and scientific progress (see Franklin 1996, p. 166). This new glamour, together with the longing for a child represented as a basic need that needs to be satisfied like hunger or thirst, constitutes a powerful support for couples seeking treatment for infertility. In the face of this medically and socially constructed need, options like heterologous insemination or adoption have barely had a chance (see, e.g., Snowdon and Green 1997).

In contrast to such a biologistic view is a sociological account of the desire to have a child. According to Elisabeth Beck-Gernsheim (1993), the reference to nature becomes more and more questionable. Rather than being a natural desire, the wish to have a child refers to the fact that anonymity, impersonality and lack of emotionality, which are characteristic of daily life in modern societies, make the relationship to a child something special. Since this wider context of women's desires has rarely been reflected on, reproductive medicine was able to construct the image of being the 'last and only hope' for women or couples classified as infertile. Hope is the central metaphor by which the business proceeds.

My point is not to question the suffering of women or couples desperately wanting a child. But if this suffering is a condition that is not only due to infertility or genetic problems but which is heavily influenced by social factors, then medico-technical interventions are not the only way to overcome it. As has already been said, heterologous insemination is much more efficient, much less expensive and much safer for women and future children. Since IVF has become such a highly symbolic technique, however, such methods are perceived as barely more than a bad replacement of IVF for couples who cannot afford this cost intensive treatment (see Nisker 1996).

The fact that heterologous insemination or egg donation are not only restricted legally in many countries, but also not very well accepted among couples with fertility problems, points to a genetic ideology that is tightly connected to ART and supported by the growing recognition of the human genome project. The increasing importance of such genetic ideology can be related to individualisation and other social phenomena accompanied by it. When larger social structures decay and the stability of traditional institutions is waning, then genes and the germ-line can be seen as symbols representing more stable structures and relations compared to modern social relations. Genes and the germ-line are the concepts by which similarities and alliances are defined. In the context of reproductive and genetic technologies they may not only become new centres for feelings of togetherness and mutual responsibility, but also (post-)modern icons symbolising family bonds, lineage and kinship. In this respect, reference to genetics may take the place of more traditional representations of family bonds, and may provide the modern individual with the impression of embeddedness in larger structures, now scientifically defined by experts in genetics. At the same time, genetic selection and genetic manipulation become material practices of self-production and self-composition.

A final reason why the new reproductive technologies have become so important in personal and public perception is that they have taken over the function of a ritual that marks the transition from one phase of life into the other: from being a childless women to becoming a mother, and from being a couple to becoming a family. In modern societies with family structures falling apart, this important transition in the life of a women or a couple is no longer bound to rituals like marriage-in-white, the moving of the wife to the home of her husband, etc. It has, therefore, been suggested by Lenzen (1993) and Franklin (1996) (amongst others) that medically assisted conception and childbirth ensure that these events are enacted as dramatically as possible, in order to mark the step from one stage of life to another.

In this sense, the new reproductive and genetic technologies not only stand for the treatment of infertility and the prevention of children with inherited diseases, but also for the control of procreation and the genetic endowment of one's progeny. With this implicit goal, reproductive and genetic technologies conform perfectly to the socially expected self-management that includes the management of bodily functions and future health. In times when unlimited health becomes more and more important in highly competitive job markets, and social security systems are in crisis, the ability to function according to the needs of the market becomes enormously important. Our increasing ability to manipulate not only single physiological reactions but also bodily functions from the beginning to the end of life changes our understanding of the physical basis of human existence: the body becomes a project, an object that can be technically and rationally designed and subordinated to human will. It is transformed into a material object of self-design. The body becomes a field of action that is alienated from the conscious self. The new genetic and reproductive technologies become a symbol for medical and social self-commitment to subordinate not only external, but also internal human nature to scientific and medical progress (see Kollek 1996).

5 The social role of discourse on ethics

The conclusion that can be drawn from this is that living conditions in modern societies are structured in such a way that they demand, support, promote and consolidate reproductive and genetic technologies. In individualised societies, rational control of the self becomes the leading paradigm. The authority that tells us what to do and how to behave is no longer located in external institutions but shifted 'from without to within' (see Beck and Beck-Gernsheim 1994; Giddens 1991 and 1994; and Heelas 1996). Reproductive and genetic technologies fit in perfectly with this demand for self control. What we experience today is a major social and cultural change driven by biomedical technologies enabling us to control our biology to a far greater extent than ever possible before. Development and implementation of new medical and other technologies, however, are interdependent processes. New technologies are products and instruments of social needs, interests and conflicts. In this sense, they are cause and effect at the same time.

From the very beginning, the new reproductive and genetic technologies were accompanied by controversy. It is one of their most characteristic properties. These controversies were and are seen as an obstacle for the undisturbed unfolding and expansion of medical potential and economic power. During the last decade, many philosophers and theologians became interested in biomedical ethics. A new profession, the 'bioethicists' emerged. Different institutions were founded to establish professional education and research in biomedical ethics, and ethics became more and more institutionalised.

On the one hand, this institutionalisation can bee seen as a sign of the growing awareness of ethical questions and problems associated with new developments in reproductive medicine and genetics. On the other hand, it can also be interpreted as the response of democratic liberalism to a growing social criticism of genome research and the new reproductive technologies, in which many different groups participated. But whereas the first discussions were characterised by a plurality of voices and arguments coming from different groups and experiences, such as handicapped people, feminists, theologians, activists from grass roots health movements, and so on, today's discourse is more and more dominated by philosophers and the logic of philosophical ethics. This has certainly contributed to the clarity of arguments. But it has also had the result of streamlining the different voices participating in public discussion for and against human engineering by assisted reproduction and genetics. 'For the biomedical sciences the solution which became'—according to Hilary Rose—'increasingly clear over the course of the eighties was the deeper institutionalisation of "ethics" as a means of guiding public regulation' (1994, p. 179). Today, there is definitely a danger that the so-called principlism dominates discussions and becomes a tool to silence public controversies without solving or eliminating the problems provoking them (see Kollek and Feuerstein 1999).

156

The importance and political dynamite of this type of bioethics reasoning and discourse is largely underestimated. At first glance, it seems to contribute to the social closure of conflicts, but at the same time it opens up new spaces for medico-technical developments and their implementation. New procedures, which are more far-reaching than established ones, are then legitimised by existing practices, without challenging them seriously, as is happening currently with pre-implantation genetic diagnosis, germ line interventions and cloning of human embryos for so-called therapeutic reasons.

This would not have been possible without the management of acceptance by the dominant discourse on ethics (see Feuerstein and Kollek 1999). Its consists of a well-designed strategy of self-restriction. Scandalous applications of IVF, like fertilising menopausal women or lesbian couples by IVF, are excluded, and genetic diagnosis should—according to dominant rules and guidelines—only be applied for the prevention of diseases (or embryos affected by it), and not for selection of desirable traits, although it is almost impossible to draw a clear cut line between these two categories. Accordingly, embryos should not be created for research purposes only, but research may be done on so-called surplus embryos.

By such rules, bioethics has in fact had the effect of setting some limits to the application of biomedical technology. But these restrictions have neither been very efficient nor very lasting. First, they do not consider the problems and shortcomings of daily medical practice. Second, biomedical ethics itself is very flexible. Construction of bioethical norms occurs not in conflict, but in touch with public discourse, although this has been criticised by Mieth (1997) amongst others. In doing so, bioethics is highly successful. But since bioethical norms are continuously altered as a reaction to public and professional discourse and, in addition, to the needs of science and the economy, their erosion is pre-programmed once a new technique appears on the market. This can be observed very well in the debate on cloning. What we experience in this public space cleared of conflicts by dominant bioethical discourse is something that the German philosopher Gernot Böhme (1998) has called 'a normalization' of new techniques. By this normalization 'the technological undermining of the common', which constitutes morality, looses its original explosiveness.

If we do not agree with changes seen in the context of reproductive and genetic technologies, we should examine critically measures for what counts as acceptable, and put forward our own. The most relevant question, however, that still needs to be explored is therefore: how do we want to live? As individuals, as society, as global communities? Do the new technologies conform to these goals? What kind of technical, social, political alternatives do we have, and how can they be promoted? If we really want

157

to have choices and to be free in our decisions about our own future and that of our children, then such equivalent alternatives need to be developed, implemented and available.

Notes

1. Lesley Brown was the mother of Louise Brown, the first 'test tube' baby.
2. Data from the German state Nordrhein-Westfalen, according to publications of the Huntington Self-Help Group. (Huntington-Kurier Nr. 1/1997, p. 4, Deutsche Huntington Hilfe e.V. (ed.), Duisburg).
3. See *Die Zeit,* issue of 10 December, 1998.
4. See the different contributions in Kettner 1998
5. Cited by Stanworth 1987, p. 15.

References

Andrews, L. B., Fullarton, J. E., Holtzman, N. A. and Motulsky, A. (1994), *Assessing Genetic Risks*: *Implications for Health and Social Policy*, National Academy Press: Washington D.C.

Badinter, E. (1998), 'Mutterschaft und medizinisches Handeln', *Lexikon der Bioethik*, Vol. 2, Gütersloh, pp. 722–724.

Bauman, Z. (1996), 'Morality in the Age of Contingency', in Heelas, P., Lash, S. and Morris, P. (eds), *Detraditionalization. Critical Reflections on Authority and Identity*, Blackwell: Oxford.

Beauchamp, T. L. and Childress, J. E. (1994), *Principles of Biomedical Ethics*, Oxford University Press: New York.

Beck, U. (1992), *Risk Society: Towards a New Modernity*, Sage: London.

Beck-Gernsheim, E. (1993), 'Health and Responsibility—From Social Change to Technological Change and Vice Versa', in Haker, H., Hearn, R. and Steigleder, K. (eds), *Ethics of Human Genome Analysis: European Perspectives*, Attempto: Tübingen, pp. 199–217.

Beck, U. and Beck-Gernsheim, E. (1994), *The Normal Chaos of Love*, Polity Press: Cambridge.

Beck, U. and Beck-Gernsheim, E. (1996), 'Individualisation and "Precarious Freedoms": Perspectives and Controversies of a Subject Centered Sociology', in Heelas, P., Lash, S. and Morris, P. (eds), *Detraditionalization: Critical Reflections on Authority and Identity*, Blackwell: Oxford.

Berger, P., Berger, B. and Kellner, H. (1974), *The Homeless Mind: Modernization and Conciousness*, Vintage: New York.

Black, R. B. (1991), 'Women's Voices After Pregnancy Loss: Couples' Patterns of Communication and Support', *Prenatal Diagnosis,* Vol. 9, pp. 795–804.

Black R. B. (1994), 'Reproductive Genetic Testing and Pregnancy Loss: The Experience of Women', in Rothenberg, K. H. and Thomson, E. J. (eds), *Women & Prenatal Testing: Facing the Challenges of Genetic Technology*, Columbus: Ohio, pp. 271–290.

Böhme, G. (1998), *Ethik im Kontext*, Suhrkamp: Frankfurt.

Clarke, A. J. (1997), 'The Genetic Dissection of Multifactorial Disease: The Implications of Susceptibility Screening', in Harper P. S. and Clarke, A. J. (eds), *Genetics, Society and Clinical Practice*, pp. 93–106.

Danner Clouser, K. and Gert, B. (1990), 'A Critique of Principlism', *Journal of Medicine and Philosophy*, Vol. 15, pp. 219–236.

De Toqueville, A. (1969), 'Of Individualism in Democracies', in Meyer, J. P. (ed.), *Democracy in America*, Vol. 2, Doubleday: New York.

Donnai, P., Charles N. and Harris, R. (1981), 'Attitudes of Patients after "Genetic" Termination of Pregnancy', *British Medical Journal*, Vol. 282, pp. 621–622.

Edwards, R. G. (1998), 'Introduction and Development of IVF and Its Ethical Regulation', in Hildt, E. and Mieth, D. (eds), *In Vitro Fertilisation in the 1990s: Towards a Medical, Social and Ethical Evaluation*, Ashgate: Aldershot, pp. 3–18.

Feuerstein, G. and Kollek, R. (1999), 'Flexibilisierung der Moral. Zum Verhältnis von biotechnischen Innovationen und ethischen Normen', in Hradil, S., Gunz, M. and Honegger, C. (eds), *Kongreßband I des Freiburger Kongresses der DGS, ÖGS und SGS*, in press.

Fletcher, J. F. (1988), *The Ethics of Genetic Control: Ending Reproductive Roulette*, New York.

Fox, R. (1994), 'The Entry of U.S. Bioethics Into the 1990s: A Sociological Analysis', in DuBose, E. R., Hamel, R. P. and O'Connell, L. J. (eds), *A Matter of Principles? Ferment in U.S. Bioethics*, Trinity Press International: Valley Forge PA, pp. 21–71.

Franklin, S. (1996), *Embodied Progress: A Cultural Account of Assisted Conception*, Routledge: London and New York.

Gert B., Culver C. M. and Danner Clouser, K. (1997), *Bioethics: A Return to Fundamentals*, Oxford University Press: New York.

Giddens, A. (1991), *Modernity and Self-Identity: Self and Society in the Late Modern Age*, Polity Press: Cambridge.

Giddens, A. (1994), 'Living in a Posttraditional Society', in Beck, U. and Giddens, A., *Beyond Left and Right: The Future of Radical Politics*, Stanford University Press: Stanford, pp. 56–109.

Heelas, P. (1996), 'Introduction: Detraditionalization and Its Rivals', in Heelas, P., Lash, S. and Morris, P. (eds), *Detraditionalization: Critical Reflections on Authority and Identity*, Blackwell: Oxford.

159

Hepp, H. (1994), 'Ethische Probleme am Anfang des Lebens', in Honnefelder L. and Rager, G. (eds), *Ärztliches Urteilen und Handelns. Zur Grundlegung einer medizinischen Ethik*, Insel: Frankfurt, pp. 237–283.

Kaye, H. L. (1992), 'Are We the Sum of Genes?', *Wilson Quarterly*, Vol. 16 (Spring), pp. 77–84.

Kettner, M. (ed.) (1998), *Beratung als Zwang: Schwangerschaftsabbruch, genetische Aufklärung und die Grenzen kommunikativer Vernunft*, Suhrkamp: Frankfurt.

Knorr-Cetina, K. (1997), 'Sociality with Objects: Social Relations in Postsocial Knowledge Societies', *Theory, Culture and Society*, Vol. 14, No. 4, pp. 1–30.

Kollek, R. (1996), 'Metaphern, Strukturbilder, Mythen. Zur symbolischen Bedeutung des menschlichen Genoms', in Trallori, L. N. (ed.), *Eroberung des Lebens: Technik und Gesellschaft an der Wende zum 21. Jahrhundert*, Verlag für Gesellschaftskritik: Wien, pp. 137–153.

Kollek, R. and Feuerstein, G. (1999), 'Bioethics and Antibioethics in Germany: A Sociological Approach', *International Journal of Bioethics*, in press.

Kreuz, F. R. (1996), 'Attitudes of German Persons at Risk for Huntington's Disease Toward Predictive and Prenatal testing', *Genetic Counselling*, Vol. 7, No. 4, pp. 303–311.

Kurinczuk, J. and Bower, C. (1997), 'Birth Defects in Infants Conceived by Intracytoplasmic Sperm Injection: An Alternative Interpretation', *British Medical Journal*, Vol. 315, pp. 1260–1265.

Lenzen, D. (1993), *Krankheit als Erfindung—Medizinische Eingriffe in die Kultur*, Fischer: Frankfurt.

Lippman, A. (1991), 'Prenatal Genetic Testing and Screening: Contructing Needs and Reinforcing Inequities', *American Journal of Law and Medicine*, Vol. 17, pp. 15–50.

Lloyd, J. and Laurence K. M. (1985), 'Sequelae and Support After Termination of Pregnancy for Fetal Malformation', *British Medical Journal*, Vol. 290, pp. 907–909.

Marteau, T. M. and Drake, H. (1995), 'Attributions for Disability: The Influence of Genetic Screening', *Social Science and Medicine*, Vol. 8, pp. 1127–1132.

McFarlane, A. (1979), *The Origins of English Individualism: The Family, Property and Social Transition*, Cambridge University Press: New York.

Mieth, D. (1997), 'Ethische Probleme der Erforschung des menschlichen Genoms', in Petermann, F., Wiedebusch, S. and Quante, M. (eds), *Perspektiven der Humangenetik*, Schöningh: Paderborn *et al.*, pp. 177–194.

Nippert, I. (1997), 'Auf dem Weg zum Wunschkind? Einstellungen zur vorgeburtlichen Diagnostik in Deutschland und Europa', *Die Frau in unserer Zeit*, Vol. 3, pp. 23–32.

Nippert I. (1998), 'Wie wird im Alltag der Diagnostik tatsächlich argumentiert? Auszüge aus einer deutschen und einer europäischen Untersuchung', in Kettner,

M. (ed.), *Beratung als Zwang. Schwangerschaftsabbruch, genetische Aufklärung und die Grenzen kommunikativer Vernunft,* Campus: Frankfurt am Main, pp. 53–172.

Nisker, J. (1996), 'Rachel's Ladder or How Societal Situation Determines Reproductive Therapy', *Human Reproduction,* Vol. 11, No. 6, pp. 1162–1167.

Parsons, E. and Atkinson, P. (1993), 'Genetic Risk and Reproduction', *The Sociological Review,* Vol. 41, No. 4, pp. 679–706.

Pfeffer, N. (1993), *The Stork and the Syringe: A Political History of Reproductive Medicine,* Polity Press: Cambridge.

Pfeffer, N. and Woolett, A. (1983), *The Experience of Infertility,* Virago: London.

Robertson J. A. (1992), 'Ethical and Legal Issues in Preimplantation Genetic Screening', *Fertility and Sterility,* Vol. 57, pp. 1–11.

Rose, H. (1994), *Love, Power and Knowledge: Towards a Feminist Transformation of the Sciences,* Indiana University Press: Bloomington.

Sandelowski, M. and Jones, L. C. (1996), 'Healing Fictions: Stories of Choosing in the Aftermath of the Detection of Fetal Anomalies', *Social Science,* Vol. 42, No. 3, pp. 353–361.

Shiloh, S. (1996), 'Decision-making in the Context of Genetic Risk', in Marteau, T. M. and Richards, M. (eds), *The Troubled Helix: Social and Psychological Implications of the Next Human Genetics,* Cambridge University Press: Cambridge, pp. 82–103.

Sjögren, B. and Uddenberg, N. (1988), 'Decision Making During the Prenatal Diagnostic Procedure. A Questionnaire and Interview Study of 211 Women Participating in Prenatal Diagnosis', *Prenatal Diagnosis,* Vol. 8, pp. 263–273.

Snowdon, C. and Green, J. M. (1997), 'Preimplantation Diagnosis and Other Reproductive Options: Attitudes of Male and Female Carriers of Recessive Disorders', *Human Reproduction,* Vol 12, No. 2, pp. 341–350.

Stanworth, M. (1987), 'Reproductive Technologies and the Deconstruction of Motherhood', in Stanworth, M. (ed.), *Reproductive Technologies: Gender, Motherhood and Medicine,* Polity Press: Cambridge, pp. 9–25.

Turner, L. (1994), 'Problems Surrounding Late Prenatal Diagnosis', in Abramsky, L. and Chapple, J. (eds), *Prenatal Diagnosis. The Human Side,* pp. 134–148, London

Von Gontard, A. (1986), 'Psychische Folgen des Schwangerschaftsabbruchs aus kindlicher Indikation', *Monatsschrift Kinderheilkunde,* Vol. 134, pp. 150–157.

Waldschmidt, A. (1998), *Selbstbestimmung in Gesundheitsversorgung und Rehabilitation—Theoretische Grundlegung. Forschungsbericht,* Universität Dortmund.

White, G. B. (1998), 'Crisis in Assisted Conception: The British Approach to an American Dilemma', *Journal of Women's Health,* Vol. 7, No. 3, pp. 321–328.

White van Mourik, M. C. A., Connor, J. M. and Ferguson-Smith, M. A. (1992), 'The Psychosocial Sequelae of a Second-trimester Termination of Pregnancy for Fetal Abnormality', *Prenatal Diagnosis,* Vol. 12, pp. 189–204.

Comment: *Transcending the either/or: Can bioethics be critical?*

Hub Zwart

1 Introduction

Regine Kollek's paper is interesting, even fascinating, and I agree with many of the things she says. Yet, the genre conventions of giving comments force me to be critical, rather than enthusiastic, and to point to the weaker, rather than to the stronger aspects of her paper. I will comply with these conventions, of course, but not without first having complimented her on her achievements. Moreover, I will not merely respond to this particular paper by Regine. Rather, I will regard it as a specimen of a particular kind of discourse, for this enables me to raise some issues of broader concern, rather than mere textual ones. The paper contains many interesting details, but I will concentrate my response on two important issues. First, I will draw attention to Regine Kollek's critique of the standard account usually accompanying the development and introduction of new technologies. Notably, I will concentrate on the concepts of *free choice* and *biological need*. Subsequently, being a bioethicist myself, I will comment on Regine Kollek's critique of the social role and astonishing career of bioethics.

2 The standard account and the attitude of suspicion

In dealing with the first issue, I will proceed in a 'dialectical' manner. First, I will summarise the standard account as criticised by Regine Kollek. Subsequently, I will summarise Regine Kollek's critique. Finally, I will bring forward my own criticism of her critique.

As pointed out in Regine Kollek's paper, the standard account that usually accompanies the development and introduction of new biotechnologies consists of two basic claims. In the first place, it is claimed that

163

the use of these new technologies, like for example IVF, results from free and rational choice, that these technologies increase the individual's ability to shape her own biography and structure her own life. A second important justification for introducing these technologies is that they actually respond to a pre-existing need or demand. Or, to put it more precisely, it is claimed that procreation, i.e., giving birth to a child that is genetically one's own, constitutes a biological need, something like an unstoppable desire or force, a biological destiny, a vital necessity.

Now, as Regine Kollek rightly points out, these claims must be regarded as highly problematic. Why? Because rather than being solely the outcome of free choice, the act of applying for IVF is often motivated to a considerable extent by social expectations and internalised ideals. The applicant may actually (whether she is aware of it or not) be responding to the strong symbolical meanings attached to these interventions. Indeed, the glamour and prestige of modern medicine may well enable the individual involved to dramatise important life events, such as giving birth. Furthermore, Regine Kollek emphasises that the desire to give birth to a child genetically one's own should not be regarded as a *biological* need, but rather as a socially and culturally constructed one, a need that proves itself to be historically flexible, responding to, and shaped by, temporary social expectations, changing over time.

Although I tend to agree with the basic import of Kollek's critique, I have serious problems with the *ethical implications* that seem to evolve from it. Notably, my problem concerns the false dichotomy on which her critique apparently relies, namely the one between biological need and social expectation. On the one hand, it must be emphasised that most if not all socially constructed needs do have a biological or physical correlate. These needs are socially *shaped*, rather than created *ex nihilo*. Nevertheless, I agree with Regine's claim that in order to understand the inherent logic of human desire, social construction is more important than biology. We are cultural beings, living in an ever-changing world of symbolical meanings and social expectations. There are no purely biological needs. Even the intake of food and water, for example, is cultivated and ritualised—we do not live by bread (and water) alone. The question, however, is: what are the implications when it comes to assessing the significance of these culturally shaped needs from an ethical point of view? Are socially constructed needs less important, less legitimate, less urgent than biological ones? Can we say that needs become less important the more socially constructed they are?

No! To begin with, the very distinction between biological and socially constructed needs is flawed, as was already pointed out. Moreover, even those needs that can be said to be highly constructed and culture-dependent can still be of dramatic significance to the individuals that happen to cherish them. They may even prove to be astonishingly durable, and the effort to realise them may be regarded as extremely worthwhile. They may well be experienced as more important even than food and drink. In short, what does it mean, ethically speaking, when we replace the phrase *biological need*, as it occurs in the standard account, by the phrase *socially constructed need*, as it occurs in Regine Kollek's paper? The fact *as such* that social expectations and symbolical meanings affect our choices, does not, in and of itself, decrease their ethical significance. It does not make these choices arbitrary, capricious, flexible, suspect, or less real. A socially constructed need can indeed be a very important and legitimate one—even more so if we realise that *all* needs are socially constructed, to a greater or lesser extent.

3 The astonishing career of bioethics

Regine Kollek's rather critical account of the social role of bioethics is a familiar and partially valid one. Indeed, it has been suggested before that, rather than challenging new technologies, bioethics in fact promotes their social acceptance, notably by streamlining and pacifying social controversy. And it has often been argued that bioethics is in fact a new form of bureaucratic professionalism, that social controversies find themselves increasingly dominated by a new bioethical logic, with the result that the original explosiveness of these controversies is dramatically reduced. Bioethics, it is said, refuses to reflect on its own premises, and eventually facilitates the introduction of new technologies by manipulating public debate. Finally, there is a slippery-slope aspect to bioethics. For although initially certain scandalous applications are excluded, gradual erosion of these restrictions is pre-programmed and eventually, bioethics aims at the normalisation of these technologies.

As I said, this type of criticism is well-known, and I have voiced it myself on one or two occasions. It must be taken very seriously, no doubt. Nevertheless, I think we should be somewhat more precise and careful in our self-criticism. Regine Kollek presents us with a rather gloomy picture of bioethics *as a whole*, bound to trigger suspicion and resentment. But is this picture realistic, reliable and fair? No, it is not! It is based, once again, on a false dichotomy, an unsatisfactory either/or. This time, the dichotomy consists of the claim that the basic objective of bioethics is *either* to challenge and block the development and introduction of new technologies, *or* to promote and facilitate their social acceptance. It is a dichotomy somewhat similar to the Dutch version of the famous dictum *Stand and deliver!*—namely *Either your money or your life!* Somehow, there must be a way to escape from both alternatives and to secure a middle-ground.

Indeed, there is, I would say, a middle-position, one that neither aims at merely inciting public fear or suspicion, nor at simply clearing the ground for scientific optimism—and I will refer to it as *critical alertness*. It involves an attitude of sensitivity and alertness, rather than suspicion, both to the risks and to the possibilities of these new technologies. In a way, Kollek is right, and we bioethicists *must* be aware of this risk of becoming an ideology, a new form of bureaucratic professionalism, etc.—but this is not, I would say, our inevitable fate or destiny. Rather, it is my contention that a legitimate and philosophically acceptable form of bioethics is possible, one that proceeds in a methodologically sound and well-considered manner and aims at recognising both the truths and the fallacies at work in scientific optimism as well as in public fear.

The principlistic approach elaborated by Beauchamp and Childress and others often serves as a scapegoat for the kind of criticism articulated by Regine. The criticism is basically correct insofar as these principles are regarded as a kind of technical equipment, ready-at-hand, allowing us to solve all our problems, even the tragic ones. However, the use of principles is legitimate, I would say, insofar as they are regarded as hermeneutical tools, rich in content, with a long history, allowing us bring some structure into the problem situations we find ourselves in. If we need principles, that is, we also need to know what principles *are*. When Regine Kollek emphasises the importance of paying attention to the paradoxical nature, the social dimension of our problems, etc., my response would be that this is precisely what we, as bioethicists, must try to do.

I suspect, moreover, that her critique relies too much on a certain version of what has been called the 'dialectics of enlightenment', a form of criticism that (rather monotonously) tries to point out that freedom is really coercion, that democracy is really totalitarianism (thus blurring the distinction between both), that progress is really repression, etc.—a form of criticism, in short, that evolves out of a mood of chronic suspicion. Instead, I would advocate (as I said) an attitude of critical alertness to the presence both of instances of coercion and of possibilities for choice, that is, a more precise, more detailed, more sensitive form of reflection, not an apocalyptic and chronically distrustful one, but a reflection based on the willingness to reflect on the phenomena as they really emerge, shaping and changing our world—a reflection that is sensitive both to the predictable and to the unexpected, and that is situated on the boundary between philosophical anthropology and ethics. What do I mean by that?

4 Philosophical anthropology and ethics: Or, some dramatic transitions in the history of bodily life (in outline)

Bioethics is a form of applied ethics, but the term 'applied ethics' may be somewhat misleading insofar as it suggests that we already have at our disposal a ready-made ethic, a kind of technical tool waiting to be applied. In reality, bioethics is (or ought to be) a much more inductive form of philosophical reflection. We do not know what ethical concepts or ethical principles really mean until we start applying them. Application is a creative process, a practice of discovery. Concepts and principles are not to be applied in a mechanical or quasi-automatic manner. Rather, they tend to be affected by the application process itself and tend to become more and more fleshed-out as they find themselves exposed to real-life phenomena. Moreover, the world we live in is constantly changing, and this means that even those concepts and principles that have managed to establish themselves in a more or less canonical form will sooner or later find themselves challenged again by new experiences and developments.

This does not mean, however, that the history of bioethics proceeds in a completely chaotic and random-like fashion. To begin with, some discoveries are more significant than others. The discovery on which Immanuel Kant insisted, namely that persons are to be respected rather than manipulated, must be regarded as an irreversible one, a discovery that really made a difference, an instance of moral progress that changed our moral world. Moreover, although the concepts and principles of ethics often find themselves challenged by new technological developments and scientific discoveries, this does not mean that they simply have to adapt and accommodate themselves to the new circumstances. In some cases, we rather expect them to offer serious resistance. But in any case, in order to provide a critical comment on technological and scientific developments, we must be aware of the basic tendencies at work in these developments and be informed about them as detailed and precisely as possible. In short, the Kantian claim that we are *either* involved in anthropology (collecting and analysing the actual, empirical facts) *or* in autonomous, normative ethics, must give way to a continuous interaction between inductive research and normative analysis.

Regine Kollek points out, for example, how the formerly inseparable process of conception, pregnancy and birth suddenly finds itself divided into scientifically and technically distinguishable stages. What used to be an integrated, spherical whole is transformed into a series of units that can be manipulated separately from one another. In this manner, biotechnology no doubt has a profound impact on the way we experience our pregnancies, as well as other important life events. Many similar examples may be added. Geneticalisation will affect our concept of disease, organ donation

167

will affect the way we experience the integrity of our bodies, sex-change operations will affect the way we experience our sexual relationships, etc. What we learn from these and similar examples is that a philosophical anthropology that has the objective of determining once and for all the essential structure of human existence is out-dated. The basic structures of human existence are flexible, profoundly historical, and sensitive to technological and scientific developments. The way we experience our bodies, our pregnancies, our sexual life, etc., is bound to change over time—a process, moreover, which is well-documented in literary, scientific and other archives. The contours of our anthropological self-image change as new ethical questions emerge. And whereas, on the one hand, the actual power of medicine over bodily life has increased dramatically, new forms of dependency and new physiological limits are being discovered as well. We have to reflect on and incorporate these developments in our diagnoses in order to make them more adequate and precise. But this does not mean that bioethics becomes uncritical and apologetic. Rather, we must cultivate what I referred to as an attitude of alertness, both to the risks and to the possibilities inherent in these developments. For moral criticism remains rhetorical as long as detailed insight into the phenomena at hand is lacking.

Comment on *Technicalisation of human procreation and social living conditions*

Barbara Maier

1 Introduction: Why *make* babies?

The main reason for 'making' babies by reproductive medicine's assistance is the infertility of one or both partners. But nowadays, a second reason is becoming more important: the control of the possible genetic heritage that would-be parents at risk could transfer to their offspring. This can be controlled to a certain extent. The desire for a child, or a healthy enough one, seems the promoting factor for acknowledging reproductive medicine's legitimation also in cases of pre-implantation genetic diagnosis (PGD).

The intensity of the desire for a child and the suffering induced by remaining childless against one's will are assumed to be legitimate reasons for reproductive interventions. What does then suffering mean? In the case of infertility, self-discrimination, discrimination of the infertile partner and social discrimination on the grounds of psychosocially predominating loss experiences (loss of an acceptable self- or body image, of status, self-confidence, loss of control over desire-fulfilling potential) make infertile people become patients with an 'illness' others do not understand.

A special kind of suffering occurs in cases where people are diagnosed (in accordance with existing indications) with 'bad' genes that in procreation might be transferred to their offspring.

The situation of 'carriers' is thus especially problematic. The risk of transferring a genetic disorder to their offspring and thus acting unlovingly makes them feel in some sense guilty and obliged to submit to prevention. They are supposed to be ready to undergo what is offered by reproductive medicine combined with PGD in order to qualify in advance as parents the way society expects them to be to achieve knowledge about their own status in order to avoid not only affected but also carrier-offspring. Carrier children, again, would probably face the same problems their parents have

169

at that time. So the 'making' of babies, feasible to a certain degree, seems to be highly desirable: for whom and at what cost?

2 Technology is much more than technique[1]

This is especially true for biotechnical developments, as Regine Kollek has impressively shown in her paper. Social structures (social structuring) correspond(s) to bio(technical) medicine and both influence each other in promoting an image of human beings and of lifestyle that could be characterised as *'possessive individualism'*.

Possessive individualism is at work in reproductive medicine as well and this in a rather specific way. Reproductive medicine is available in most western countries. The legitimation for the intervention of reproductive medicine seems increasingly provided by the (more and more individualised) desire for a child (see Mieth 1995).

The increase of the potential of desire fulfilment and the decrease of binding potential in relationships (provoked by social destruction as well as by biotechniques) in modern societies fit in completely with the concept of autonomous expression of the self—even in reproductive matters.

Procreation becomes more self-expression than the expression of a lived relationship. To this extent, perfect procreation is crucially important for self-esteem. The individual is responsible for the outcome of the offspring and especially the woman is often blamed for having ignored outcome controlling technologies.

Out of prejudice, disabled children are even assumed to result from parental ignorance. Their parents are blamed for their existence and held responsible by society for the children's handicaps. Reproductive and genetic enlightenment force us to know and to react according to the knowledge available to us (see Beck-Gernsheim 1993). Fate is not part of one's life any more.

So biotechnical medicine corresponds with the concept of the self in modern societies. Bioethics seems to be in search of this correspondence, too—appeasing the dangerous potential biotechnical possibilities might have and often even ignoring the contradictions in which biotechnologies sometimes involve the people concerned as well as society.

As an illustration, here is an example: whereas prenatal diagnosis (PND) entails the possibility of conflict between interests of mother and 'her' developing fetus, PGD at least offers a medical escape from this. The relational potential (even when this is going to be destroyed) is evident in the first case and neglected in the second. The result is a dilemma faced by people who intensely long for a child and at the same time have to be prepared to let embryos be discarded because they are not qualified to be transferred to the woman's womb.

Those who are aware of this face a double loss, which psychologically is not so easy to overcome.

3 The modification and *transformation potential* of reproductive and genetic technologies for individuals as well as for society

1. The meaning of being (and possibly remaining) childless or being at risk of having a handicapped child for one's concept of oneself and one's role in society is essentially altered by the existence of reproductive and genetic technologies. Their persuasive potential is evident when acceptance of childlessness or solidarity with handicapped people decreases in society.
2. Medically and socially *constructed needs* (having a child, or having a perfect one) develop into *rights* and subsequently into *duties*. The right to procreate seems to correspond with the duty to have assisted reproduction if you are not able to procreate by yourself, or with the duty to undergo PGD if you are a member of a risk group. Responsible procreation then means technically controlled reproduction. Without using technology, infertility or a handicapped child will be ascribed by society to the couples who neglected their duty: to procreate by assisted reproduction under the control of PGD.
3. The transformation potential is especially evident when looking at bonding processes and parent-child relationships. The individual desire for a child (or for a healthy one) is the focus of reproductive interventions that push aside questions of changing established relationships (especially the character and formation of relationships) by reproductive and genetic medicine.
4. Nowadays we experience modification and even transformation in the perception as well as in the conditions of human existence—in procreation as well as in assisted procreation reproductive medicine. Commodification and commercialisation of people and embryos may lead to the undermining of relationships and their relevance in society.
5. Biotechnologies have a transforming potential for medicine itself: healing and helping suffering people are held up against screening and preventing (not only diseases but also affected human beings). If PGD becomes more and more available in the future, it will certainly also be on offer for infertile people without special genetic risks.
6. Anticipating future possibilities, IVF might be considered to be the usual method of procreation because of better, improved control compared to so-called old fashioned spontaneous procreation.

Reproductive and genetic medicine could in this way be presented as a necessity for a healthy 'new' generation after a genetic check-up (see Kass 1972).

For an illustration of what an elaborated PGD could bring to future generations, see the vision that Ernst Peter Fischer (1995) has critically elaborated as an experiment of extrapolation into the future. Following Isaiah Berlin (1994), who was convinced that there is nothing more destructive for human life than a fanatical belief in the perfect life, he depicts the following vision.

Starting with the early 90s the following tendencies are already at work.

> Young educated middle class couples of today (the early 90s) represent . . . the first generation which is—thanks to reliable contraception and prenatal diagnosis—able to choose concerning their offspring. These possibilities of choice, as restricted as they might be, seem to have brought a subtle but significant change in attitudes toward children. Whereas in the past, would-be parents hoped and prayed for a healthy and talented baby, couples of the present generation very obviously expect that their child will be a 'perfect baby'. They take quite some burdens upon them, even an abortion, to avoid having a child which is handicapped or even has the 'wrong' sex. The introduction of testing for hereditary diseases and genetic dispositions will undoubtedly increase this struggle for the 'perfect baby' of the well-off middle classes. (Ibid.)

On the other hand, birth control, prenatal diagnosis and abortions are rather rare amongst the poor and economically disadvantaged. Those, who in a hostile world are forced to fight for their survival, frequently have neither the energy nor the educational background to think about such luxury as the procreation of a 'perfect baby' (Bishop and Wadholz 1991).

If would-be parents were to be offered the options for certain character-features or skills of their potential children, they would probably select socially desirable ones. They would opt for rather similar ones despite confessed pluralism and individualism. The thereby resulting children would have similar qualities, skills etc. That renders them, the qualities as well as the children, less valuable because everyone is in possession of these qualities. In addition, as time passes, socially desirable qualities might change. How would skills in sports be advantageous when sports have stopped to attract people in a certain society? How is one to use cultural achievements in a society addicted to TV and computers? In this way, gifted, genetically endowed people would experience a deep disappointment. Fischer draws the conclusion: the most perfect baby, the most 'designed' one, would be the most disappointed and disappointing adult (see Fischer 1995).

To the extent that the autonomy of would-be parents seems to increase, the future autonomy of their potential children decreases. For the 'perfect child', only the options that their parents have chosen for them remain. That cannot really be called having options at all. No human being is ever provided with less liberty. The perfect baby is perfectly unfree as an adult. 'Tailor-made children' are those deprived of their uniqueness and at the same time of their potential to live creatively. They have to function according to their parents will—without any chance to escape (see Fischer 1995).

4 Reproductive and genetic technologies: are they really beneficial to women? Do they really promote reproductive autonomy?

The possible implications that IVF/ICSI (which also underlie procedures for PGD) might have, raise doubts about the beneficence of assisted procreation.

4.1 Medical implications

Severe hyperstimulation syndrome is seldom, but sometimes life threatening.

Multiple pregnancies, as a result of problematic transferential practice, might cause pre-term deliveries and pre-term birth with physical implications for the children, and developmental handicaps. But there are also social implications that triplets, quadruplets, etc., have for parents and their families.

4.2 The psychosocial implications

Work on the psychosocial implications should take into account the experiences of women who have undergone reproductive interventions (see Maier 1997).

a. The 'logic', the structure, and the dynamics of IVF/ICSI, including the fact that it is a condition for PGD, influence infertile people or those at risk of having a handicapped child.
    Do they impose a bearable risk on women, who are probably placing themselves at risk, e.g., by PCO-syndrome, which might mediate severe hyper-stimulation syndrome?

173

Is it really of benefit to a woman to be treated for a male's 'disease'?

Is it far better for a woman to undergo IVF treatment in order to avoid a handicapped child than to abort such a child? At present, PND is still recommended after PGD—because, as yet, the latter is not reliable enough.

The price to be paid for all this is high—especially for the women.

b. For the infertile couple, IVF is something that they cannot perform on their own and for which they need medico-technical help. Given their lack of reproductive power, their own procreation has to be passed on to reproductive medicine. This might cause further deterioration of self-confidence and self-esteem.

IVF involves placing one's trust in a technically induced process, which to a large extent no longer lies in the hands of the couples involved and often cannot be influenced by them. For them, IVF means being dependent on reproductive technologies and facing their own insufficiency to conceive, or have a sufficient healthy child. It also means being judged inadequate as a result of the diagnostic process.

c. In spite of well-known low success-rates (IVF 20%, ICSI 25%, cycles for PGD 25%), people undergoing IVF have high, unrealistic expectations of becoming pregnant. These expectations are probably induced by the high pressure induced by being childless or having a handicapped child. When great expectations become frustration following unsuccessful IVF procedures, the emotional balance of the woman, the man, and the couple are threatened.

d. To what extent and in what ways do IVF procedures influence women, men, and their relationship with their potential children? To what extent, and regarding which features, does PGD (in particular) shape the relationship of would-be parents to their potential children?

Because a pregnancy might be terminated after the results of amniocentesis or chorionic villus sampling, such procedures engender a more emotionally distant relationship between the mother and the embryo-fetus than is usual. Pregnancies before such testing might be termed 'tentative pregnancies' (Katz-Rothman 1989), until the tests fail to reveal any genetic abnormality or disease. However, that a mother accepts a child only on the condition that he or she is sufficiently healthy and genetically well endowed might damage the relationship between the mother and the potential child.

Is the integrity of the mother-child relationship not also at stake in PGD cases? Would not the selection of embryos that this involves mean that children who learn of this gain the impression that they owe their own lives to being genetically qualified enough to become accepted by their parents? Reproductive technologies promote tendencies towards conditional parental acceptance. Could not such tendencies, in turn, encourage the withdrawal of resources at the end of life on the basis that a person's state of health is of less importance the older he or she is? The beginning and end of life are two completely different dimensions. I would not like to equate them. But a society that makes decisions about the beginning according to special conditions might perceive the same conditional framework at the end—especially under the pressure of scarce resources, etc.

e. People undergoing IVF procedures often do not speak about them, avoid families with children and concentrate only on their longing for a child. Reproductive medicine, as a purely medical answer to the complex problems of infertile couples, cannot claim to represent the only and sufficient problem-solving strategy for them. On the contrary, it sometimes increases their difficulties—as has been described above.

No psycho-social counselling is available for the majority of couples who ultimately remain childless after technical intervention has failed.

f. IVF/ICSI (also when performed for PGD) has a potential to instrumentalise and depersonalise. Depersonalisation occurs when the procedures damage women's bodies as well as their relationships with their partners and children.

Feminists question the treatment of women for male infertility. Should medical treatment involving multiple risks for women be allowed for male infertility (as in ICSI) or for the sake of PGD?

Many of the procedures involve selection. PGD involves embryo selection, PND is used for fetal control (and also for the control of PGD results) and, in multiple pregnancies, fetal reduction might become 'necessary' in order to rescue the pregnancy as such and prevent additional risks for the mother.

4.3 Questions about reproductive autonomy

The first question is, 'Whose autonomy should materialise in which context?' The second question is, 'How might an uncritical perception of autonomy develop into subtle control mechanisms undermining liberal societies?'

Autonomy is the highest ranking of the shared values in Western societies (see Beauchamp and Childress 1994). It means self-conception and self-creation and, in consequence, responsibility for self-development in several aspects of life.

Rational decision making is the basis of this project. And 'the rational' seems to be instantiated by the 'scientific-technical.' To control one's own life is an essential task of modern life. We desire to extend our control of our offspring when our control of our own lives is threatened. It is true that we are nowhere as vulnerable as we are in our children.

We seem to have less control of our children with respect to their lives, education and behaviour—due to our concern with self-development (possessive individualism). But to compensate for this, we try to gain control over their genetic endowment according to our genetically reductionist image of humankind. Genes are modern icons that are held to guarantee the future of children and oblige their parents not so much to educate them as to follow the rules of biotechnology.

Are we psychologically and socially prepared to opt for or against using these technologies? Is having options the only and adequate way of exercising autonomy? Are we not, when opting for technological reproduction, under the control of experts rather than expressing our autonomous choice? Are the options really at our disposal? Who really possesses the mental and analytical ability to opt for or against controlling offspring, judging, or accepting them? Are the pre-conditions for opting as equal for educated people as for uneducated ones, for the rich as for poor, etc.?

5 Ethical relevance of medical indications

The assessment of technology must not only recognise indications but also focus on the development of shifts in indications. IVF was originally introduced to 'treat' tubal blockage. Indications, nowadays, have changed. IVF/ICSI is also performed for 'idiopathic' sterility, whatever is meant by this.

IVF/ICSI might even be performed when non-medical reasons call for it, e.g., the social development of postponing pregnancies later in life (due to the better education of women as well as the lack of kindergartens).

The questionable indications for the genetic check-up of embryos by PGD, which involves healthy women in IVF procedures, should raise an intensive debate on the indications for which IVF-PGD should be available in order to avoid the discrimination against people affected by diseases or disorders, as well as the discrimination against carriers who find themselves on the indication list.

Medically persuasive (i.e., persuasive in relation to criteria of objectivity and feasibility) and coercive tendencies are inevitable. At first glance, PGD seems to be restricted to certain medical indications. These are thought to be medically objective, but in reality they are also shaped by the social framework. Which genetic diseases (or disorders) should be considered to be indications for medical intervention and which not? Would that be dependent on viability or providability of treatment? Would not the extent to which handicapped children will be socially accepted and respectfully treated in the society where they and their parents live also probably count?

Social forces must not be underestimated in accepting or denying indications for PGD. This dimension should be analysed and critically examined in the course of introducing ethical dimensions into evaluation processes.

6 The social 'design' and the biomedical 'design'

The social and biomedical 'designs' are compared in different contexts, but seldom sufficiently differentiated. Social expectations change the social design of individuals. However, they are influences on living subjects, who are—more or less—capable of adopting or rejecting designing moments/features/forces. Discussion and argumentation are possible in principle, whereas 'biomedical designing' (as far as it is or ever will become feasible) subjects human beings to a basically determined state.

The illusion of the abolition of contingency and finitude attributes responsibility to designers (parents who desire to design their children and the designing 'medical engineers'). The self-understanding of human beings in our culture and living structures, their 'humanity', has depended, up until now, on the personal concept of being born and raised by identifiable parents who have accepted them as they are—without being basically determined or chosen under certain conditions (see Wucherer-Huldenfeld 1994).

7 Bioethics' role and the assessment of technology

Assessment of the technology of biotechniques is necessary for the evaluation of the social implications of available and applied technologies. But there is often a methodological prejudice when the assessment of technology and its relationship to bioethics are discussed.

H. ten Have (1995) warns of the degradation of bioethics to another problem-solving strategy comparable to the strategies of technology itself. To this extent, bioethics also leads to what Regine Kollek, from a sociologist's perspective, called 'the normalisation of new techniques,' the mental, moral and cultural preparation of acceptance of basically life-changing technologies.

Images of man and nature, as well as values that have until now been shared, are undermined in advance, not even questioned, but pushed aside by created needs and the provocation of demandable, because technically materialisable, rights.

Following their intrinsic logic, technologies create a kind of moral codex about how prospective parents have to perceive their duties in order to receive the help of technology for a perfect baby.

It seems to me that revelation of the unquestioned (but very questionable) adaptation of human decisions and acts, as well as the conditions for (reproductive) technologies, is most important. 'Technological fixes' decrease human autonomy while pretending to increase it by providing more options. The presuppositions of these options have to be examined and must not be taken as given without discussing the implications they have. The assessment of technology should take up the task of revealing new dimensions of responsibility. Aiming at an equivalence of available knowledge and consequences of our actions according to knowledge, even if we do not achieve this, we should strongly question the goals of applied reproductive technologies.

8 Final remarks

What are biotechnologies doing with us and to us, to our children, to the relationships we live in or leave and to solidarity and humaneness?

What are the criteria for living satisfactorily as a human being? And where do the criteria stem from?

What is demanded is not repair ethics, the task of which is to appease the contradictions biotechniques provoke, but innovative creative ethics (see Mittelstrass 1991), which asks questions about our image of humankind and meets the challenge to reveal the contradictions in which we get involved by overexpanding our autonomous choices concerning future generations.

Note

[1] See Dyson 1995.

References

Beauchamp, T. L. and Childress, J. F. (1994), *Principles of Biomedical Ethics*, Oxford University Press: New York.

Beck-Gernsheim, E. (1993), 'Prädiktive Medizin: Ist Wissen besser als Nichtwissen?', in *Psychosomatische Gynäkologie-Geburtshilfe*, Springer: Berlin/Heidelberg.

Berlin, I. (1994), *Den Ideen die Stimme zurückgeben*, Fischer: Frankfurt a. Main.

Bishop, J. E. and Waldholz, M. (1991), *Landkarte der Gene*, Droemer Knaur: München.

Dyson, A. (1995), *The Ethics of IVF*, Mowbray: London.

Fischer, E. P. (1995), 'Perfekte Menschen in perfekter Gesellschaft. Über die Freiheit, sich ein vollkommenes Baby aussuchen zu können, und einige Widersprüche, auf die man dabei trifft', *Recht auf Kinder—Recht auf Eltern. Autonomie, Pluralismus und die Fortpflanzungsmedizin*, Loccumer Protokolle Vol. 58, pp. 75–88.

Kass, L. R. (1972), '"Making Babies"—The New Biology and the Old Morality', *The Public Interest*, Washington, pp. 18–56.

Katz-Rothman, B. (1989), *Schwangerschaft auf Abruf: Vorgeburtliche Diagnose und die Zukunft der Mutterschaft*, Metropolis: Marburg.

Maier, B. (1997), 'The Effects of IVF on the Women Involved', in Hildt, E. and Mieth, D. (eds), *In Vitro Fertilisation in the 1990s: Towards a Medical, Social and Ethical Evaluation*, Ashgate: Aldershot, pp. 187–194.

Mieth, D. (1995), 'Ethische Fragen der Fortpflanzungstechnologie', in Tinneberg, H.-R. and Ottmar, C. (eds), *Moderne Fortpflanzungsmedizin: Grundlagen, IVF, ethische und juristische Aspekte,* Thieme: Stuttgart/New York.

Mittelstrass, J. (1991), 'Auf dem Wege zu einer Reparaturethik?', in Wils, J.-P. and Mieth, D. (eds), *Ethik ohne Chance? Erkundungen im technologischen Zeitalter.* (Ethik in den Wissenschaften 2), Attempto: Tübingen, pp. 89–108.

Ten Have, H. (1995), 'Medical Technology—Assessment and Ethics: Ambivalent Relationships', *Hastings Center Report,* Vol. 25, No. 5, pp. 13–19.

Wucherer-Huldenfeld, A. K. (1994), Ursprüngliche Erfahrung und personales Sein. Ausgewählte philosophische Studien. I. Anthropologie. Freud. Religionskritik.

Part Five

MORAL REASONING IN APPLIED ETHICS

Moral reasoning in applied ethics: The place of moral philosophy in the ethical discussion concerning reproductive medicine and human genetics

Marcus Düwell

Introduction

The aim of this paper is, in many ways, difficult to achieve. The object is to clarify the position and the role of moral-philosophic considerations in dealing with problems in applied ethics. The topic is neither solely of moral-philosophical nature, nor is it concerned with the clarification of a bioethical issue itself. Rather the methodical connection of several dimensions of ethical reflection is my concern. The difficulty is that the perspective from which the methodical connection is looked at changes according to which position in moral-philosophy is taken. The thematic focus of the *European Network for Biomedical Ethics* will be the starting point for a general reflection on this methodological problem. To begin with, I will present some complexities of problems that are especially important for the *Network*. In a second step, I will discuss some possibilities for constructing ethical theories. The specific ethical approach is not so important; rather, the position and understanding of the role of justification in the respective approach is the focus of attention. In this process, the possibilities for presenting the specific problem area from the perspective of different ethical theory-building concepts should become clear.

1 Reproductive medicine and molecular genetics: areas of ethical problems

During the conception of the *European Network for Biomedical Ethics*, we were most concerned with bringing together and connecting the numerous isolated ethical discussions concerning reproductive medicine and molecular genetics. We had the impression that essential moral aspects of problems in biomedical ethics would be neglected, if the close association of technical possibilities and research development in medical areas were not recognised. Therefore, any ethical evaluation would fall short of its goal if these connections were not considered.

1.1 Ethical problems of in vitro fertilisation

The ethical evaluation of *in vitro* fertilisation and the following embryo transfer (IVF/ET) already raise a host of questions. It would be very short-sighted to reduce the ethical question to whether or not artificial insemination should be allowed at all. There are hardly any fundamental objections concerning technically assisted fertilisation that are independent of the consideration of the implications that the development and application of this technique would have. On the other hand, the fact that there are no fundamental objections does not mean that it is morally allowed.[1] The problem area is to be described as follows:

1. What are the *psychological and social consequences* for the woman who takes advantage of these techniques? This is a continuing problem because their low success rate brings unavoidable stress. In connection with this, other questions arise concerning counselling. Does counselling provide sufficient clarification of the problem? Are alternatives to assisted procreation presented? How are they presented, and what is the scope of their presentation?

2. What is the *moral status of pre-embryos, embryos and fetuses*? This question comes up in connection with cryopreservation, the production of surplus embryos, and research on embryos considered necessary for the continuing development of IVF.

3. Is it only *morally permissible* to offer couples technical means of fulfilling their wish for a child, or do they have a justified *right to one*? This problem implies the following: in case there is a right, society could be obligated to continue IVF development, which would have to have recourse to embryo research.

Whether society has an obligation to the couple, depends on the moral status of (pre-) embryos. If the embryo has rights, there will be a conflict of rights. If the protection status of the embryo is lower, such an obligation becomes conceivable. This latter case would also imply that the necessary financial means should be made available. However, to justify such an obligation it would first be necessary to show that no other moral responsibility has higher priority. If we assume that the (pre-)embryo deserves no moral protection, the assumption that IVF is allowed could legitimise continued development.

In order to ground an *obligation on the part of society* to make IVF/ET available and to continue developing the techniques, one would have to presuppose that a positive right exists. I will define positive and negative rights in the following way: a negative right exists when I have a justified claim not to be hindered in a certain action. Others are obliged not to harm me or hinder me in my action. On the other hand, a positive right implies my justified claim to support in reaching my goal.[2] This distinction is not the same as 'Doing and refraining from doing'. Protection of a negative right can require action as well. There is, however, a difference according to the recipients of both kinds of rights. A negative right is addressed to each agent. If I have the right not to be killed, everybody has the obligation to act according to that. But a positive right to education, for example, is not correlated to an obligation for everybody to teach me. The positive right is addressed to the community or to specific institutions.

Even if assisted procreation can be morally justified, requiring society to further develop techniques and offer them to the public remains to be justified. If there is no right to one's own child and if the (pre-)embryo deserves protection, at least at a reduced level, it would be difficult to legitimise the use of embryos in research for the development of IVF. If, however, there is such a right, a lower moral status of the embryo could legitimise such an obligation of society. On the presupposition that there are strong arguments for the existence of that right, embryo research for the development of IVF would be only forbidden if the embryo had full moral status. In that case there would be a conflict of rights, but on the presupposition of a full moral status of the embryo the right of existence of the embryo would be of higher importance than the right to have a child.

4. Another dimension of IVF/ET development concerns the *effects it has on our lives*. It is difficult to formulate these effects, but they are undoubtedly important.[3] From a cultural-historical point of view, conception and pregnancy have been seen as a process that the woman experiences in a special way, in that the process itself is uncontrollable. The naturalness of pregnancy has traditionally implied the woman's passivity, which as an attitude has often ended in the death of the woman and the fetus. The woman's social dependence was and still is significantly related to this attitude. Many cultures compensate for this dependence by idealising the mother role. Given this background, the advent of technology in this natural experience seems to be an act of liberation. In the past, medical technology has basically served to control the birth process and its

burdens. Nevertheless, fifty years ago Horkheimer and Adorno (1969) showed that the technical control of human nature releases a potential that can lead to ever more subtle coercion. Later, Michel Foucault made the same point. Domination of the human body by external forces is not the only concern. Rather, as Foucault describes in *La Historie de la sexualité*, since the late Roman Empire the body has increasingly become an object of self-control, an object of mistrust. In the 20th century, the woman's body is viewed increasingly as an object of technical intervention and public observation (see Duden 1991). In connection with our work, we ask whether women perceive themselves as free from natural forces through the use of technology and whether the traditional, cultural-historical association of 'woman' with 'passivity' and 'nature-bondage' is being reproduced. In the case of intra-cytoplasmatic sperm injection (ICSI), a male weakness has been used as a reason for technological intervention in the female's body. This can be considered not only as a medical intervention, but also as a cultural intervention based on the associations it evokes.

These observations alone are not enough for a moral judgment. I am only interested in pointing out the central theme of how awareness changes. Public discussion and pictures presented by the media are less influential in shaping cultural awareness, regardless of whether they are experienced by one or several women. The mere knowledge of the various technological possibilities for intervening in conception and pregnancy changes the subjective relationship we have to this dimension of human existence. Reaching an ethical evaluation of these aspects is difficult, because such an evaluation must first be worked out hermeneutically. Many such descriptions seem to be speculative. It is also not directly apparent how these changes in dimensions of awareness can be evaluated ethically.

1.2 Ethical problems of pre-implantation genetic diagnosis

The four complexes of problems described above arise when IVF/ET is viewed simply as a technique for treating infertility. The complexities of the relevant aspects increase, however, as soon as the possibilities of *molecular medicine* are considered in relation to IVF. Then questions come up that are beyond the scope of the aforementioned problem complexes. Since pre-implantation genetic diagnosis (PGD) enables genetic diagnosis before the beginning of a pregnancy, it seems to present an important alternative to prenatal diagnosis (PND). Regarding morality, the following points of view seem to be especially relevant.

PGD can increase the couple's ability to decide autonomously. At risk couples can, if they are willing to take on the difficulties of IVF, have a higher degree of security that certain genetic diseases will not be passed on. This increases the number of options. A choice is created that excludes the problems of PND and a possible abortion. At the same time, however, there is a fundamental change in moral points of view in comparison to PND.

The first point of view again concerns the *moral status of the embryo and fetus at different stages of development*. In simplified terms, I presume that in PGD a totipotent cell would be used. This is not the case in certain methods and applications of PGD (see de Wert 1998). How should one evaluate this?[4] If only persons are granted moral relevance, then there is no immediate relevant difference between discarding a fertilised egg and an abortion in an advanced stage of pregnancy. Personal characteristics such as self-consciousness, freedom and the ability to act cannot be inferred in either case. Nor is there any difference in the evaluation of PND and PGD, if we assume that at the time of fertilisation a single zygote becomes entitled to all moral rights. From either ethical position, there is no difference in regard to the moral status of pre-embryos, embryos and fetuses. When weighing up PGD and PND, only the burden on the affected woman is important in the first case. In the second case, weighing up would be unnecessary at all.

1.2.1 The moral status of the embryo in the context of the argument for human rights of Alan Gewirth

There have been several attempts to say that the embryo indirectly deserves moral protection. These attempts refer to the fact that the embryo has the *potential* to develop into a person, or that there is an *identity* or *continuity* between the person and the embryo he or she once was. This leads to different consequences. One side argues that a being who is related to the person through potentiality, identity or continuity should be treated as a person himself. The consequence of this position is that the woman and the embryo/fetus have the same moral status in case of a conflict in the pregnancy. The other side argues that embryos deserve a lower degree of protection because only agents have full moral status. In any case it is not evident how one can argue for the moral status of the embryo without referring to its potential to develop into a person. If the embryo is seen only from the perspective of its actual characteristics, there is no obvious special characteristic that is of specific moral relevance in comparison to the characteristics of other entities. But if the moral importance of the embryo is legitimate only from the perspective of this potentiality, then an entity that has moral relevance only by virtue of its potentiality to become a person has a different moral status to that of an entity that is a person.

D. Beyleveld argues in his paper in this volume against this kind of argumentation. The gradualistic concept I am referring to here does not always involve the argument of proportionality that A. Gewirth uses in his

Reason and Morality (1978, pp. 121ff.). The principle of proportionality means that human rights can be possessed in degrees related to the degree to which the relevant features of agency are realised by a being.[5] Beyleveld is right in arguing that this principle is invalid. A different argument is the principle of potentiality for which K. Steigleder argues. Steigleder shows that embryos and fetuses deserve moral protection, but in a different way from agents. One can show that agency is the constitutional point for morality as such, insofar as only agents can understand moral norms and protect each other. By means of the argument Gewirth presents, one can also show that each agent has a right to the generic features of agency.[6] If that is the case, one has to ask what relevance this argument for a supreme principle of morality has for concrete moral judgments. For that question it is important to understand that agency is an ability that develops and depends on special characteristics of our being as a body. To this extent, agency is internally connected with elements that precede our actual or dispositional abilities to act. And if agency is the central element of morality, as Gewirth has shown, then it is—as K. Steigleder (1998) says— 'morally significant' that the embryo has the potential to develop into an agent. But that moral significance is on a different level and binding in a different way from the rights that are directly derived from the moral principle. A different proposal for an argumentation for the moral status of an embryo/fetus is the argument via the principle of precaution presented by D. Beyleveld. He argues that the supreme principle of morality shows what rights an agent has, but the question is: Who is an agent? About that question we cannot be sure. We have no metaphysical foundation for the existence of another agent. To the extent that we accept the high moral importance of the protection of an agent, we must be careful, if we cannot be sure whether some entity is an agent or not. And thus—Beyleveld argues—the principle of precaution is a reason for us to protect embryos and fetuses. So far Beyleveld. I think that it is correct that the principle of precaution is important for the application of the Gewirthian moral principle, but I cannot see that it is especially relevant for the case in question. Beyleveld only refers to the general metaphysical uncertainty of the existence of another agent. But in that respect, there is no difference between fetuses, animals, and other entities. Beyond the general metaphysical problem we have no evidence for a special uncertainty concerning the agency of an embryo. That means that we must give the same level of protection that we have to give to the embryo to animals, stones, landscapes, computers and bottles of wine as well. Doing that, however, would be a way of showing that the supreme principle of morality is not applicable. The specific status of a human embryo is not to be understood by looking only at its actual capacities. We can only understand it if we see the embryo in the development of the specific features that are so important for being a possessor of the moral rights. I cannot go into detail now. But I think that we can also only understand our various conflicts concerning the use of embryos and fetuses if we make the assumption that these possess moral importance, but of another kind than the moral right of the pregnant woman.

1.2.2 A comparison between prenatal diagnosis and pre-implantation genetic diagnosis

A comparison of PGD and PND shows two major differences. First, in PGD the diagnosis and decision to implant or discard an embryo is carried out on an early embryo or a pre-embryo. At first sight, the gradualistic concept of protecting the embryo seems less of a problem. On the other hand, how can we describe the conflict situation? With PND, a diagnostic technique is offered that is carried out when there is already a pregnancy. This means that the embryo/fetus deserves protection and this conflicts with the right to self-determination of the mother. The woman has the last say because the embryo is a part of her. The partner's responsibility arises from his relationship to her. We can differentiate several viewpoints from which a decision can be made. It is decisive that an abortion can be legitimised only in relation to the pregnant woman. The conjectured condition of the future child is only relevant in as far as the woman anticipates her future life and its associated burdens. Only the conflict between the fact that the embryo deserves protection and the woman's right to self-determination, coupled with the assumption that the rights of an individual who has full moral status outweigh the derived moral status of the embryo, provide a foundation for the moral imperative that leaves the decision to the woman.

With PGD, however, there is no pregnancy, and thus that specific conflict is eliminated. It must be reasoned that the woman and (since couples usually claim the services of PGD) the couple not only have the right to decide against a particular pregnancy, but even more, that they have a positive right to have a child without certain handicaps. However, this reasoning does not establish a right, as opposed to the reasoning leading to a free decision in the case of PND.

The moral evaluation would be different, however, if we could show that the moral status of the early embryo or pre-embryo is significantly different from that of the later embryo. Within the scope of a gradualistic concept concerning the moral status of the embryo, the question would be whether the differentiation of the fertilised cell is at all morally relevant. This reasoning could refer to the consideration that there is no such identity relationship between the pre-embryo and the future person as exists with the embryo and the fetus. An ontological identity is first established after the completion of the differentiation between embryo and placenta, or possible multiple embryos. The completion of identity formation in this context is certainly an important point in the gradualistic concept. However, this break cannot be construed to mean that a person holds rights immediately after it occurs. Despite that, the break is significant. Whether this point is then so significant that there is no moral status before its completion is another question.

Along with these questions, which are connected with the moral status of the embryo, there are a number of fundamental questions that concern the entire area of early genetic diagnosis. What is the legitimate subject of a diagnosis that is coupled with an abortion or the rejection of a pre-embryo? Certainly it can be reasoned that only the woman (and secondly her partner) can be the subject who decides. However, the possible moral perspectives for her decision have not been named. In our context, it is relevant that the decision to subordinate the embryo's protection can be legitimised only by the woman's rights. This could occur if a severe handicap is expected, a handicap that would be a burden for the woman and/or the couple. However, where we draw the limit is of central importance. Since no medical definitions that could help us set limits are available, the question becomes which handicaps can be considered unreasonable. We could reason that each woman must decide for herself. But we have to consider the enormous pressure accompanying such a decision. Not only the individual woman faces pressure. But it is irrefutable that a discussion of which cases should be cases of genetic diagnosis will have consequences for the social recognition of people with the specific disabilities discussed. The social context in which the decision is made is also of vital importance for the ethical discussion. The individual right of the woman is the major reason to substantiate a free decision. At the same time, numerous factors influence the freedom of the decision. At the latest, the question of which cases physicians should recommend for genetic diagnosis is the point where a break occurs. Here the individual decision meets the public discussion about disabilities. It seems obvious that the mere existence of the possibilities of genetic diagnosis changes social awareness and the individual experience of pregnancy. There is, for example, a notorious discrepancy between the number of pregnancies estimated to involve genetic risk and the number of children born with genetically related disabilities. In addition, dealing with genetically disabled children is increasingly becoming a factor in the decision. There is hardly any doubt that these factors are important both socially and ethically. This sketch of the problem area gives rise to the following ethical questions.

1. What is the moral status of the (early) embryo and the fetus?
2. Which interests and rights are involved in the decision-making process and and how should they be weighed up?

3. What is the relationship between the individual decision-making process and the social context, and this from two perspectives:
   a. in relation to the social influences on the woman's decision and
   b. in relation to the effects of the existence of the possibilities of genetic diagnosis on social acceptance of disabilities?
4. Is it possible to make an ethical evaluation of changes that are connected to reproductive medicine and early genetic diagnosis?

2 Moral philosophy and applied ethics

From a moral-philosophical perspective, even my attempt to describe the problem area is biased. I have inserted a number of assumptions into the description. Now we need to elucidate this process in terms of methods and moral philosophy. In addition, alternative ways to tackle the problem must be confronted. I will pursue three topics.

1. Coherence.
2. Moral rights.
3. Social ethics and normative ethics.

2.1. Coherence

I have supposed that moral rights and duties, the moral status of embryos, and moral evaluation can be argued about through reasoning. Up to now, I have mainly pointed out what consequences result from different normative preconditions. Basically, this has been a descriptive and hermeneutical process. We start with a problem that has come up in the discussion and work out normative preconditions that are the basis of the moral judgment expressed. In the next step, we try to describe coherent evaluation possibilities starting from expressly or implicitly assumed moral convictions. Two criteria can be applied to this procedure: the *internal coherency of the moral judgment*, and the *completeness of the problem description*. The meaning of such an inspection is the question that logically follows. Although internal coherence is an essential prerequisite for any ethical reflection, it is obviously neither adequate for grounding a moral standard nor for backing up a recommendation for action. We can try to back up those convictions that are based on moral judgments by extrapolating them from our daily moral convictions. Beauchamp and Childress (1994) introduced their four 'Principles of Biomedical Ethics' in this sense. Using these principles, one ought to be able to structure the lines of argument in a discourse, to comprehend conflicts, and to facilitate medical-ethical argumentation. This approach is so attractive, because it is built on moral convictions present in everyday life. It seems acceptable to anyone doubtful about the possibilities of moral reasoning. Furthermore, it is attractive to those who view moral reasoning as possible, but doubt that a real public consensus about moral fundamentals is possible. John Rawls (1993) advocates looking for an overlapping consensus that is substantiated by differing normative general theories. This is not a substitute for moral-philosophical discourse, but the latter loses its importance in clarifying controversial questions. The theory of Beauchamp and Childress and the 'overlapping consensus' of Rawls appeal to those who are attempting to reach an effective social consensus. There are, however, some basic problems to this approach. The first problem is which point of view should be chosen. The structure of the problem area is based on this perspective. The Beauchamp/Childress approach, for example, was criticised, because the choice of principles and the contents are arbitrary (see Clouser and Gert 1990). As a matter of fact, the details covered in the consensus are obscured rather than clarified by the principles. The principles are really formal compromises that create the impression of unity. Because of the obscurity of the principles and their position in the overall complex of moral argumentation, the problem shifts, with the interpretation and evaluation of the principles becoming the actual task of ethical reflection. This approach reflects only the convictions of individual persons or social groups. Its contribution to the critical clarification of controversial questions is therefore doubtful.

The status of the results of such coherency tests is thus unclear. It is always possible that the basic moral convictions could be false. Obligations cannot be identified using this method. This is even more disturbing when the results of such a consensus are made law and become binding for all members of society. The basis of the obligation has not itself been grounded. The coherency test cannot even substitute for a legitimation of that kind of obligation that is the result of a political dispute, the result of a democratic decision-making process. Political decisions, however, take into account only majority opinions. It is not the task of moral experts to achieve political consent. In politics, there are no moral experts, only representatives of the people. And it is not apparent why there should be departments and institutes for ethicists, ethical research projects or ethical dissertations to achieve this. In this respect, ethicists would be wise to limit themselves to their expert function. Their competence goes only as far as their theoretical claims can be justified. It is not their task to function as a substitute for political decision-making processes.

However, ethics is gaining in political and social importance because of the claim to moral legitimacy made by modern constitutional states. Human dignity, human rights and duties to assist other humans are normative concepts used to ground legitimacy in social discussions. Whoever wants to help infertile couples by means of IVF or to help at risk couples by genetic screening, asserts his or her moral intentions, at least rhetorically. In addition, whoever sees this assistance as a social task claims, implicitly, that there are such things as public duties. These duties justify the use of public funds to develop the corresponding technical aid.

This all means that moral claims are a part of our communication about the responsibilities and aims of medical technology. This is also true when there is a sceptical attitude toward moral claims and when the discussion is limited in terms of morality. Even if the attitude exists that the legitimacy of a technique cannot be judged as binding in each case, there seems to be minimal agreement that these techniques can only be applied after free and informed consent. It is exactly this position of appearing to be the only remaining generally accepted moral conviction in a pluralistic world that gives the notion of informed consent such central importance. How is the demand that informed consent be respected validated? If it is claimed that the right to self-determination legitimises informed consent, then the validity of this right is claimed implicitly. However, if informed consent is viewed simply as a practical instrument to regulate a conflict, its central importance is no longer anchored. After all, there are other means of regulation. It then follows that the general acceptance of informed consent can be shown to exist only as long as the right to self-determination is generally recognised. If that is not the case, then its acceptance cannot be morally required.

Because of the obvious presence of moral arguments in social discourse, it seems reasonable to assume that the task of medical ethics is to examine critically the validity of those arguments. Thereafter, however, medical ethics is not responsible for creating a consensus. Instead, it is limited to exploring the possibilities for argumentation. In limiting itself to these tasks, medical ethics fulfils an important political function, an argumentative function that politics cannot fulfil. Politics, on the other hand, not ethics, is responsible for arriving at a consensus and reaching a compromise. Exactly that which distinguishes politics from ethics, is what gives ethics its political function. If ethics tried to be a pseudo-political institution, an unavoidable problem would arise: not all social groups would be represented. Educational prerequisites would exclude this possibility. Ethics would then become the agent of obscure interest groups.

In order to enter the medical-ethical discussion about the validity of moral judgments in relation to medicine, ethics must have a basic attitude of openness to moral cognitivism. Ethicists must at least consider it possible to validate moral judgments through reasoning. Otherwise the argumentation process has little meaning. Ethics would then lose its function as the theoretical reflection on our moral convictions and experience.

In our context, when ethics tries to question the validity of moral judgments, it is confronted with claims. Like Gewirth, I too would like to talk about 'moral rights' in the sense of 'claim rights'.[7] Rights then mean justified moral claims. Moral claims are very closely related to our problem. In describing the problem, I questioned whether couples have the right to have a child, whether they have the right to a healthy child, and to what extent the embryo and fetus have rights.

If the discussion does away with moral rights, then the problem description would have to replace the word 'rights' with 'interests'. It follows that there would be no conflicts of rights, but only conflicts of interests. Conflicts of interest, though, are not *ipso facto* moral conflicts. A's interests are simply placed beside B's interests. The conflict would first be moral if A's interest was related to B's by demanding that B respect and take into account A's interest, and if A thought that he was entitled to this respect. A's demand would be a moral claim because he maintains that he possesses the corresponding right. Of course, we could choose different terminology, but the question would remain the same.

If we sacrifice the idea of moral (claim-)rights, the demand for an *impartial consideration of interests* suffers on two counts. First, it is not clear why interests should be considered impartially. We cannot conclude this simply from the fact that there are interests. On the other hand, talking about impartial consideration of interests does not provide criteria for deciding which interests deserve consideration and which do not. Therefore, an examination of rights provides a more suitable framework for understanding moral conflicts. At the same time, the status of rights is uncertain. R. Brandt maintains (in a simplified version) that awarding someone a right means, in certain societies, that it is reasonable for that person to be strongly motivated to assert his claim priority in a conflict (see Brandt 1992, p. 187). This view, however, levels the claim to validity, which is connected to the assertion of a right, in comparison with other claims. 'Strong motivation' is also possible in other cases, not just in the case of rights. From a moral perspective, a special priority is accorded to rights, in as far as moral rights have a claim to priority when one's own interests oppose social convention or even the law. The claim to prior consideration alone leads to a corresponding character of duty, simply from the concept of rights.

J. Habermas (1996, p. 222) doubts that rights have a genuine moral nature. Rights in the sense of human rights are, according to Habermas, intrinsically juridical in nature. Human rights have been fought for historically, and in modern constitutional states all citizens have been granted basic rights. When inborn rights are mentioned in classical human rights declarations, it does not mean they have been placed at our disposal by the state. They have been fought for and won throughout history. But which human claims and interests deserve to be granted to each and everyone? Since this is not *ipso facto* clear, human rights themselves give rise to the question of which potential rights should be established as legal norms. We discuss moral rights as soon as questions of legitimisation of human and citizens' rights appear.

By bringing rights into the area of morals, I will in no way challenge the establishment of legal norms. I will, instead, show that the reason for legitimisation lies in the moral realm. Only if it makes sense to talk about moral rights is it at all apparent why reflection on the right to life of an embryo is a question of ethics. If we understand rights only as juridical concepts, the question of ethics arises only in terms of the establishment and interpretation of legal regulations. Then it has little meaning, whether ethicists or general philosophers approve of or deny the right of life to embryos.

The mere discussion about the different claims of moral rights brings up the need for justification. Since a moral right makes a claim that can be critically applied to juridical rulings and conventions, it follows that justification of the moral right cannot originate from referral to existing conventions and laws. Making a moral claim itself refers to the question of which rules and principles can prove its justification. Consequently, when we attempt to understand what makes up a moral conflict, we reason. Applied ethics cannot avoid questions of moral reasoning.

2.3 Social and normative ethics

Up to this point, I have not shown that the process of moral reasoning can be carried out successfully. Neither do I intend to show this. I consider moral reasoning, as presented by A. Gewirth, to be successful, but I will not demonstrate that in this paper. Something else is more important. I wanted to point out the status of the question of moral reasoning within the framework of applied ethics. An ethics of principles, which I support, is often faced with prejudices. It is viewed as empty and formalistic, as *deductive* and insensitive to certain *contexts of action*. It is also seen as incapable of respecting the concreteness of situations of action. None of this is true.

Criticism of Gewirth's position as lacking content and being formalistic is clearly false. The highest moral principle, the Principle of Generic Consistency *(PGC)*,[8] demands respect for the necessary features of agency. Therefore the principle has *ipso facto* content. But it is more important to me to show how reasoning with a moral principle can be brought together with social contexts. In addition, I want to show that its application is not carried out deductively.

In the new ethical discussion, the ethics of principles is compared to a comprehensive *ethics of the good life* (see Krämer 1992). The relationship between these two dimensions can be seen as *competitive* or *complementary*. We can try to interpret all ethical problems by asking how it is possible to lead a good and successful life. Ethical problems then become disputes over what a good life is. This position presents two problems. First, moral obligations cannot be derived from the essential elements of a good life. The mere fact that elements are identified obliges no-one to behave accordingly. Secondly, an ethics of the good life has problems with pluralistic life-styles. It has difficulty recognising that there are different morally acceptable life-styles, because it claims to solve moral conflicts by showing what the elements of binding life-styles are.

If the relationship between normative ethics and the question of the good life is understood as complementary, these problems disappear. The task of normative ethics is to show which moral rights and duties exist. By showing which rights can be justified and which actions are morally allowed or forbidden, a space is opened for actions that are not subject to moral obligations. The area of moral rights is not only anchored, but it is at the same time limited. By a strict moral-philosophical examination of normative claims, an inflationary expansion of moral rights into all areas of human life can be prevented. In this way, an area in which questions about the good life have their place is described. Morality claims primary consideration in shaping human life. But it does not eliminate the need to ask which elements belong to a good life. However, it does take the moralising out of this question.

Now, from the perspective of an ethics of moral rights, it is not necessary to see the relationship between the two areas as one in which normative ethics identifies and protects several basic rights while everything else is morally neutral. An ethics of principles is even more necessarily a social ethics. This is connected to our basic understanding of applied ethics. An ethics of principles can carry out strict moral reasoning only at a general level. But applied ethics does not proceed deductively. There is no deductive relationship between the general moral principle and its application in a concrete context of action. This has far-reaching consequences for our topic. In the problem I described at the beginning, I tried to show that, in regard to morality, the psycho-social stress of IVF, the practice of counselling for PND, and the discussion of the concept of disability relating to possible indications for PND are morally meaningful. Within the framework of an ethics of principles, the task of applied ethics is, first, to give the most comprehensive description possible. Second, it should make judgments on the basis of the moral principles that have been justified.

Gewirth's position gives rise not only to the question of which rights are directly touched upon when this technique is applied. Also important is how effectively it can be guaranteed in the long term that individuals will be aware of their rights, that they are protected in the long term, and that a social climate is created that makes the protection of these rights possible. This formulation is relatively vague. The vagueness, however, results from the fact that the application of moral principles to concrete situations means that only a few actions look directly moral or immoral. As soon as one is faced with the complex connections of a modern society, the social-ethical dimension of the protection of moral rights gives rise to such high complexity and depends on so many factors that applied ethics becomes a difficult business. The more complex relations are, the more prerequisites for validity arise in any one concrete case. In applied ethics as in social ethics, we are concerned with understanding the social context and effects of new medical techniques, as well as judging them on the basis of what is moral-philosophically provable. The validity of the concrete moral judgment depends on two factors. Firstly, it depends on how well and how thoroughly the connections of the situation of action are described, and secondly, on the success of the moral-philosophical reasoning.

The connection between normative ethics and social ethics is conceived in a completely different manner in many liberal concepts of ethics. From the *liberal point of view*, only those actions are morally dubious or forbidden that directly threaten the freedom of another. This genuinely moral dimension is understood as an area in which only categorical arguments count. If this is not the case, only practical or social-political problems arise. If the moral area is understood in this sense, a connection to social ethics is not possible.

The question of moral reasoning is also relevant to which dimensions can play a role in moral evaluation at all. From a liberal point of view, the social conditions for the use of IVF and molecular medicine are the subject of ethical reflection only in a limited form. From my own reflection, it is exactly the degree of generality in moral reasoning that makes it necessary to connect it with a comprehensive understanding of the concrete context. Normative ethics, therefore, unavoidably becomes social ethics. From this conception of the relationship between moral reasoning and social ethics it becomes evident that it is important whether the technical possibilities of reproductive medicine and molecular medicine influence the subjective awareness and experience of pregnancy. However, moral relevance must necessarily be less precisely formulated as the direct application of the moral principle of the rights of individuals.

3 Final remarks

I have tried to describe the problem area of our network and to point out ways of approaching moral evaluation. In doing so, it was important for me to show that in all approaches to ethical evaluation in applied ethics, prerequisites pertaining to the task of ethics are laid down that are based on fundamental concepts of moral philosophy. Applied ethics and bioethics cannot bypass questions of moral reasoning. At best, they can presuppose that it is impossible to solve questions of moral reasoning rationally. Then the necessary consequences should be drawn and no more attempts to claim the existence of moral obligations should be made. But then no claims can be made for self-determination, there can be no duty to help, and no demand for informed consent as a moral demand. I suspect that moral conflicts could not even be described.

The anchoring of moral principles must once again refer to the complex process of application in a society where the different contexts of action are difficult to understand. A simpler path for clarifying moral conflicts would only be possible if we refused to recognise this complexity. However, it would certainly not be the best path.

Notes

[1] Concerning the moral implications of IVF/ET, see Hildt and Mieth 1998.

[2] The relation between positive and negative rights is explained in Gewirth 1996, pp. 31–70.

[3] In the papers of Regine Kollek and Jean-Pierre Wils in this volume you will find some examples.

[4] For the new German debate concerning the moral status of the embryo see Rager 1996; Kaminsky 1998; Engels 1998; Junker-Kenny 1998; Düwell 1999; and Steigleder 1999.

[5] Some critical remarks are to be found in Hill 1984.

[6] For a short overview of the argument, see the paper by Beyleveld in this volume.

[7] Representing this position are Gewirth 1978 and 1996; Beyleveld 1991; and Steigleder 1999. On the concept of moral rights, see also Hohfeld 1964; and Almond 1991.

[8] 'Act in accord with the generic rights of your recipients as well as of yourself' (Gewirth 1978, p. 135).

References

Almond, B. (1991), 'Rights', in Singer, P. (ed.), *A Companion to Ethics*, Blackwell: Oxford, pp. 259–269.

Beauchamp, T. L. and Childress, J. F. (1994), *Principles of Biomedical Ethics*, Oxford University Press: New York and Oxford.

Beyleveld, D. (1991), *The Dialectical Necessity of Morality: An Analysis and Defense of Alan Gewirth's Argument to the Principle of Generic Consistency*, Chicago University Press: Chicago.

Brandt, R. (1992), 'The Concept of Moral Rights and Its Function', in Brandt, R., *Utilitarianism and Rights*, Cambridge University Press: Cambridge.

Clouser, K. D. and Gert, B. (1990), 'A Critique of Principlism', *Journal of Medicine and Philosophy,* Vol. 15, pp. 219–236.

De Wert, G. (1998), 'Dynamik und Ethik der genetischen Präimplantations-diagnostik—Eine Erkundung', in Düwell, M. and Mieth, D. (eds), *Ethik in der Humangenetik: Die neueren Entwicklungen der genetischen Frühdiagnostik aus ethischer Perspektive*, Francke: Tübingen, pp. 327–357.

Duden, B. (1991), *Der Frauenleib als öffentlicher Ort. Vom Mißbrauch des Begriffs Leben*, Fischer: München.

Düwell, M. (1999), 'Präimplantationsdiagnostik—eine Möglichkeit genetischer Frühdiagnostik aus ethischer Perspektive', in Düwell, M. and Mieth, D. (eds), Von der Prädiktiven zur Präventiven Medizin—Ethische Aspekte der Präimplantationsdiagnostik. *Ethik in der Medizin,* Band 11, Supplement 1, pp. 4–15.

Engels, E.-M. (1998), 'Der moralische Status von Embryonen und Feten—Forschung, Diagnose, Schwangerschaftsabbruch', in Düwell and M., Mieth, D. (eds), *Ethik in der Humangenetik. Die neueren Entwicklungen der genetischen Frühdiagnostik aus ethischer Perspektive*, Francke: Tübingen, pp. 271–301.

Gewirth, A. (1978), *Reason and Morality*, Chicago University Press: Chicago.

Gewirth, A. (1996), *The Community of Rights*, Chicago University Press: Chicago.

Habermas, J. (1996), *Die Einbeziehung des Anderen: Studien zur politischen Philosophie*, Suhrkamp: Frankfurt a. Main

Hildt, E. and Mieth, D. (1998) (eds.), *In Vitro Fertilisation in the 1990s: Towards a Medical, Social and Ethical Evaluation*, Ashgate: Aldershot.

Hill, J. F. (1984), 'Are Marginal Agents "Our Recipients"?', in Regis Jr., E. (ed.), *Gewirth's Ethical Rationalism: Critical Essays with a Reply by Alan Gewirth*, Chicago University Press: Chicago, pp. 180–191.

Hohfeld, W. N. (1964), *Fundamental Legal Conceptions*, Yale University Press: London and New Haven.

Horkheimer, M. and Adorno, Th. W. (1969), *Dialektik der Aufklärung. Philosophische Fragmente*, Suhrkamp: Frankfurt a. Main.

Junker-Kenny, M. (1998), 'Der moralische Status des Embryos im Kontext der Reproduktionsmedizin', in Düwell, M. and Mieth, D. (eds), *Ethik in der Humangenetik: Die neueren Entwicklungen der genetischen Frühdiagnostik aus ethischer Perspektive*, Francke: Tübingen, pp. 302–324.

Kaminsky, C. (1998), *Embryonen, Ethik und Verantwortung: Eine kritische Analyse der Statusdiskussion als Problemlsungsansatz angewandter Ethik*, Mohr Siebeck: Tübingen.

Knoepffler, N. (1999), *Forschung an menschlichen Embryonen: Was ist verantwortbar?* Hirzel: Stuttgart/Leipzig.

Krämer, H. (1992), *Integrative Ethik*, Suhrkamp: Frankfurt a. Main.

Rager, G. (1996), 'Embryo—Mensch—Person: Zur Frage nach dem Beginn des personalen Lebens', in Beckmann, J.P. (ed.), *Fragen und Probleme einer medizinischen Ethik*, de Gruyter: Berlin/New York, pp. 254–278.

Rawls, J. (1993), *Political Liberalism*, Columbia University Press: New York.

Steigleder, K. (1998), 'The Moral Status of Potential Persons', in Hildt, E. and Mieth, D. (eds), *In Vitro Fertilisation in the 1990s: Towards a Medical, Social and Ethical Evaluation*, Ashgate: Aldershot, pp. 239–246.

Steigleder, K. (1999), *Grundlegung der normativen Ethik. Der Ansatz von Alan Gewirth*, Alber: Freiburg i.Br./München.

Comment: *Ethics, normativity and hermeneutics*

Paul J. M. van Tongeren

The very interesting paper by Marcus Düwell consists of two parts. In the first part, the author gives a description of the problem area, or even areas in the plural. He makes some fine distinctions between different questions, and in particular gives a clear presentation of the interrelatedness of these questions—and thus of the complexities of the problems under discussion.

In the second part of his paper, Düwell pleads for a specific kind of moral reasoning in applied ethics. With this he distances himself from at least two other positions: first from a purely descriptive ethics, which would not be practical enough, and secondly from a political pragmatic decisionism, which—I presume—could be called too practical.

The specific kind of moral reasoning he pleads for is conceived as the validation or justification of normative positions by way of a theoretical founding of them and of their presuppositions. Moral judgments are conceived of as being judgments about moral claims, and moral claims are claims that should be explained and justified in terms of moral rights and duties.

If I summarise it in this way, we still do not know what 'moral' means, or what makes judgments, claims, rights and duties into moral ones. There might be an answer to this in Düwell's paper, but one that is—in my opinion—problematic. I will come back to this at the end of my comment.

So, to resume and conclude this very brief summary: the first part of the paper is descriptive and preparatory, and this part is called 'hermeneutical'. The second part of the paper could be characterised as being 'meta-ethical' insofar as it discusses the terminology and methodology of a normative and applied ethics. So we have to some extent a hermeneutical and meta-ethical paper in which a plea is made for a normative ethics. The normative ethics advocated is, furthermore, taken in a rather narrow sense, i.e., it is conceived as a theory of norms and principles and their theoretical justification. I call this a rather narrow conception because I think that there is more normative ethics than just the theoretical foundation of norms, that even a hermeneutical ethics can have normative force, and thus that normativity should not be reduced to the validation of norms. I will

201

come back to this point as well, since my comments and questions will all be related to Düwell's conception of normative ethics. I will raise three questions or points of comment, the last being the most elaborated and critical.

1. The final part of Marcus Düwell's paper is about the relation between normative ethics and social ethics and about the status and role of normative ethics in applied ethics. Applied ethics is—according to Düwell—the application of normative ethics to a specific area, by means of the interpretation of the meaning of the justified norms for the relevant situation and conditions. We are warned that this application is not just a matter of simple deduction, but rather a matter of explanation, translation and interpretation. I would say that the best term to summarise this explanation, translation and interpretation is 'hermeneutics'. It might be relevant to be reminded of the fact that Gadamer (1975, pp. 290ff.) stresses precisely the *'subtilitas applicandi'* as being central to his conception of hermeneutics.

2. Secondly, if one does agree with this account and interpretation of Düwell's paper, i.e., if applied ethics should be acknowledged as being hermeneutical as well, I wonder whether this should not have serious consequences for the theory that was situated between the hermeneutical first part, and the applied and as such hermeneutical last part, i.e., for the normative ethics itself! For, at least from a hermeneutical perspective, it will be difficult to explain how this normative ethical theory in which moral rights are established and justified, and which is embedded in a hermeneutical framework, could possibly not be hermeneutical itself. Let me—briefly—explain what I mean: I interpreted Düwell's 'social ethics' as the interpretation of norms (rights, duties, principles), i.e., as the establishment of their meaning in terms of the given historical and cultural situation. Well, if such an interpretation is necessary in order to find out what those norms (etc.) mean, then what could a theory be that abstracts away from the historical and cultural situation and conditions? To put it differently, should we not acknowledge that as soon as we concentrate on the meaning of the concepts used in any theory, we are unavoidably drawn into the hermeneutical dialogue, or even into the conflict of interpretations (I refer to the contribution of Jean-Pierre Wils in this same volume). If we want to understand what we mean by what we say, we cannot avoid the hermeneutical arena, even if according to some people this is a swamp.

3. My third and final question (but there might be a few final questions) regards Marcus Düwell's interpretation of morality in terms of justified claims, or even his identification of morality with justified claims that certain interests be respected; i.e., with rights (and their corresponding duties).

This implies at least two characteristics. First, morality is in this conception only something between people (or—if you want—between

202

such beings that have rights); i.e., it is a social thing. And secondly, morality has to do with obligations and prescriptions, obligations and prescriptions that seem to be extremely binding, they overrule other preferences or inclinations and oblige one to obey them.

In the first place, I have the impression that this conception of morality looks very much like the narrow liberal one, from which Düwell says he wants to distance himself. Both seem to restrict morality to what interferes with the freedom of the other or the justified claims for respect that people have on one another. And both seem to speak in categorical terms.

In the second place, I cannot help being reminded, especially by this last characteristic, this identification of morality with obedience to categorical principles, of what Nietzsche writes about Kant: 'Kant . . . suggest[s] with [his] morality: "what deserves respect in me is that I can obey—and you *ought* not to be different from me"' (1966, p. 187). In another of his writings, Nietzsche points to this same feature as one that is characteristic for the Germans. If I quote from this text as well, it is on the condition that the reader (and certainly Dr. Düwell) accepts that I do not mean this as an argument *ad hominem.* I mean I would not dare to quote the beginning of this second text if it were to be taken as meant in a personal sense. The text begins like this: 'A German is capable of great things, but it is improbable he will do them: for, as befits a sluggish spirit, he obeys whenever he can' (Nietzsche 1982, p. 207). I do want to quote some more from this text, because here Nietzsche suggests a contrast between the Germans and the Greeks, with which he indicates another conception of morality.

> Now, if a nation of this sort [he has listed various characteristics of the Germans] concerns itself with morality, what morality will it be that will satisfy it? The first thing it will certainly require is that in this morality its heartfelt inclination to obedience shall appear idealised. 'Man has to have something which he can *obey unconditionally*'—that is a German sensation, a German piece of consistency: it is to be encountered at the basis of all German moral teaching. [And then follows the other conception:] How different an impression we receive from the whole morality of antiquity! All those Greek thinkers, however varied they may appear to us as individuals, seem as moralists like a gymnastics teacher who says to his pupil: 'Come! follow me! Submit to my discipline! Then perhaps you will succeed in carrying off a prize before all Hellenes'. Personal distinction—that is antique virtue. (Ibid.)

Is not a conception of morality that excludes this kind of virtue too narrow? And does not Marcus Düwell exclude it from morality where he at least suggests that morality should be restricted to the area of moral rights and duties, in order—as he puts it—'not to eliminate the need to ask which elements belong to a good life, however, [to] take the moralising out of this question'?! Would it not be more adequate to acknowledge the moral significance of other appeals than only those that can legitimately be posited as obligatory for everyone, or than only those that concern justified respect for the interests of others?

I think this is also—and even especially—true in the framework of our problem-area concerning new technologies for human procreation and related issues. It is precisely morally relevant that we concentrate on questions like these: What do we make out of ourselves? How do we realise ourselves in the way we deal with our own lives, our own bodies, our own preferences, inclinations, etc., in the way we use technology or let technology take over? How do we deal with chance occurrences, for example, or how do we make ourselves more or less skilled and ready to deal with such occurrences?

What exactly is the point in—as Marcus Düwell advocates—taking moralising out of these questions? Is what he suggests not begging the question? For moralising about these questions would only be dangerous if it meant phrasing them in terms of (universal) rights and duties. But it is—in my opinion—this restrictive interpretation of morality that is the problem, as it prevents the acknowledgement of the moral significance of these and many other aspects of our lives.

References

Gadamer, H.-G. (1975), *Wahrheit und Methode: Grundzüge einer philosophischen Hermeneutik*, Mohr: Tübingen.

Nietzsche, Friedrich (1966), *Beyond Good and Evil: Prelude to a Philosophy of the Future* (translated by W. Kaufmann), Vintage: New York.

Nietzsche, Friedrich (1982), *Daybreak: Thoughts on the Prejudices of Morality* (translated by R. J. Molligdale), Cambridge University Press: Cambridge.

Comment: *Moral experience and rationality*

Roberto Mordacci

1. It is certainly a good strategy to consider the moral questions posed by reproductive medicine and molecular genetics together. No doubt, the issues surrounding artificial procreation are exacerbated by such techniques as PGD and in general by the possibility of studying and modifying the DNA of human embryos in the earliest phases of their development. An increasing number of opportunities for observation and intervention surround fertilised human eggs nowadays and the interests of several persons are involved in the evaluation of what should and could be done with them.

It is nevertheless true that posing such questions exclusively in terms of interests already introduces a prejudice into their possible solutions. It is assumed, for example, that interests describe the basic elements of moral reasoning and that, consequently, any application of practical reason will be, fundamentally, a weighing of those interests against each other. This approach limits rather severely the range of solutions that can be achieved: for example, it is hardly plausible, within such a perspective, to argue for the inviolability of one special interest over the others, because a mass of critical interests (of different individuals or even within the same subject) will probably always outweigh any particular interest of a single individual (or a single personal interest confronted with a number of others). Therefore, there will be only *prima facie* interests, and particular interests will always rank lower than the sum of many individual interests together. This is how a certain kind of utilitarianism tries to make sense of its account of ethical life, that is, by expressing its basic elements in terms that predetermine both the description of morality and the available forms of moral reasoning, moral norms and moral solutions. But is the basic assumption really granted? Do we really need to pose moral questions in the area of reproductive and molecular medicine in terms of interests? In other words, is the utilitarian/consequentialist conception of practical reason true or at least necessary?

The first thing we may say is that such a picture of moral reasoning seems too simple to reflect the complexities of ethical life: the discussion about the possibility of altruism by such different authors as Thomas Nagel (1970) and Bernard Williams (1973) has shown, if anything, that the image of a completely egoist agent is the description of an unbearable ethical life, and that the inherent structure of agency implies a reference to the interests of the others such that rational action requires a step (whether a Kantian or a Humean one does not matter here) beyond the self towards the other. And any picture of moral life exclusively in terms of interests is inevitably too self-centred for that.

Second, as Marcus Düwell rightly observes, such a way of conceiving moral reasoning does not recognise the difference between the dynamics of practical reason and the process of political deliberation: in fact, while consensus among the interested parties is the foundation of legitimacy, ethical consistency is a complex issue in which reason plays a fundamental role and consensus is not the basis but the hoped for result of sound argument. The assignment of a merely political role to ethical argumentation is only one of the consequences of taking an impersonal point on view on moral life, as if an ethical problem was a matter of conflict between completely determined sets of individual interests, constituted and defined before meeting others. According to this perspective, morality looks like the attempt to reconcile projects that are defined in advance as completely non-related to each other and therefore basically hostile to each other.[1] Furthermore, the place of such a meeting is the public arena, so that 'public ethics' is viewed as a necessary resource for making it possible for opposing views to live together. But what if we consider an individual who is in his formative years and who is looking for a confrontation on what *really* matters, who wants to be helped in giving a *form* (a kind of coherence, if you like) to his interests and desires, and is given instead, by so-called 'ethics', nothing more than a set of procedural rules, e.g., that one should not violate the privacy of others with inappropriate questions?

2. The typical and quite justified strategy at this point, against the limits of consequentialism, is to try to show that moral conflicts are better represented in terms of rights (and, correspondingly, of duties) than in terms of interests, and that moral problems are to be solved by trying to find the strongest obligation or the most inviolable right, or an acceptable (reflective) equilibrium between minor infringements of various duties and rights. We do have some preconceptions concerning what should and should not be done, and the scope of moral reasoning is intended to define a hierarchy of duties or at least a framework of inalienable rights for any rational agent. The result of such work is supposed to achieve *theoretical* consistency between moral beliefs and considered judgments and *pragmatic* consistency between principles and actions.

Justified moral claims are therefore, in the perspective suggested by Gewirth (1978), prior to any convention and laws and have to be argued for on the basis of a general principle of reason (what Gewirth calls the 'Principle of General Consistency') concerning respect for every rational agent and essential goods needed to act. Social ethics is the result of many forces, but moral reasoning itself is among them and, as far as ethics is concerned, rational considerations are able to show, at least, that one or more policies, for example, are not consistent either with the principles that pretend to have generated them or with other fundamental principles based on rights. We may say that, in this perspective, moral rationality can at least show where and when the claim of consistency is not met by individuals or societies in their norms or their practices. This is not irrelevant, if we consider that a genuine moral conflict arises where each proposed path pretends to be justified in its claims (otherwise, we do not have a conflict but only different and often quite compatible moral options): a perspective based on the analysis of rational action in terms of conformity to a general principle will suggest that if our present moral convictions lead us to contradictory behaviour or inconsistent thought, we'd better reform our moral system or the theory that we claim justifies our deliberative processes. This may have revolutionary implications for both individual and social life, and in this case it is not just a matter of comparing the consequences of action but, so to say, of guaranteeing the conditions that make human rational action itself possible.

Granted all this, such a perspective still has to face a more radical set of objections, those suggested, for example, by the arguments proposed by Bernard Williams[2] and others against the very idea of a moral theory.[3] The basic objection is that ethical consistency is not the same thing as logical consistency, and that therefore ethical life is not measured in the degree of logic it deploys, because it is far more complex than any reasoning could ever succeed in justifying adequately. Moral experience is made up of desires, thoughts and emotions that cannot be explained nor taken into account in a theory-like approach. This means that the reasons for action do not always or necessarily lie in the realm of moral theory or morality, especially if these are conceived as basically centred on duties and obligations. There are a number of considerations that are important for an individual and a social ethical life and that cannot be described in terms of rights or obligations; nonetheless, such aspects as emotions (e.g., shame, guilt, regret), luck, motivations, unexpected negative outcomes of previous well-intentioned actions, dispositions of the body and psychological reactions in the circumstance are ineluctably parts of an individual's life, which condition his perception of his and the others' life and therefore of the situation as a whole.

It is not that the system of morality or the language of obligation is flawed or systematically wrong; it is rather that the perspective of a whole life (in order to try to live an overall good life) requires us not to overlook what the agent has actually gone through, his personal history, because it is this that determines the moral tone of his actions, which cannot be judged too abstractly. This should give a less dramatic role to formal arguments and in particular to morality as a framework of rules of thought and principles of action. On the other hand, this should not lead, as with Williams, to a sceptical position in ethics, such that truth (e.g., the truth of a connection between a principle and its consequences) does not matter to ethics; the awareness of the limits of formal rationality should make us realise that any reduction to principles leaves a part of the actual lives of persons outside the moral picture. These lives nonetheless are wholes that cannot simply erase from a final view of themselves (a view that must, if any view can, be called a *moral* view)—all that is not comprised in the language of rights and obligations.

3. A more precise critique of the picture of moral reasoning suggested by Düwell, and developed by Beyleveld and Gewirth, might take the approach of a defence of certain implications of the perspective of a good life, that is, of the point of view of an Aristotelian ethic (in a rather loose sense), based more on the notions of virtues and character, rather than on the rightness of actions *per se*. This should not be understood just as the choice of a field in the debate. Aristotelian ethics has its own faults and shortcomings, and some of them have been indicated by Düwell himself: the difficulty of determining the essential features of a good life and the consequent problem of pluralism. To this, one might argue that it might be possible to sketch out the essential features that *any* form of a good life cannot do without (rather than doing more or less the same regarding the essential features of action), so that we can reach a point of view from which some forms of life just cannot be good for *any* human being; having said this, we might as well agree that all the rest is freedom.

The real problem is rather that of the foundations of ethics, and in particular the connection between a plausible description of a specifically human form of life (and therefore of some traits suggesting a vague idea of what we mean by 'human nature' or just 'human') and normative ethics. The question of social ethics and its relation to normative ethics goes a step farther. Issues concerning human nature, or the notion of person or human dignity, are obviously fundamental in applied as well as in general ethics, as is also witnessed by the fact that the vexed question of the status of the human embryo is at the top of the list of the issues surrounding artificial procreation and molecular medicine. This is at the same time a moral and an ontological question, and it is very difficult to distinguish rigidly between descriptive and normative aspects of it. I will not pursue that question any further here, but it is clear that some kind of (implicit or explicit) theory describing the central features of a distinctively human life is connected with both the question of how to treat human embryos and the foundations of norms, rights, duties, and even interests. What happens quite often is that an implicit image of humanity underlies many ethical theories, which therefore do not provide an adequate foundation for their basic principles (such an objection concerns some forms of utilitarianism and liberalism or rights-based ethics as well). It is obvious that the picture sketched by Düwell cannot just be charged with incompleteness (any theoretical proposal can), if anything, for reasons of space. What I would like to do is rather to suggest a different perspective on ethics, so that these problems can be faced on a different battlefield.

4. Rights-based ethics traces a distinction between normative and social ethics. The first deals with those concepts that form the basic elements of ethical argumentation such as moral rights, fundamental duties, human dignity and so on; such a level of discourse grounds the legitimacy of acts, and ethical consistency is defined as consistency between justified principles and choices, or as consistency between justified claims/rights and actions. The context of actions, the texture of social, historical and personal commitments and expectations is to be completely described in order to formulate an appropriate judgment in applied ethics, but this is rather a complement to ethical argumentation than a formative part of it; the context does not substantiate the normative force of deliberation, but rather has the role of giving content to the rather formal and abstract principles to which the argument appeals. Using a different terminology, we may say that the first part covers what may be called 'morality' in the sense of a structured framework of obligations and rights,[4] while the second should serve as a more complete description of ethical life, integrated with all the elements of the social and historical context. What remains unclear is what normative role, if any, ethical life has when confronted with the requirements of morality; if, for example, the complexities of a particular situation for a particular subject seem to give an acceptable meaning to the infringement of a particular obligation, would this infringement be acceptable as *moral* behaviour? Would it count simply as a fault or would it receive a coherent sense in the light of the life of that person?

One may say that the perspective of rights seems protected against such an objection. Rights, and especially basic ones (and in particular so-called negative rights), are different from duties in the sense that they seem to raise a protective wall around the subject rather than asking him to perform certain actions. In this sense, it seems easier to claim that there are inviolable rights that no whole-life perspective can allow to be violated even in a single instance in a lifetime.[5] But it is a commonly shared opinion (and an easily justifiable one) that there is a systematic correlation between duties and rights such that any right of a person raises a claim towards an other subject, thus generating a corresponding duty. Thus, at least in the case of duties to others (but, I would argue, also in the case of duties to oneself), the main thesis of the existence of basic rights stands together with its implications for duties, and there seem to be good reasons for recognising that especially stringent obligations exist, such as those connected with fundamental rights, so that it is hardly possible to imagine a situation justifying their infringement. So far, some (but very few) rights may be basic for elaborating a morality that would have to be, more or less, a common shared feature of any conception of the good life.

The point is rather how to give proper justification to such a claim of reason to establish the foundation of morality; this is undoubtedly connected with the inquiry concerning human nature, and the main issue here is whether we should consider, in a comprehensive picture of it, not only transcendental traits (the Kantian route) but also empirical ones (the Humean route), and how many or which ones of the latter. I cannot pursue that task here, but it might be suggested that a conception of ethics enabled to take these aspects into account should not be limited to the consideration of the rightness of acts, but should rather be concerned with the *meanings* conveyed by certain kinds of acts, so that the historical situation of the subject comes into the picture; to give just a hint, this is essentially a hermeneutical task. As a concluding remark, I will try to illustrate this point very briefly.

5. If we take as one of the aims of ethical inquiry (even in applied ethics) the attempt to give foundation and content to the idea of ethical life (or the good life), moral rights seem to come one step too late, because they seem to be based on a fixed knowledge of human nature. This may be inevitable and even correct; but it seems that our description is reductive if we reduce humanity to the traits coverable by rights and duties, and ethical life to the protection of rights and the compliance with obligations. What does ethical life look like if the only things we see are possible violations of basic rights or infringements of fundamental principles or duties? Does it not look like something rather unattractive, where the relationship between human beings has an unbearably defensive tone? Is not this a *legal* image of humanity? What we expect from ethics is not only (or not even fundamentally) protection: that we expect from law.[6] We expect ethics to help us discover what is worth being pursued for me, as a human being and as the particular human being that I am. We would like to be helped to see what would make more sense, what would make our actions meaningful and

coherent with what we desire most (and not abstractly consistent with some general principles), and what would enable us to express meanings in our gestures that convey a content for a communicable meaningful life even in the presence of misfortune or disabilities. Here comes the point made by good life ethics: human life needs to make sense (and *therefore* to be good) rather than be simply protected. It is of course true that protection and mutual respect are prerequisites for any possible sense, but that is not the whole story and probably not what we most care about.

Rights-based ethics can of course concede that our description of ethical life must be more complete than is allowed for by rights and duties alone. But if the language of normative ethics is made up only of duties and rights, could we ever *see* anything else in ethical life? How can we describe what rights cannot see and, what is more important, how can we understand its normative force? For example, how could we take into account emotions like guilt, regret and shame, and most of all expressive actions, which convey a vague, rather fuzzy but in the end not empty notion of what a good life might look like? So, our description of ethical life and of moral experience, to be decently complete, must probably start again from the beginning and ask which meanings certain actions, gestures and practices have for us (now, here); and rights, in their turn, might be thought of as one way to protect the possibility that a human life can have a meaning (not just to protect an individual entity as such empty of meaning) or even to prevent certain kinds of meanings (racism, violence, cruelty, irresponsibility, etc.) from fixing their hold on a particular life.

Notes

[1] Needless to say, such an implicit picture of human life is basically derived from Hobbes, whose influence on modern moral philosophy is never stressed enough.

[2] See especially Williams 1965. For the critique of morality and moral theory see Williams 1985.

[3] For a reconstruction of this debate and a pro-theory perspective see Louden 1992.

[4] This is the usage adopted mainly by Williams, especially in Williams 1985. It is used here only as a convenient expression to indicate a particular conception of the moral life, but Williams' usage is not really justified, in that it does not cover the common usage of the term.

[5] Would this be really different from the attempt to sketch out the basic features of any form of the good life? Although methodologically very similar, such an attempt would be different from the appeal to the principles governing rational action because it would need to take into account more fully the personal,

historical and emotional aspects of a whole life rather than the formal structure of action *per se*.

6   I suspect modernity draws this approach from a rather Hobbesian perspective on human life and, therefore, on ethics itself.

References

Gewirth, A. (1978), *Reason and Morality*, University of Chicago Press: Chicago.

Louden, R. B. (1992), *Morality and Moral Theory: A Reappraisal and Reaffirmation*, Oxford University Press: New York.

Nagel, T. (1970), *The Possibility of Altruism*, Clarendon Press: Oxford.

Williams, B. (1973), *Problems of the Self*, Cambridge University Press: Cambridge.

Williams, B. (1985), *Ethics and the Limits of Philosophy*, Cambridge University Press: Cambridge.

Part Six

LEGAL REGULATION OF ASSISTED PROCREATION, GENETIC DIAGNOSIS AND GENE THERAPY

Legal regulation of assisted procreation, genetic diagnosis and gene therapy

Deryck Beyleveld and Shaun Pattinson[1]

This report describes the legal regulation of assisted reproduction, genetic diagnosis, and gene therapy within the countries of the EU, and presents a framework for classifying the moral and philosophical issues. It has two parts.

In the first part, we describe the regulation of assisted reproduction, embryo research, cloning, germ-line gene therapy, pre-implantation genetic diagnosis (PGD), and prenatal diagnosis (PND) and abortion. Where legislation exists, it typically prohibits reproductive cloning and germ-line gene therapy, either prohibits non-therapeutic embryo research or subjects it to conditions (such as a 14 day cut-off point), permits abortion and PND, and regulates those assisted reproductive techniques that involve the storage or use of embryos outside the body. However, there is far less convergence on issues such as the permissibility of PGD, and the use of medically assisted reproduction by single women and homosexual couples.

In the second part, we outline a framework for understanding the moral and philosophical issues raised by these regulatory approaches. This framework classifies positions according to the level of non-derivative or intrinsic moral status granted to the embryo or fetus (hereafter embryo-fetus), and the ground offered for this level of intrinsic moral status, thereby highlighting the extent of dissensus in this area.

We conclude by selecting a number of issues that could usefully be addressed by future research.

1 Eligibility criteria for access to assisted reproduction

Table 1

Country	Legislation	Legislative Criteria	Eligibility	Techniques Subject to the Eligibility Criteria
Austria	Act No. 275 of 1 July 1992.[2]	Must be a married couple or stable heterosexual cohabitee, and be deemed able to provide a satisfactory home for the child (s. 2(1)).[3] All other treatments for infertility must have proved unsuccessful or be considered hopeless.[4]		Artificial insemination, IVF, GIFT, & embryo transfer.[5]
Belgium	None.[6]	Not applicable (hereafter N/A). In practice, assisted reproduction is available for single and lesbian women at more than five Flemish centres.[7]		N/A. No information on the techniques that are subject to eligibility criteria in practice.
Denmark	Law No. 499 of 12 June 1996 on Biomedical Research. Law No. 460 of 1997 on Medically Assisted Reproduction.[8]	None.[9] In practice, treatment is restricted to women who are (a) married or have been cohabiting for 3 years;[10] (b) under 37 years at the time of entry onto the waiting list; (c) without children; &		Artificial insemination, IVF, and directly related techniques.[11] There are a few provisions in relation to practitioners concerning information and consent with regard to assisted reproduction

216

		(d) have a medical need for treatment.	generally (ss. 23 & 24 Law No. 460).[12] These provisions are not concerned with eligibility as such.
Finland	None.[13]	N/A.	N/A.
	Proposed legislation exists.[14]	The proposed legislation restricts access to couples who are married or cohabiting, who are involuntarily childless or whose offspring are likely to inherit a serious disease. Also, the woman must be under 50 years old.[15]	The proposed legislation covers artificial insemination, IVF, and related techniques.[17]
		In practice, assisted reproduction is, at present, only offered to married couples and heterosexual cohabitees.[16]	No information on the techniques that are subject to eligibility criteria in practice.
France	Law 94-654 of 29 July 1994.[18]	Must be (a) a couple consisting of a man and a woman; (b) alive, i.e., posthumous insemination is prohibited; (c) married or able to prove at least 2 years cohabitation; and (d) of reproductive age (Art. L-152-2).[19] Treatment is only to be provided to alleviate infertility or to avoid the transmission of a par-	(a) Clinical & biological practices for IVF; (b) transfer of embryos; (c) artificial insemination; and (d) all techniques having similar results that use assisted reproduction outside of the natural process (Art. L-151-1).[21]

		ticularly serious disease (Art. 8).[20]	
Germany	Embryo Protection Act 1990.	None.	Any technique involving the *in vitro* production or use of an embryo (s. 1).
	IVF is also covered by guidelines of the Federal Physicians' Chamber.[22]	The legislation is supplemented by guidelines of the Federal Physicians' Chamber, which require physicians to ensure that the couple are in a stable relationship. These guidelines state that, in principle, access should be restricted to married couples. A specific committee has the power to consider the case of unmarried persons. So, in practice, assisted reproduction is typically offered to married couples only.[23]	
Greece	No specific legislation.	N/A.	N/A.
	However, s. 59 of Law 2071 of July 1992 provides for a presidential decree that will regulate the establishment and function of units for artificial fertilisation. This decree has not yet been issued.[24]	In practice, assisted reproduction is only offered to married couples and heterosexual cohabitees.[25]	No information on the eligibility criteria that are used in practice.

Ireland	None.[26]	N/A.	N/A.
	Assisted reproduction is carried out under guidelines of the Medical Council.[27]	Under the guidelines, IVF may only take place with married couples.[28]	No information on the eligibility criteria that are used in practice.
Italy	None.[29]	N/A.	N/A.
		Code of Medical Deontology 1995 (which provides guidance for physicians) prohibits insemination outside stable heterosexual couples, after the death of one of the partners, and for elderly women, and prohibits any form of surrogacy.[31] Also, under the Code, IVF is only available where there is a medical need for treatment.[32]	The techniques covered by the proposed legislation include IVF, artificial insemination, and related techniques.[35]
		Some clinics in Italy were, however, among the first to treat post-menopausal women.[33]	In practice, Catholic hospitals, subject to Vatican instruction, do not perform IVF, although some undertake GIFT.[36]
	Proposed legislation exists.[30]	Under the proposed legislation, access to assisted reproduction is granted to married or stable heterosexual couples of potentially fertile aged 52 or less (Art. 5).[34]	

Luxem-bourg	None.	N/A.	N/A
		In practice, no assisted reproduction services are available.[37]	
Netherlands	Hospitals Act.	None.[39]	No information.
	Decree on IVF Planning 1989.[38]	In practice, most IVF centres adopt an age limit of 40 for the woman.[40]	No information on the eligibility criteria used in practice.
Portugal	None.[41]	N/A.	N/A.
		In practice, offered to stable heterosexual couples.[43]	In practice, there is currently only limited provision for donor insemination, IVF, & GIFT.
	A Draft Bill is currently under consideration.[42]	No information about the techniques covered by the Draft Bill.	No information on the eligibility criteria imposed under the Draft Bill.
Spain	Law 35 of November 1988. Unimplemented, due to challenge as unconstitutional on enactment. Therefore, the provision of assisted reproduction is currently subject to professional self-regulation.[44]	None. Under s. 6 'every woman' is eligible for treatment as long as she provides her written consent, is at least eighteen, and is mentally competent.	Unimplemented law covers IVF, GIFT, artificial insemination, and related techniques.
Sweden	Law No. 711 of 14 June 1988 on	Donor insemination and IVF are restricted to	IVF, artificial insemination, and

	IVF. Law No. 1140 of 20 December 1984 on Insemination.[45]	married couples or cohabitees who have been in a relationship for at least 2 years (s. 2 Law No. 1140, & s. 2 of Law 1988, respectively).[46] The couple must be unable to have children by natural means.[47]	related treatments.
UK[48]	Human Fertilisation and Embryology Act 1990.	Account must be taken of the welfare of any child who will be born or affected as a result of treatment (including the need for a father of any child born as a result of treatment): s. 13(5). In practice, clinics often use criteria based on age, medical history, duration of infertility, and likelihood of success.[49]	A licence is required for treatments or procedures that involve (a) creation, storage, or use of embryos outside the body (ss. 3(1), 1(2) & 1(3)); or (a) storage or donation of gametes (s. 4(1)).

Increased public awareness of medically assisted reproduction has brought with it a growing demand for these services. This demand, operating in an area of limited resources and great moral controversy, has resulted in access to these services being subject to limitation, often in the form of legislative eligibility criteria.

Table 1 shows diverse legislative criteria.[50] At one extreme is legislation, like the French legislation, which effectively prohibits the use of assisted reproduction for homosexual couples, single women, non-cohabiting heterosexual couples, surrogate women, and post-menopausal women.[51] Where the couple seeking access to assisted reproduction is unmarried, both the French and Swedish legislation require cohabitation for at least two years, whereas in Austria no specific period of cohabitation is required.

A much more permissive approach has been adopted by the UK Act, which provides for any woman to have treatment, provided that account is taken of the welfare of any child who will be born or affected as a result of the treatment. This includes consideration of the need for a father of any child born as a result of treatment, which places a heavier burden on non-heterosexual couples, but does not exclude anyone.[52] Like the Danish legislation, the unimplemented Spanish law is even more permissive, because it explicitly states that 'every woman' is eligible for access to assisted reproduction.

Since the Spanish law has not yet been fully implemented, the *de facto* position in Spain is shaped by non-legislative mechanisms, such as professional guidelines, rather like countries such as Belgium, Greece, Finland, Ireland, Italy, and Portugal, which have no legislation governing access to assisted reproduction. This does not mean that assisted reproduction is available to everyone in those countries. In fact, even where legislative eligibility criteria exist, clinics often have discretionary power to impose additional eligibility requirements. What this means is that, in some countries, harsh *de facto* eligibility criteria apply. For example, in Ireland assisted reproduction is only offered to married couples; in Belgium, Finland, and Greece, access is restricted to married or cohabiting heterosexuals; and in Luxembourg, no such services are offered at all (see Schenker 1997, p. 174).

Overall, the countries of the EU impose three levels of legislative eligibility criteria on those who are not part of a heterosexual couple: either the eligibility criteria exclude such persons from access to assisted reproduction (e.g., France), place harsher requirements on them (e.g., UK), or provide such persons with equal opportunity of access (e.g., Spain). Further, where non-heterosexuals are excluded, there is often a requirement that the heterosexual couple be married or cohabiting for a stated period. And, the eligibility criteria applied in practice are often far stricter than the legislative position would imply.

However, legislative eligibility criteria are not applied to all medical assistance to reproduce. For example, in the UK the need to consider the welfare of any potentially affected child only applies to treatments or procedures that involve the creation, storage, or use of embryos outside the body, or the storage or donation of gametes. This means that many assisted reproductive techniques, such as artificial insemination and gamete intra-fallopian treatment (GIFT) using non-donated gametes, are not subject to legislative eligibility criteria.

Similar limitations apply to the legislation of other countries. For example, the Austrian, Danish,[53] French, German, Spanish, and Swedish legislation cover IVF, artificial insemination, and directly related techniques only. This means that many medical responses to infertility are not subject to legislative eligibility criteria, including

(a) surgical repair of damaged fallopian tubes;
(b) general practitioner advice; and

(c) the prescription of drugs to maintain and procure pregnancy.

So far we have concentrated on those countries that have legislation governing access to assisted reproduction. Legislative assemblies have not, however, been particularly quick or successful in their attempts to introduce legislation. This is not because assisted reproduction is thought to be uncontroversial or to lack priority. It is because it has proven to be too controversial. For example, since the rejection of the first proposed legislation fifteen years ago, Italy has found itself unable to reach sufficient political consensus for legislative intervention.[54] Belgium has faced similar difficulties—as illustrated by the refusal of the King to sign the Abortion Act in 1990 (see Schotsmans 1998, p. 2). Ironically, as a result, both Italy and Belgium are, by default, among the most permissive countries in Europe.

In such countries, specific legislation is not likely to be absent for long—for example, Portugal is likely to enact legislation in the very near future—but its present absence does show that assisted reproduction can be successfully regulated by non-legislative means and it shows that the controversiality of assisted reproduction is not simply a matter of the newness of the techniques.

1.2 Embryo research

Table 2.1

Country	Legislation	Legality of embryo research
Austria	Act on Procreative Medicine No. 275 of 1 July 1992.[55]	Embryo research is prohibited, though examination and treatment may be allowed if it is necessary to achieve a pregnancy (Art. 10).[56] There is a fine for violation.[57]

Belgium	None.[58]	Embryo research is permitted by default.[60]
		In practice, only two of the Free Universities undertake embryo research.[61]
		The Committee of Medical Ethics of the National Scientific Research Fund recommends that embryo research should seek to enhance the chance of implantation in the uterus and not be performed after 14 days.
	Proposed legislation exists.[59] Law No. 499 of 12 June 1996 on Biomedical Research.	Under Art. 5 of the proposed legislation, the creation of embryos *in vitro* for scientific research is prohibited, except: (a) after a decision of a special commission, conforming to the procedure in Art. 10(1); (b) where the research cannot be done using supernumerary embryos; and (c) all the other provisions of the proposed law are fulfilled. Thus, the creation of embryos for research will be allowed, subject to certain conditions.[62]
Denmark	Law No. 460 of 1997, on Assisted Reproduction, ss. 25–28.	The collection and fertilisation of eggs for research is allowed under certain conditions, such as the agreement of a regional ethics committee.[63]
		Research must seek to improve IVF techniques.[64]
		Fertilised eggs can only be kept *in vitro* up to 14 days (excluding any periods of cryopreservation).[65]
		Fertilised eggs subjected to research cannot be transferred to the womb, unless this can happen with no risk of transferring genetic diseases, malformations, etc. (Ch. 4(3)/(4)).[66]
		Research involving the fusion of genetically different embryos or parts of embryos is not permitted.[67]

Finland	Act on Medical Research No. 488 of 1999.[68]	Embryo research is permitted under licence up to 14 days after fertilisation (excluding periods of cryopreservation) (s. 11). The consent of the gamete donors has to be obtained in writing (s. 12).

Creation of embryos for research is prohibited. Fertilised eggs that have been subject to research cannot be transferred to the womb, and they are not to be kept alive for more than 14 days after fertilisation. The maximum time limit for cryopreservation of embryos to be used for research is 15 years after which the embryos are to be disposed of (s. 13).

Violation of ss. 11 or 13 is sanctioned by up to 1 year imprisonment or a fine (s. 25). Violation of s. 12 is sanctioned by a fine (s. 27).[69] |
| France | Law 94-654 of 29 July 1994 & Decree 97-578 of 28 May 1997, which form part of the Public Health Code.[70] | *In vitro* conception of human embryos for research is prohibited (Art. L-152-8).[71]

In 'exceptional' circumstances, the couple may permit studies to be carried out on the embryo, provided they give written consent, and the studies have a medical purpose, do not impair the embryo, and have the approval of the Comité National d'Ethique (Art. 152-8).[72] Thus, only non-destructive (therapeutic) research is possible.[73]

Any embryo research must have a direct advantage to the embryo concerned or contribute to the improvement of medically assisted reproduction techniques.

Research is limited to the seventh day after fertilisation.[74]

Any violation of the law is severely sanctioned (7 years imprisonment and FF 700,000 penalty).[75] |

Germany	Embryo Protection Act 1990.[76]	It is an offence to
		(a) fertilise a human egg for any purpose other than to start a pregnancy in the woman who produced the egg (Art. 1(2));
		(b) use an embryo for any purpose other than its maintenance and healthy development (Art. 2(1)); and
		(c) separate and use totipotent cells of an embryo for research and diagnosis.[77]
		Thus, non-therapeutic embryo research is prohibited.
		Violation of the law is severely sanctioned by imprisonment up to 3 years or a fine (s. 2).[78]
Greece	None.	Embryo research is permitted by default.[79]
		The Greek Central Council for Health has recommended that research on embryos should be permitted only during the first 14 days from fertilisation (excluding any period of storage).
Ireland	The Eighth Amendment to the Constitution (Art. 40.3.3).[80]	Implicitly prohibited.[81]
		Also, practically impossible because the Medical Council's ethical guidelines require all embryos to be transferred to the woman's body.[82]
	No specific legislation.	No research is being conducted on human embryos.[83]
Italy	None.	Embryo research is permitted by default. Most is performed with the aim of improving the success rate of IVF/GIFT.[85]
	Proposed legislation exists.[84]	The proposed legislation prohibits the production of embryos for research, along with all non-therapeutic embryo research.[86]
Luxembourg	None.	No embryo research is being performed.

Netherlands	None.[87]	Embryo research is permitted by default. The Health Council has recommended that an embryo should not be grown *in vitro* beyond 14 days following fertilisation.[89]
	Proposed legislation exists.[88]	The Dutch government is currently preparing a law that is in tune with this recommendation.[90]
Portugal	None.[91]	Embryo research is permitted by default. The National Council of Ethics for the Life Sciences has declared that the production of embryos for research is 'ethically unacceptable'.[92]
Spain	Law 35 of November 1998. Challenged as unconstitutional on enactment.[93]	Under the unimplemented law, research is permitted on non-viable embryos up to 14 days after fertilisation, provided the parties concerned give their written consent (ss. 15(1)/(3) & 20). Research can only be conducted on viable embryos if it is applied research of a diagnostic character or if it has a therapeutic or prophylactic purpose, and the non-pathological genetic patrimony is not modified (s. 15)(2)). A committee reviews each proposal.[94] Research must have a purpose laid down in s. 16, such as the improvement of the techniques of assisted reproduction, or increasing knowledge about infertility, gene and chromosome structure, contraception, or the origin of genetic and hereditary diseases.

Sweden	Law No. 115 of 14 March 1991 on Research or Treatment with Fertilised Human Eggs.[95]	Surplus embryos may be used for research with the consent of the couple undergoing treatment (s. 1).[96] Embryos that have been subjected to experiments must be destroyed at the end of the 14th day (s. 2).[97] No gametes or embryos that have been the subject of research can be transferred to the woman's body (s. 4).[98] The research must be related to the improvement of IVF techniques and approved by an ethics committee.[99]
UK	Human Fertilisation & Embryology Act 1990.	Research on embryos is permitted under licence up to the appearance of the primitive streak or up to 14 days after fertilisation, whichever is the earliest (ss. 1(3)(a) & 1(4)). The creation of embryos specifically for research is permitted under licence (Sch. 2, para. 3(1)). Any research must be 'necessary or desirable' for promoting advances in the treatment of infertility; congenital disease; miscarriage; conception; or gene/chromosome abnormalities (Sch. 2, para. 3(2)).

Legal regulation of embryo research seeks to balance respect for nascent human life with the benefits that can be produced by advances in scientific knowledge. Given the emotive nature of embryo research, it is no surprise to discover that this regulatory balance is far from uniform. In fact, all possible regulatory approaches can be seen in the EU. This is displayed in Table 2.2 overleaf.

Table 2.2

Legislative Approach		Non-Legislative Approach	
Permitted subject to conditions	Prohibited (unless therapeutic)	Permitted by default	Prohibited by default
Denmark	Austria	Belgium	Ireland
Finland	Germany	Greece	Luxembourg
France (exceptionally if non-impairing)		Italy	
		Netherlands	
		Portugal	
Spain			
Sweden			
UK			

A minority of EU countries—Austria and Germany—prohibit embryo research by legislation; the majority of those with legislation permitting it subject to a number of conditions. For example, the Danish, Finnish, Spanish, Swedish, and the UK legislation permit embryo research up to 14 days after fertilisation, and French legislation permits embryo research which doesn't impair the embryo in 'exceptional' circumstances (but only up to 7 days after fertilisation). After this period, the destruction of the embryo is typically required (France being an exception). Moreover, where embryo research is permitted, the purposes of such research are often prescribed. For example, as table 2.1 shows, the Spanish and UK legislation require embryo research to be for a purpose laid down in the legislation.

Where no specific legislation has been enacted, embryo research is either permitted or prohibited by the legal and cultural tradition of the individual country. For example, in Ireland, the Medical Council's ethical guidelines require all embryos to be transferred to the woman's body (see MacKellar 1997, p. 17), and the Eighth Amendment to the constitution also implicitly prohibits embryo research by declaring that

> [t]he State acknowledges the right to life of the unborn and, with due regard to the equal right to life of the mother, guarantees in its laws to respect, and, as far as practicable, by its laws to defend and vindicate that right.

Consequently, in Ireland, no research is being conducted on human embryos. In contrast, in countries such as Belgium, Greece, and Italy embryo research is permitted in the absence of any relevant legislative response.

The European Convention on Human Rights and Biomedicine could have a dramatic effect on these countries. Article 18(1) of this Convention states that

> [w]here the law allows research on embryos in vitro, it shall ensure adequate protection of the embryo.

The term 'adequate protection' is not defined. So for those countries unable to make a reservation by invoking their pre-existing law under Article 36, signing the Convention might have the effect of hindering (or perhaps even prohibiting) embryo research. Indeed, Article 18(2) states that '[t]he creation of human embryos for research purposes is prohibited'.

1.3 Cloning

Table 3

Country	Legislation	Legislative provisions concerning clonin additional to those addressing embry research
Austria	Act No. 275 of 1 July 1992.[100]	Cloning is indirectly prohibited.[101]
Belgium	None.	None.
	Legislation covering medical ethics including cloning is currently being considered by Parliament.[102]	

Denmark	Law No. 499 of 12 June 1996 on Bio-medical Research. Law No. 460 of 1997 on Assisted Reproduction.[103]	Research on, and assisted reproductive treatment with the aim of, producing genetically identical individuals is prohibited, as is nuclear substitution.[104]
Finland	Act on Medical Research No. 488 of 1999.	Conducting medical research for the purpose of facilitating the cloning human beings is a criminal offence and sanctioned by up to 2 years imprisonment or a fine (s. 26).[105]
France	Laws 94-653 and 94-654 of 29 July 1994.[106]	The embryo research that would be necessary to clone a human being is prohibited (see above, 1.2). Thus, human cloning is implicitly prohibited.[107] The Consultative National Ethics Committee for Health and Life Sciences (CCNE), in its Opinion No. 54 of 22 April 1997, opposed the production of identical human beings.[108] It also recommended that the ban should be made more explicit when the legislation is revised in 1999.[109]
Germany	Embryo Protection Act 1990 (s. 6).	It is an offence to create an embryo that is genetically identical to another embryo, fetus, or any living or dead person.[110] The Act does not define the term 'genetically identical'.[111]
Greece	None	The Greek Central Council for Health has recommended that assisted reproduction should not be used for the creation of genetically identical human beings.[112]
Ireland	None.	The legal position is uncertain.[113]

Italy	Ministerial Decree of 5 March 1997.[114] Such decrees have legal force for only 90 days unless converted by a vote of Parliament, which did not happen here.[115]	The decree prohibited all forms of experimentation and intervention aimed at (even indirectly) cloning a human or animal.[116] The National Bioethics Committee (CNB) has expressed the view that cloning should be prohibited.[117]
Luxembourg	None.	None.
Netherlands	None. Proposed legislation exists.[118]	The Dutch government proposes to prohibit the cloning of human beings, but permit the use of cloning techniques in embryo research (before 14 days after conception) in forthcoming legislation.[119]
Portugal	None.[120]	The National Council of Ethics for the Life Sciences has expressed its opinion that the cloning of human beings is 'ethically unacceptable' and must be prohibited'.[121]
Spain	Law 35 of November 1998 (s. 20), and Title V of the Penal Code (s. 161(2)).[122]	It is a criminal offence to create identical human beings, by cloning or other procedures aimed at race selection.
Sweden	Law No. 115 of 14 March 1991.	Embryo and oocyte cloning is implicitly prohibited with criminal sanctions.[123]
UK	Human Fertilisation & Embryology Act 1990.	Licences are required for the nuclear substitution of an embryo (s. 3(3)(d)), and for the creation of an embryo outside of the body (ss. 3(1)(a) and 1(2)), where an embryo is defined as a live egg that has been fertilised or is in the process of fertilisation (ss. 1(1)(a) and (b)).

The regulation of human cloning—the deliberate creation of a human being that is genetically identical to another human being or has the same nuclear gene set as another human being—is patchy.[125] Where legislation within the EU countries does address cloning, it is often influenced by the previous scientific orthodoxy that cloning by nuclear substitution would be done either by replacing the nucleus of an embryo, or replacing the nucleus of an egg with a nucleus from an embryonic cell. In other words, somatic cell nuclear transfer—where the nucleus of an egg cell is replaced with a nucleus of a somatic cell taken from an adult—was not considered to be a possibility before the creation of the sheep named 'Dolly'.[126] It follows that the application of the 'Dolly technique' to human beings might evade legislative provisions that have been drafted too narrowly.

The UK legislation provides an interesting case. In addition to the licensing requirement imposed on the storage, use, or creation of an embryo outside the body, the UK legislation prohibits the granting of a licence for the nuclear substitution of an embryo. This has led the Human Genetic Advisory Commission (HGAC) and the Human Fertilisation and Embryology Authority (HFEA) to declare that, depending on the method used, cloning is either prohibited or subject to a licensing requirement.[127] Surely, it might be objected, cloning using the Dolly technique does not involve the creation of an embryo, because an embryo is defined under the Act as 'a live human embryo where fertilisation is complete', including 'an egg in the process of fertilisation'. As Dr. Wilmut and Professor Bulfield put it

> [t]he oocyte is an egg but it has not been fertilised and it never is fertilised because the nucleus is transferred to it.[128]

However, in practice, it is very likely that the term 'fertilisation' will be judicially construed to include the nuclear substitution of an egg, especially since the HFEA seems to be acting according to this construction of the term.[129]

If fertilisation includes cloning using the Dolly technique, it is interesting to note that

> [t]he HFEA's policy is that it will not license any research which has reproductive cloning as its aim. (HGAC and HFEA 1998a, paragraph 5.4, p. 11)[130]

233

What this means is that, although cloning a human using somatic cell nuclear transfer is not prohibited in the UK, insofar as it is caught by the legislation, it is just about impossible to do it legally.[131]

Another example of legislation that was clearly intended to prohibit cloning is the German Embryo Protection Act (Embryonenschutzgesetz) 1990. Section Six of this Act renders it an offence to create an embryo that is genetically identical to another embryo, fetus, or any living or dead person. Many believe that this provision is sufficient to prohibit cloning by any method (see, e.g., Winter 1997). However, the Act does not define the term 'genetically identical', so it is questionable whether it is wide enough to encompass a clone produced by somatic cell nuclear transfer whose mitochondrial DNA will not be identical to that of the nuclear DNA donor.[132] Even if it is not, given that the clear intention of this provision was to prohibit cloning by any method, and the fact that this act invokes penal sanctions for activities such as conducting embryo research, it would be extremely unwise to attempt to clone a human being in Germany.

A slightly different position exists in Spain, where the creation of identical human beings—by cloning or any other method—is a criminal offence only where it is aimed at race selection. This provision is clearly wide enough to encompass the development of any new cloning technique, and is particularly interesting because it indicates that the Spanish legislature does not find cloning objectionable *per se*, but instead objects to the racism that it can be used to express.

In general, cloning by nuclear transfer is either prohibited expressly (as in Germany) or implicitly (as in Sweden), or not addressed by the legislature at all (as in Belgium, Greece, the Netherlands, and Luxembourg). It is likely that cloning by any method will soon become illegal in just about all the EU countries, because of the pressure for a global legal ban on the development and use of this technique on human beings. In fact, ten of the fifteen EU countries have now signed the European Convention on Human Rights and Biomedicine and its additional protocol on the prohibition of cloning human beings.[133] This protocol makes what was implicit in the Convention[134] explicit by declaring that

> [a]ny intervention seeking to create a human being genetically identical to another human being, whether living or dead, is prohibited. (Article 1(1))

Since 'genetically identical' is defined as 'sharing with another the same nuclear gene set' (Article 1(2)), somatic cell nuclear transfer is included within this prohibition.

The term 'human being' is also not defined in the Convention, so the Netherlands, when it signed the Convention and its protocol, added an interpretative statement stating that

> [i]n relation to Article 1 of the Protocol, the Government of the Kingdom of the Netherlands declares that it interprets the term 'human beings' as referring exclusively to a human individual, i.e., a human being who has been born.[135]

This statement aims to make room for cloning experiments on embryos within the first fourteen days after fertilisation.

There are a number of other international instruments banning human cloning.[136] For example, in November 1997, UNESCO published the Universal Declaration on the Human Genome and Human Rights, which stated in Article 11,

> [p]ractices which are contrary to human dignity, such as reproductive cloning of human beings shall not be permitted.[137]

Also, the EC has recently passed a Directive on the Legal Protection of Biotechnological Inventions (Directive 98/44/EC), which states in Article 6(2)(a) that 'processes for cloning human beings' are unpatentable. This is very likely to act as a disincentive for commercial research and investment into cloning.[138]

1.4 Germ-line gene therapy

Table 4

Country	Legislative provisions concerning germ-line gene therapy in addition to those addressing embryo research
Austria	Act on Procreative Medicine 275/1992 prohibits germ-line gene therapy (Art. 9(2)).[139]
Belgium	None.
Denmark	Under Law No. 460 of 1997, eggs and sperm must not be genetically modified. Germ-line gene therapy is not permitted.[140]

Finland	Act on Medical Research No. 488 of 1999 prohibits research on embryos or gametes for the purpose of developing methods to alter hereditary characteristics, unless it aims to find a cure or to prevent a severe hereditary disease (s. 15). Violation is sanctioned by up to 1 year imprisonment or a fine (s. 25).
	The working group (set up by the Ministry of Justice) reporting on the use of gametes and embryos in assisted fertilisation had proposed that no gametes or embryos be used in assisted fertilisation where the genetic heritage has been modified.[141]
France	Law 94-654 of 29 July 1994 prohibits germ-line gene therapy and germ-line genetic manipulations.[142]
Germany	Embryo Protection Act 1990 explicitly prohibits germ-line gene therapy (Art. 5(1)/(2).)[143]
Ireland	None.
Greece	None.
Italy	None.
Luxembourg	No information.
Netherlands	None.
	The Health Council has recommended a moratorium on human germ-line gene therapy.
Portugal	None.
Spain	Under s. 15(2)(b) of the unimplemented[144] Law 35 of November 1998, research on viable embryos can only be conducted where 'the non-pathological genetic patrimony is not modified'.
Sweden	Under Law 115 of 1991, research to develop techniques for achieving hereditary alterations (germ-line interventions) is forbidden (s. 2).[145]

UK	Under the Human Fertilisation and Embryology Act 1990, a treatment licence cannot 'authorise altering the genetic structure of any cell while it forms part of an embryo' (Sch. 2, para. 1(4)), and the same is true of a research licence, 'except in such circumstances (if any) as may be specified in or determined in pursuance of regulations' (Sch. 2, para. 3(4)).

Like cloning by nuclear transfer, germ-line gene therapy—which involves modifying genes so that they can be passed on to future generations—has not yet been successfully performed on humans and has a consensus against its use. Consequently, where germ-line gene therapy and its associated research is addressed by legislation, it is either prohibited or heavily restricted.

The Austrian, Danish, French, German, and Swedish legislation expressly prohibit germ therapy. Even the usually permissive UK Act prohibits germ-line gene therapy, and permits its associated research only where it is allowed by regulation. However, no such regulation currently exists.

Slightly different approaches are adopted by the Spanish and Finnish legislation. The Spanish legislation prohibits embryo research where the non-pathological genetic patrimony is modified, and the Finnish legislation goes further by explicitly permitting germ-line gene therapy where it aims to find a cure for, or prevent, a serious hereditary disease.

Germ-line gene therapy might also be permitted by default in some countries that have no specific legislation. Such countries include Belgium, Greece, and Italy.

Once again, the European Convention on Human Rights and Biomedicine might have an effect on this, because Article 13 declares,

> [a]n intervention seeking to modify the human genome may only be undertaken for preventive, diagnostic or therapeutic purposes and only if its aim is not to introduce any modification in the genome of any descendants.

Where a signatory country does not, or is unable to, make a reservation under Article 36 in regard to this provision, it would appear that germ-line gene therapy is prohibited.

As with cloning, the prohibitive inclinations of the European Convention are shared by many other international instruments. For example, Article 24 of the Universal Declaration on the Human Genome and Human Rights states that the International Bioethics Committee of UNESCO should contribute to dissemination of the principles set out in the Declaration and make recommendations to the General Conference

> in particular regarding the identification of practices that *could be contrary* to human dignity, such as *germ-line interventions'*. (Our emphasis)[146]

Also, Article 6(2)(b) of the EC Directive on the Legal Protection of Biotechnological Inventions declares that 'processes for modifying the germ line genetic identity of human beings' are unpatentable.[147]

1.5 Pre-implantation genetic diagnosis (PGD)

Table 5.1

Country	Legislation	Legality of PGD
Austria	Act on Procreative Medicine No. 275 of 1 July 1992.	Implicitly forbidden, because under s. 9(1), gametes and pre-implantation embryos[148] are only permitted to be medically examined and treated to the extent necessary to establish a pregnancy.
Belgium	None.[149]	Permitted by default. A licence is required to establish a centre for genetics.[150]
Denmark	Clinical use: Law No. 460 of 1997, ss. 7 and 21.[151] Research: see Table 2.1.	Implicitly permitted.

238

Finland	None.	Permitted by default.[153]
	Proposed legislation exists.[152]	A working group report, given to the Ministry of Justice in 1997, recommended that the use of assisted reproduction should not be allowed for the purpose of choosing a child's sex or characteristics, except to avoid serious hereditary sex-related disease.[154]
France	Law 94-654 of 29 July 1994.	Authorised by a law that requires the publication of a further decree, which has not been issued. Thus, PGD is currently impossible in France.[155]
		The unimplemented law allows PGD only where (a) it is undertaken in a centre licensed by the 'National Commission of Medicine and Biology of Human Reproduction and Prenatal Diagnosis'; and (b) the couple in question provides written consent and has a high probability of producing a child with a severe and incurable genetic defect (Art. 162-17).[156]
Germany	Embryo Protection Act 1990.	It is an offence to fertilise a human egg for any purpose other than to start a pregnancy in the woman who produced the egg.[157] Also, the removal of a totipotent cell is prohibited.[158] Thus, PGD is implicitly prohibited.
Greece	None. [159]	Permitted by default.[160]
Ireland	None.	Any diagnosis of the pre-implantation embryo is implicitly prohibited, as the Eighth Amendment states, '[t]he State acknowledges the right to life of the unborn and, with due regard to the equal right to life of the mother, guarantees in its laws to respect, and, as far as practicable, by its laws to defend and vindicate that right'.

239

Italy	None.	Permitted by default.
Luxembourg	No information.	No information.
Netherlands	None.	Permitted by default.[161]
		Clinical research will fall within the forthcoming Medical Research Involving Human Subjects Act.[162]
Portugal	None.	No information.
Spain	Law 35 of November 1998. Since this was challenged as unconstitutional on enactment, the provision of PGD is currently subject to professional self-regulation.	Permitted under the unimplemented law. Assisted reproduction is expressly allowed for the prevention and treatment of illnesses of a genetic or hereditary origin (s. 12(1)). However, genetic selection for non-pathological characteristics is prohibited (s. 13).
Sweden	Law No. 115 of 14 March 1991.	Permitted only for the diagnosis of serious, progressive, hereditary disease that leads to premature death and for which there is no cure or treatment. [163]
UK	Human Fertilisation and Embryology Act 1990.	Permitted. Research licences can be granted for any activity that is 'necessary or desirable' for the purpose of 'developing methods for detecting the presence of gene or chromosome abnormalities in embryos before implantation' (Sch. 2, para. 3(2)(e)).
		Embryos that have been the subject of research may not be returned to the womb (s. 15(4)).

Unlike cloning and germ-line gene therapy, there is no consensus against (or, for that matter, in favour of) genetic diagnosis of the oocyte or non-implanted embryo. Consequently, all four regulatory approaches to PGD are displayed throughout the EU. That is,

Table 5.2

Legislative Approach		Non-Legislative Approach	
Permitted	Prohibited	Permitted by default	Prohibited by default
Denmark	Austria	Belgium	France (until
France (unimplemented law)	Germany	Finland	1994 law imple-
		Greece	mented)
		Italy	
Spain (unimplemented law)		Netherlands	Ireland
		Spain (until	Luxembourg
		1988, law	
Sweden		imple-	
UK		mented)	

Countries whose legislation permits PGD vary greatly in the level permissiveness.

The UK licensing authority, in accordance with the permissive legislation under which it operates, has licensed four centres to undertake PGD and its associated research. It has, however, advised the clinics that it licenses that sex selection for social reasons is unacceptable (see HFEA 1998, paragraph 7.20, p. 45).

An example of the restrictive legislative approach can be found in the German Embryo Protection Act (EPA).[164] Under the EPA, it is an offence to fertilise a human egg for any purpose other than to start a pregnancy in the woman who produced the egg. Also, no embryo research is permitted—an embryo being defined as an egg from the time of fertilisation (uniting of the nuclei) and any totipotent cell. This has lead many commentators to suggest that diagnosis of cells after they lose their totipotency is not forbidden by the EPA.[165] Nevertheless, the clear intention of the EPA was to prohibit PGD, and, in 1996, an application to conduct Germany's first PGD trial was rejected by a local ethics committee on legal grounds.

Whether PGD is acceptable in countries that do not have any specific legislation depends on the individual country's general legal and cultural framework. For example, genetic diagnosis of the pre-implantation embryo is implicitly prohibited in Ireland by the Eighth Amendment to the Irish Constitution.

> The State acknowledges the right to life of the unborn and, with due regard to the equal right to life of the mother, guarantees in its laws to respect, and, as far as practicable, by its laws to defend and vindicate that right.

In France, the law permits PGD, but its implementation requires the publication of a decree. Therefore,

> for the present, although preimplantation diagnosis should be authorized, its practice is currently impossible in France. (Viville *et al.* 1998, p. 1023)[166]

The Spanish law, which expressly permits the use of assisted reproduction for the prevention and treatment of illnesses of a genetic or hereditary origin,[167] has also not been implemented. But, due to a different legal and cultural climate, this has not prevented the use of the technique in Spain. Instead, it is performed subject to professional self-regulation. Interestingly, section 13 of the unimplemented law prohibits genetic selection for or against non-pathological characteristics.

Many other European countries do not have laws regulating PGD at all. For example, in Belgium, Greece, Italy, and the Netherlands, PGD is, in effect, permitted by default.

Countries that have signed the European Convention on Human Rights and Biomedicine will, however, have to take account of Article 14, which declares

> [t]he use of techniques of medically assisted procreation shall not be allowed for the purpose of choosing the future child's sex, except where serious hereditary sex-related disease is to be avoided.

No country is currently able to make a reservation to this provision based on its pre-existing law.

1.6 Prenatal diagnosis (PND) and abortion

Table 6

Country	Legislation	Legality of Abortion
Austria	S. 97 of the Penal Code.	Permitted (a) within 12 weeks after conception; (b) to protect the mother's health; (c) where the child will probably be severely handicapped; or (d) if the mother was under age at the time of conception.[168] PND is permitted for medical purposes only, with the written consent of the woman.[169]
Belgium	Law of 3 April 1990.[170]	Permitted (a) before 12 weeks, after counselling, where a doctor is convinced of the pregnant woman's distress and determination; and (b) up to birth, if the pregnancy would threaten the health of the pregnant woman, or there is a substantial risk that the child, if it were born, would have a serious and incurable disease.[173]
Denmark	Pregnancy Act 1973.[171] *Research:* Law No. 499 of 12 June 1996.[172]	Permitted (a) on demand (and for free) within the first 12 weeks; (b) after 12 weeks, where there are social reasons, the cause was rape or incest, or where the child is in danger of hereditary problems or sickness during the embryonic stage; and (c) up to birth, if a serious risk exists for the health of the woman.[174]

243

	Clinical use: Regulated by administrative guidelines.[175]	PND is permitted for women over 35 years and women with a risk of hereditary diseases.[176]
Finland	No information.	Permitted (a) before 12 weeks, if two physicians consider that the circumstances of the woman would place considerable strain on her, the pregnancy was caused by rape, the parents are severely limited in their ability to care for the child, or there is reason to believe that the child would be born retarded or would have or develop a serious illness or serious defects; (b) between 12 and 20 weeks of gestation, subject to the permission of the National Board of Medico-Legal Affairs; (c) before 24 weeks, subject to the permission of the National Board of Medico-legal Affairs, if tests show the fetus is seriously ill or has a serious physical deformity, and (d) up to birth, where the woman's life or health is endangered.[177]
France	Law 94-654 of 29 July 1994, forming part of the Public Health Code. Decree No. 95-559 of 6 May 1995. Decrees 97-578 and 97-579 of 28 May 1997.[178]	Permitted (a) before week 10 on demand (Art. L-162-16 of the Public Health Code);[179] and (b) up to birth, if two physicians conclude that the pregnancy endangers the life of the woman, or the child to be born will, most probably, be affected by a particularly serious incurable disorder recognised as such at the time of diagnosis (Art. 13).[180] PND procedures must be preceded by 'medical genetic counselling', fulfilling certain stated aims (Art. L-162-16).[181]

244

Germany	Criminal Code (s. 218).	Abortion is a criminal offence under s. 218, but the physician performing the abortion will not be prosecuted

Germany — Criminal Code (s. 218).

Abortion is a criminal offence under s. 218, but the physician performing the abortion will not be prosecuted

(a) up to the first 12 weeks, where the women has had counselling not later than 3 days before the termination (s. 218(a)(1));

(b) up to birth, where there is a risk to the woman's life, or a risk of permanent/serious physical or mental injury to the woman; which could not be averted by any other means (s. 218(a)(2)).[182] In practice, the risk of mental injury to the woman is interpreted to encompass abortion following PND, the emphasis being placed on the pregnant woman rather than the fetus.[183]

The pregnant woman does not commit an offence under s. 218 if the abortion is performed by a physician under 22 weeks, and if the woman has received counselling prior to the abortion (s. 218(a)(4)). Also, under this provision the court can refrain from convicting a pregnant woman, who was experiencing a situation of serious hardship at the time of the abortion.[184]

Greece — Law 1609/1986 on Abortion.[185]

Ministerial decision A3B/oik 2799/25.2.87.[186]

Law 1036/1980 on 'Family Planning'.[187]

1985 Decision of the Central Council of Health.[188]

Permitted where

(a) the embryo is less than 12 weeks old;

(b) there are indications, based on PND, that the embryo to be born will suffer from a serious abnormality and the pregnancy has not passed the 24th week of gestation;

(c) the pregnant woman is at risk of death or serious damage to her physical or mental health; or

(d) pregnancy results from rape or incest.[189]

PND must take place in a state, university, or armed forces hospital.[190]

245

Ireland	The Eighth Amendment to the Constitution (Art. 40.3.3).	The Supreme Court has interpreted the constitution as prohibiting abortion, unless there is a real and substantial threat to the life of the mother.[191]
Italy	Legge No. 194/78 of 22 May 1978, Sull'interruzione Volontaria Della Gravidanza (i.e., law on the voluntary interruption of pregnancy).[192]	Abortion on demand is available within the first 12 weeks and 6 days of pregnancy, after which abortion can only be requested where (a) the continuation of the pregnancy or delivery could endanger the woman's life; (b) the fetus has malformations so serious that the woman's psychological or physical well-being is endangered, or if her well-being is endangered by other pathological processes; or (c) the pregnancy is the result of rape.[193]
Luxembourg	Title of legislation unknown.	Permitted (a) before 12 weeks, if the pregnancy would threaten the woman's physical and mental health, is the result of rape, or if there is a substantial risk that the child, if it were born, would be very sick or be physically or mentally seriously handicapped; and (b) after 12 weeks, only if two medical doctors ascertain that birth of the child presents a serious risk to the health of the pregnant woman or the child to be born.[194]
Netherlands	The Pregnancy Termination Act 1981.[195]	Permitted up to 24 weeks, if there is a danger to the woman and she has an authentic desire to terminate.[196] In practice, this permits abortion on demand up to 24 weeks gestation.

Portugal	Arts. 140, 141, and 142 of the Penal Code.[197]	Permitted (a) within 12 weeks, if there are medical indications that it will remove the danger of death or of serious and irreversible damage to the pregnant woman's physical or psychological health; (b) up to 16 weeks, if there are serious indications that the pregnancy is the result of crime against 'sexual freedom and self-determination', (c) up to 24 weeks, if there are indisputable medical reasons indicating that the unborn child has a serious incurable disease or congenital defect, and (d) up to birth, if it is 'the only way to remove' the danger of death or of serious and irreversible damage to the pregnant women's physical or psychological health.[200] Also, (e) the physician who approves the abortion cannot perform it; (e) the written consent of the pregnant woman is required; and (f) where the abortion is performed under (c) above, a technical commission of certification is needed.[201]
Spain	Art. 417 bis of Law 9 of 5 July 1985 (part of the Penal Code).[198] Royal decree No. 2409 of 21 November 1986.[199]	Permitted (a) during the first 12 weeks, if the pregnancy is the result of a previously declared rape; (b) during the first 22 weeks, if two specialists who are not performing the abortion diagnose a serious physical or mental abnormality/handicap; and (c) up to birth, to avoid a serious threat to the life or (physical or mental) health of the woman, if stated in a report submitted by a medical specialist who cannot be the physician performing or supervising the abortion.[202]

		If an abortion is performed where none of these conditions exist, the woman will not be prosecuted. The person conducting the abortion in such circumstances might, however, be prosecuted (Art. 145).[203]
Sweden	Abortion Act of 1995.	Permitted (a) up to 18 weeks; (b) up to the end of the 22nd week, if sanctioned by the National Board of Health and Welfare (and only when there is no reason to believe that the fetus is viable); and (c) up to birth, where the pregnancy might gravely imperil the woman's life or health or the fetus is so gravely damaged that it is not viable.[204] All pregnant women are offered information on abortion, and PND.[205]
UK (excluding Northern Ireland).[206]	Abortion Act 1967 (s. 1(1)), as inserted by s. 37 of the Human Fertilisation and Embryology Act 1990.	Permitted (a) up to 24 weeks, where the continuation of the pregnancy will involve risk, greater than if the pregnancy were terminated, of injury to the woman or her family; and (b) up to birth, to save the life of the woman, to avoid permanent injury to her physical or mental health, or to avoid the birth of a severely handicapped child.

The legality of PND is largely dependent on the legality of abortion within particular jurisdictions, and abortion is the most comprehensively regulated area falling within the terms of this report. All but one of the fifteen member states of the EU have specific legislation. Ireland is the exception, as abortion is covered by the constitution rather than legislation, and the constitution (as interpreted by the Supreme Court) prohibits abortion unless there is a real and substantial threat to the life of the pregnant woman.

Thus, with the exception of Ireland, all EU countries have decriminalised abortion where certain conditions are satisfied, up to a specific period of gestation—the most permissive being the legislation of the UK and the Netherlands, which in practice allow abortion on demand up to 24 weeks gestation. In Austria, Belgium, Denmark, Finland, Germany, Greece, Luxembourg, and Portugal, abortion is generally restricted to gestational development of less than 12 weeks. In France the period is ten weeks, in Italy, up to 12 weeks and 6 days, and, in Sweden, the period is up to 18 weeks.

Within these countries, abortion is available for specific reasons beyond this period of gestation. For example, abortion is permitted up to birth to protect the mother's life in all EU countries. For our purposes, it is interesting to see that diagnosis of a serious genetic condition,[207] following PND, provides grounds for abortion. In fact, abortion following PND is permitted

(a) up to birth in Austria, Belgium, Denmark, France, Italy, and the UK;
(b) up to 24 weeks in Finland, Greece, the Netherlands, and Portugal;
(c) up to 22 weeks in Spain, and Sweden;[208] and
(e) up to 12 weeks in Luxembourg.

In some countries, use of PND is limited by other legislative conditions. For example, in France and Germany, PND cannot be used for selecting the gender of the child, except in cases of incurable sex-linked hereditary diseases (see MacKellar 1997, p. 10; and Lansac 1996, p. 1847).

In sum, abortion following the diagnosis of a genetic disorder is permitted, subject to specific conditions and gestational development, in all the countries of the EU, with the possible exception of Ireland.

2   Pro-life, pro-choice, and compromise positions

Having reviewed the legal position within the EU countries, we will now develop a framework for analysing the moral and philosophical issues.

In another paper in this volume, one of us offers a three-fold ideal-typical description of the political landscape.[209] This classifies the political landscape according to the level of intrinsic moral status granted to the embryo-fetus—that is, according to the moral status that is granted to the human embryo and fetus (hereafter embryo-fetus) by virtue of the characteristics possessed by it.

The first position, the 'pro-life' position, is characterised as granting full moral status to the embryo-fetus from the moment of conception. The second, the 'pro-choice' position, is depicted as granting no intrinsic moral status to the embryo-fetus, until at least birth. The third, the 'compromise' position, represents the view that the intrinsic moral status of the embryo-fetus increases with gestational development until it obtains full moral status at birth or beyond. In other words, the political landscape is classified according to whether intrinsic moral status is denied to the embryo-fetus (the 'pro-choice' position), granted in full to the embryo-fetus (the 'pro-life' position), or granted on a gradualist scale (the 'compromise' position).

This framework can be applied to the regulation of human reproduction, genetic diagnosis, and gene therapy only insofar as such regulation has implications for the embryo-fetus.[210] Its application is, however, far from straightforward, because the classification leaves open the possibility that the embryo-fetus might have moral status that is indirectly derived from the moral status of those with intrinsic moral status (hereafter vicarious moral status). This is especially important for the 'pro-choice' position, because it means that this position does not commit its supporters to the idea that anything can be done to the embryo-fetus with impunity.[211]

Each of these positions has implications for the regulation of the techniques under discussion. A regulatory structure adopting the 'pro-life' position would characteristically prohibit any non-therapeutic interference with the embryo-fetus. There is one possible exception to this, and that is where the 'pro-life' position is underpinned by a moral theory that aggregates or averages the interests of those with intrinsic moral status. For example, if it is possible to adopt a utilitarian position that grants full moral status to the embryo-fetus from conception, such a position could permit non-therapeutic interference with the embryo-fetus where the interests of a being with full moral status are outweighed by the aggregate (or average of the) interests of other beings with intrinsic moral status. We are not sure whether any such moral theory exists.

A 'pro-choice' regulatory structure would permit such interference, unless its restriction is necessary to protect the legitimate interests of those with full moral status; whereas the 'compromise' position would prohibit such interference except where it is necessary to protect the moral status of those with higher moral status.

For present purposes, we will concentrate on the implications of this classificatory framework for PGD and abortion.

With PGD, it is characteristically intended that the oocyte or pre-implantation embryo will be rejected if the diagnosis were to indicate the presence of an undesired gene or chromosomal abnormality. This is important, because, with the exception of the PGD technique of polar body biopsy on the first polar body, which is performed on a sister cell of the oocyte, all PGD is performed on the pre-implantation embryo. Therefore, with this exception, a non-utilitarian 'pro-life' proponent would be opposed to PGD. The 'pro-life' position's opposition to PGD is strength-ened where the technique involves the removal and consequential destruction of totipotent cells (as in blastomere biopsy), which some would argue are individual embryos.

A regulatory structure adopting the 'pro-choice' position has the potential to be far more permissive. Since this position does not grant the embryo-fetus intrinsic moral status, it will permit PGD, unless its prohibition is necessary to protect the legitimate interests of those with intrinsic moral status. Such vicarious considerations will restrict or prohibit PGD where it threatens to inflict harm on those with intrinsic moral status that is greater than the harm that will result from denying potential parents (who also have intrinsic moral status) access to PGD. In short, a 'pro-choice' regulatory structure will start from the presumption that PGD is permitted, rebutting this presumption only insofar as the embryo-fetus is shown to have sufficient vicarious moral status.[212]

The 'compromise' position, sits between the 'pro-life' and 'pro-choice' positions only on the issue of intrinsic moral status. Although the gradualist intrinsic moral status granted to the pre-implantation embryo might be minimal it is still moral status, so the presumption of such a regulatory structure must be against the use of PGD, this presumption only being rebuttable by considerations that seek to protect the moral status of a being with higher intrinsic moral status.

The impact of these three positions on the regulation of abortion is just as complex. A non-utilitarian 'pro-life' position, being the most predictable of the three, will prohibit abortion irrespective of the gestational development of the embryo-fetus except, perhaps, where the life of the mother is in danger. In contrast, the 'pro-choice' position will permit abortion up to the gestational point where the vicarious protection given to the embryo-fetus overrides the mother's right to abort. This point will depend on the strength of the vicarious considerations, the presumption being in favour of permitting abortion. Since pregnancy is potentially very harmful to the mother, the vicarious arguments are less likely to prohibit abortion than PGD. Nevertheless, they are still capable of severely limiting its availability.

The 'compromise' position will, in addition to granting gradualist intrinsic moral status to the embryo-fetus, grant vicarious moral status to the embryo-fetus. The mother will, however, have much greater moral status than the embryo-fetus. Thus, although a 'compromise' regulatory structure would start from the presumption that abortion is prohibited, one would expect abortion to be available at least during early gestation.

2.1 Applying this framework

Before applying this framework to the regulatory positions described in Part One of this report, we need to highlight a number complications.

One complication is that where the protection offered to the embryo-fetus is 'gradualist'—where gradually greater protection is granted to the embryo-fetus as it approaches birth—this does not necessarily mean that the country in question has adopted a 'compromise' position. It might have adopted a 'pro-choice' position, because vicarious moral status can also be gradualist. For example, where an embryo-fetus is protected as a means of protecting the sensitivities of those with intrinsic moral status, if these sensitivities increase with the development of the embryo-fetus, the corresponding vicarious protection offered to the embryo-fetus will also increase.

A related complication is that it is possible for the 'compromise' position—which starts from a presumption in favour of the embryo-fetus—and the 'pro-choice' position—which starts from a presumption against the embryo-fetus—to grant the same degree of protection to the embryo-fetus. However, we suspect that in practice, the regulatory structure will tend towards its underlying presumption. That is, a 'pro-choice' regulatory structure, in practice, is likely to be more permissive than a 'compromise' regulatory structure.

Bearing in mind these complications, we offer the following line diagram for the values in Table 7 below, where the numbers represent our impression of a location on the scale from the 'pro-life' position to the 'pro-choice' position. For the reasons just given, the following attributions cannot be described as more than impressionistic descriptions of the tendency of the regulation.[213]

Pro-life	*Compromise*	*Pro-choice*
1	3	5

The country tending most strongly towards the 'pro-life' position for all the techniques under discussion is Ireland. The Eighth Amendment to the Irish Constitution encapsulates the tenets of the 'pro-life' position, as it (implicitly or explicitly) prohibits abortion (except in the extreme circumstances laid down by the constitutional court), embryo research, PGD, and PND.

The other countries are more difficult to categorise in terms of these ideal-typical perspectives. The country tending most strongly towards the pro-choice position is the UK, which permits PGD (with the exception of sex selection for social reasons), permits abortion on demand up to 24 weeks gestation, permits abortion following PND up to birth to avoid the birth of a severely handicapped child, and even permits the deliberate creation of embryos for research. The UK does, however, limit embryo research to a maximum of 14 days.

Table 7

PGD	Embryo Research	Abortion
Austria, Germany, Ireland	1. Austria, France, Germany, Ireland	1. Ireland
	2. Portugal	2. France, Italy, Luxembourg, Portugal
France (1994 law), Sweden, Spain	3. Sweden, Spain	3. Austria, Belgium, Finland, Germany, Greece, Spain
	4. Belgium, Finland, Denmark, Greece, Italy, UK	4. Sweden, Denmark, Netherlands, UK
Belgium, Denmark, Finland, Greece, Italy, Netherlands, UK		
Luxembourg, Portugal		
	? Luxembourg, Netherlands	

The Spanish legislation tends strongly towards the 'compromise' position. This legislation permits embryo research only for very limited purposes, restricts abortion during the first 12 weeks to circumstances where the pregnancy is the result of a previously declared rape; and permits abortion following PND during the first 22 weeks only where the embryo-fetus is diagnosed as having a serious physical or mental handicap.

Many of the countries are difficult to classify because they either grant 'gradualist' protection—which could be due to granting the embryo-fetus gradualist vicarious moral status or gradualist intrinsic moral status—or are *prima facie* inconsistent. By inconsistent, we mean that some countries seem to have adopted different approaches for different techniques. For

253

example, the French legislation's prohibition of non-therapeutic embryo research tends towards the 'pro-life' position, but its legislative acceptance of PGD and PND tends more towards the 'compromise' or 'pro-choice' position. Moreover, Austrian and German legislation prohibit embryo research and PGD, suggesting a tendency towards the 'pro-life' camp,[214] but permit abortion and PND, suggesting a tendency towards the 'compromise' or 'pro-choice' camp. This inconsistency appears to be the result of a clash of positions within the political arena.

Italy represents the most striking example of the effects of interaction between these positions within the political and legislative arenas. In Italy, the Catholic Church's 'pro-life' position has had enough political influence to undermine any 'pro-choice' or 'compromise' legislation in all areas except abortion. It has not, however, been influential enough to enshrine itself in legislation. Consequently, the influence of the 'pro-life' camp has created a *de facto* position that ironically appears to tend towards the 'pro-choice' camp.

Evidently, the regulatory approach is the product of various social, political, legal, and philosophical influences within a particular polity. It might be the result of a political compromise; social, historical, or cultural contingencies; or the adoption of a particular normative position.

Since this is not an empirical project, we will concentrate on analysis of the philosophical perspectives underpinning the adoption of a particular position. In other words, we are not going to examine events within the political process. Instead we will explore the types of philosophical positions that could underpin our ideal-typical pro-life, pro-choice, and compromise positions.

2.2 Grounds for possession of intrinsic moral status

There are a number of potential grounds for the possession of intrinsic moral status. The three that are particularly pertinent for our purposes are those that grant intrinsic moral status to those who are

(a) sentient; i.e., capable of experiencing pain;
(b) human; i.e., members of *Homo sapiens*, or
(c) persons/agents; i.e., able to act for purposes constituting their reasons for action.

A 'pro-life' position must ground possession of intrinsic moral status on a property gained at conception, such as being human or a potential person, if these concepts are defined in a certain way.[215] Where the latter is taken to be the ground for this position, having such potential must be held to be

254

sufficient for full moral status, rather than sufficient for moral status that is proportional to the degree of potential.[216]

A 'pro-choice' position must ground possession of intrinsic moral status on a property allegedly not possessed by the embryo-fetus, such as personhood. Obviously, the idea that the embryo-fetus has any intrinsic moral status as a potential, partial, or possible person must be rejected by supporters of the 'pro-choice' position.

The 'compromise' position must be underpinned by a theory that grounds possession of intrinsic moral status on a property/relation that is had in degrees in proportion to gestational development, possession of which in full is held to be sufficient for full moral status. Such positions include those resting intrinsic moral status on degrees of

(a) possible personhood, i.e., holding that intrinsic moral status is proportional to the degree of evidence supporting the hypothesis that a being is a person;
(b) sentience; i.e., holding that intrinsic moral status is proportional to the degree of sentience possessed;
(c) potential personhood; i.e., the view that intrinsic moral status is proportional to the degree of potentiality possessed; or
(d) approach to an attribute, such as personhood; i.e., holding that intrinsic moral status is proportion to the degree of approach to the relevant attribute.

Even a brief perusal of the national and international debate reveals rhetoric that is capable of simultaneously appealing to more than one of these positions.

At the international level, one only has to look at the pronouncements of international instruments, such as the Council of Europe's Convention on Human Rights and Biomedicine, Article 1 of which demands that parties to it 'protect the dignity and identity of all human beings'. The World Health Organisation has also adopted this type of language in its 1997 resolution, which declares that

> [t]he use of cloning for the replication of human individuals is ethically unacceptable and contrary to *human integrity and morality*. (Quoted in UNESCO 1998. Our emphasis)

Such rhetoric will appeal to those adopting any of the positions outlined above. One reason for this cross-positional appeal is that all the positions that we have outlined grant full intrinsic moral status to adult human beings, and the rhetoric used can suggest that it is the moral status of adult human beings that is being protected. Moreover, the term 'human' is ambiguous as between advocating the view that moral status rests on membership of the human race (i.e., human in the biological sense) and advocating the view that moral status belongs to persons (i.e., human in a moral sense).

This rhetorical device is standard in the language used by national bodies. For example, the published opinions of the Portuguese National Council of Ethics for the Life Sciences[217] are loaded with such phrases. In one Report, the National Council asserts that

> science does not itself represent a value that may be compared to *human* life and dignity, which it is meant to serve. (National Council of Ethics for the Life Sciences 1995, p. 3. Our emphasis)

In another, the National Council asserts

> [t]he cloning of human beings, because of the problems it raises concerning the dignity of the *human person*, the equilibrium of the *human species* and life in society, is ethically unacceptable and must be prohibited. (National Council of Ethics for the Life Sciences 1997b, p. 2. Our emphasis)

In the UK, the HGAC and HFEA (1998a, p. 16) have asserted that cloning

> raises serious ethical issues, concerned with *human* responsibility and instrumentalisation of *human beings*. (Our emphasis)

Even where the language appears to be committed to a particular stance, further analysis often reveals more universal appeal. For example, the Warnock Report, which formed the basis of the UK Human Fertilisation and Embryology Act 1990, asserts that 'the embryo of the human species ought to have a special status' (Warnock 1985, paragraph 11.7), albeit less than that of a living child or adult. *Prima facie*, this statement is gradualist, suggesting a 'compromise' position. However, notice the references to 'the human species' (suggesting advocacy of the view that intrinsic moral status is grounded in membership of the human race), and the fact that gradualist conclusions can also appeal to those from the 'pro-choice' camp (due to vicarious considerations).

What this means is that apparent consensus is often not really consensus at all.

Consequently, to some extent, it is naive to look to regulatory structures for an understanding of the various philosophical positions in play. There are of course exceptions—Ireland has clearly adopted the Roman Catholic Church's 'pro-life' position grounding moral status on being human in the biological sense. But the regulatory approaches of other EU countries are more likely to be the result of political compromises than the adoption of a theoretically pure perspective.

This point is also pertinent to the regulation of medically assisted reproduction. The techniques that legislatures have been concerned to regulate are not those of medical assistance to reproduce as such, but those that are non-traditional or have evoked, or have the potential to evoke, political tension. It is hard to imagine any other ground on which the techniques that are universally subject to legislative eligibility criteria can be distinguished from those that are not.[218]

This difference between the techniques subject to legislative eligibility criteria and those that are not certainly cannot be accounted for on the basis of financial considerations, because, to take one example, surgical repair of damaged fallopian tubes is far more expensive than donor insemination. Moreover, such a position does not seem to serve to protect the intrinsic moral status that the gamete might develop because the imposition of eligibility criteria actually prevent the gamete from developing into a being that will be granted moral status by any of the positions that we have discussed.

The divergence between the EU countries over whether those who are not part of a heterosexual couple should have access to assisted reproduction, must be the result of the same kinds of forces, or factors other than the intrinsic moral status of the embryo-fetus.[219]

In short, looking at the regulatory structures within the EU tells us more about the compromises that have or have not been made in the legislative arena or the socio-political context of the polity, than it does about the underpinning ground for possession of intrinsic moral status. It also highlights the limitations of our attempt to classify the philosophical approaches to these issues. As we stated earlier, not all the philosophical differences reduce to different perspectives on the level of, and ground for possession of, intrinsic moral status. A more comprehensive treatment of this philosophical diversity would have to classify the positions available on issues such as the availability of access to assisted reproduction, the moral status of the pre-conceptus, and the level of moral harm evoked by parental attempts to influence the characteristics of offspring.

Some of the moral issues will be raised in more detail below, but we do not present an overview of the different approaches that could be taken on these issues. Such an overview would take more time and space than we have available here, and require the development of numerous other frameworks.

We do, however, wish to make a few preliminary points. First, a framework for classifying the different approaches on the relevance of marital/relational status and sexual orientation to access to assisted reproduction will have to encompass a number of very diverse perspectives. Positions on this issue can be underpinned by theories attaching very different values to considerations such as the interests of the child, the significance of the 'standard' family, the interests of minorities, the relevance of sexual orientation, and the relevance of cultural traditions. Creating a framework that accurately captures the essence of this diversity will be no easy task.

Second, since it is usually possible to adopt a position that raises issues falling outside of any particular framework, it will be difficult to construct additional frameworks that have sufficient breath without losing their elucidatory force.

3   Conclusion

In sum, the regulation of assisted reproduction, genetic diagnosis, and genetic therapy across the EU reveals many areas of convergence and divergence. For a start, the EU countries are split between legislative and non-legislative regulatory mechanisms, and between permissive and restrictive approaches. The stringency of the approach adopted does, to some extent, seem to be consistent within each country, so that those countries that are restrictive regarding embryo research are also restrictive regarding PGD, and so on. There are, of course, exceptions. For example, all the EU countries, except Ireland, have adopted permissive legislation governing abortion and PND.[220] Moreover, cloning and germ-line gene therapy have attracted almost universal prohibition.

Analysing these issues in terms of the ideal-typical 'pro-life', 'pro-choice', and 'compromise' positions illustrates the extent to which political compromise has shaped the regulation of the techniques under discussion. This analysis has also revealed a number of potentially fruitful avenues for further study.

On an empirical level, further research could usefully address at least three issues. First, studies are needed to discover the extent to which legislatures are influenced by particular philosophical perspectives. Second, research is needed to determine whether the regulatory approaches adopted within particular countries reflect the attitudes and perceptions held by the general populace. Third, empirical research is often necessary to apply a philosophical perspective because, to take one example, the force of arguments for possession of vicarious moral status rests on empirical hypotheses.

On an analytic level, any deeper philosophical analysis must be conducted from particular philosophical positions rather than groups of philosophical positions. This is not to suggest that any further analysis must adopt one particular theory; we merely suggest that further analysis would be most profitably directed at exploring the implications of particular philosophical positions one at a time, and, indeed, we are jointly and individually currently undertaking this task with regard to Alan Gewirth's Principle of Generic Consistency *(PGC)*.[221] As we have argued elsewhere, *in its application,* this rights-based theory grants intrinsic moral status to beings that are possible agents (see Beyleveld and Pattinson 1998 and 2000),[222] and, as a result, belongs to the 'compromise' camp.[223]

There are many moral issues raised by assisted reproduction, genetic diagnosis, and gene therapy, which will be addressed differently by different moral theories.

One issue is whether there is a moral right to reproduce, and if so, what the strength of this right is and whether it includes a right of access to medically assisted reproduction.[224] There is also an issue about whether any such right is purely negative (i.e., imposing duties of non-interference only) or is also positive (i.e., imposing duties of assistance). This issue is important for determining whether access to assisted reproduction ought to be provided by the state.

Another issue requiring consideration rests on the claim that PGD is superior to PND because it avoids the thorny and emotive issue of abortion (see Beyleveld 1999). The validity of such a claim will depend on, *inter alia*, the legitimacy of abortion, the moral status of the oocyte and pre-implantation embryo, and the weight given to the fact that PGD makes it easier to influence the characteristics of one's offspring and more difficult to prevent parents acting for certain motives.

In fact, all of the techniques under discussion enable parents to influence the characteristics of their offspring. This raises the question of whether it is morally legitimate to deliberately manipulate the characteristics of one's offspring before its birth and, if so, whether this applies to all characteristics or is dependent on whether the characteristic is relevant to the possession of intrinsic moral status. Further, there is also the question whether the moral legitimacy of a parental preference for or against characteristics that are irrelevant to the possession of intrinsic moral status is dependent on the characteristic in question. For example, is it relevant that some characteristics—such as Down syndrome and Huntington's disease—hinder the future offspring's range of future purposes without affecting the offspring's possession of intrinsic moral status by virtue of being human, sentient, or an agent?[225] Also, does it matter whether the characteristic in question can be treated, or influenced by other means, such as education, after birth?

Techniques that have yet to be performed on humans, such as cloning by nuclear substitution and germ-line gene therapy, raise other issues. For example, is it morally permissible to attempt to clone a human by somatic cell nuclear transfer given that it took 277 failed attempts to clone Dolly? Is it morally permissible to attempt germ-line gene therapy on humans given the difficulties highlighted by the 'Beltseville pig' incident, where the genetic switch that was supposed to trigger the production of growth hormone was permanently switched on, resulting in an obese pig with many disorders? In short, the question is: how efficient does a technique have to be before it can legitimately be applied to create a human child?

Given the number of issues evoked by these techniques, it is not surprising to find that the EU displays such great divisions. Indeed, it is surprising to find any consensus at all.

Notes

[1]   We gratefully acknowledge the help that we received in compiling information on the relevant laws. We are especially grateful to Hille Haker (Zentrum für Ethik in den Wissenschaften, Universität Tübingen) who put a great deal of time and effort into making contacts and collating information on our behalf. Although space prevents us from acknowledging all those who helped, we would particularly like to thank Denis Cusack (Division of Legal Medicine, University College Dublin), Gilda Ferrando (Dípartimento di Diritto dell' Economia d dell' Impresa, Facultá di Economia), Tina Garanis-Papadatos (Athens School of Public Health, University of Athens), Jennifer Gunning (Cardiff Law School, University of Wales), Ramio Lahti (Faculty of Law, University of Helsinki), Salla Lötjönen (Faculty of Law, University of Helsinki), Joâo Carlos Loureiro (Centro de Direito Biomèdico, Universidade de Coimbra), Annamari Hynninen (Faculty of Law, University of Helsinki), Amelia Martín-Uranga (University of Deusto), Sabine Michalowski (Sheffield Institute of Biotechnological Law and Ethics, Sheffield University), Dietmar Mieth (Zentrum für Ethik in den Wissenschaften, Universität Tübingen), Roberto Mordacci (Unità di Etica e Filosofia, Università Vita-Salute San Raffaele), Linda Nielsen (University of Copenhagen), Guido Pennings (Free University of Brussels); Paul Schotsmans (Centrum voor Bio-Medische Ethiek en Recht, Leuven), Nina Schultz-Lorentzen (Institute of Law, University of Copenhagen), Ghislaine van Thiel (Centre for Bioethics and Heath Law, Utrecht), and Guido de Wert (Instituut voor Gezondheitsethiek, Maastrict). We also like to thank those who wrote reports, either in a language other than English or on non-EU countries, which we were unable to utilise in this report, including Janusz Balicki (Academy of Catholic Theology, Warsaw), Hans-Georg Koch (Maximum-Planck-Institut für Straftrecht, Freiburg), Josef Kure (Institute of Bioethics, Brno), Alex Mauron (Bioethics Research and Teaching Unit, Geneva Medical School, Centre Médical Universítaire), Judit Sándor (Central European University Budapest), and Günter Virt (Institut für Ethik in der Medizin, Wien). Needless to say we are responsible for any errors and omissions.

2   See Bernat 1993, p. 494; and MacKellar 1997, p. 2; and Gunning and English 1993, p. 147.

3   See Bernat 1993, p. 496; MacKellar 1997, p. 2; Schenker 1997, p. 176; and Gunning and English 1993, p. 147.

4   See Gunning and English 1993, p. 147.

5   See Gunning and English 1993, p. 147; and Bernat 1993, p. 496.

6   See Gunning and English 1993, p. 148. Article 318(4) of the Civil Code does, however, state that a husband cannot dispute his paternity if he has consented to artificial insemination or 'any other act aimed at procreation', except when the conception of a child is not the consequence of such an activity (Schotsmans 1998, p. 1).

7   Information provided by Guido Pennings.

8   Information provided by Nina Schultz-Lorentzen.

9   See Gunning 1998, p. 99.

10   See Nielsen 1996a, p. 310, and Nielsen 1997, p. 127. However, see Schenker 1997, p. 176 for a conflicting view.

11   Information provided by Nina Schultz-Lorentzen.

12   Information provided by Nina Schultz-Lorentzen.

13   Assisted reproduction is, however, subject to the general legislation on health services, which means that only authorised medical personnel can carry out fertilisation treatments (see Hynninen 1998, p. 5).

14   Proposed by a working group report given to the Ministry of Justice in 1997 (see Hynninen 1998, p. 5). The proposed bill has not been introduced into the Parliament and the project has been taken back to the Ministry for re-evaluation following the parliamentary elections in March. (Information provided by Salla Lötjönen.)

15   See Hynninen 1998, p. 5.

16   See Schenker 1997, p. 176. However, a decision was made in May 1999 to prepare legislation that would allow homosexual couples to register their relationship, which might lead to a more liberal attitude towards homosexual couples in the future. (Information provided by Salla Lötjönen.)

17   See Hynninen 1998, p. 5.

18   See Lansac 1996, p. 1843; and Gunning 1998, p. 99.

19   See Lansac 1996, p. 1843; Schenker 1997, p. 176; and Gunning 1998, p. 99.

20   See Latham 1998a, p. 95; and Lansac 1996, p. 1843.

21   See Lansac 1996, p. 1843. 'Confused' artificial insemination (with sperm from more than one man) is forbidden (Article 673-3), donor insemination is allowed only as a 'last resort' (Article 152-6), and donated embryos can only be used 'exceptionally' for couples who cannot conceive without a donor (Article 152-5) (see Sutton 1996, especially p. 43).

22   Information provided by Sabine Michalowski.

23   Information provided by Sabine Michalowski.

24 See Garanis-Papadatos 1998, p. 1; Gunning and English 1993, p. 172; and
    Nielsen 1996a, p. 309.
25 See Schenker 1997, p. 176.
26 See MacKellar 1997, p. 17.
27 See MacKellar 1997, p. 17.
28 See MacKellar 1997, p. 17; and Schenker 1997, p. 176.
29 See, MacKellar 1997, p. 18; Nielsen 1996a, p. 309; Nielsen 1996b, p. 332; and
    Gunning and English 1993, p. 155.
30 The latest proposal is the unified text of 27 January 1998, which has been
    drawn up by the Commission for Social Affairs of the Chamber of Deputies
    (see Ferrando 1998, p. 4).
31 See Ferrando 1998, p. 2; and Schenker 1997, p. 176.
    We would like to thank Roberto Mordacci for expanding our understanding of
    this Code.
32 See Ferrando 1998, p. 2; Gunning and English 1993, p. 155; and MacKellar
    1997, p. 18.
33 See Nielsen 1996a, p. 309.
34 As translated by Ferrando Article 5 grants access to

      adult couples of different genders, married or living in stable conditions,
      with a potentially fertile age and, however, not older than fifty-two.
      (Ferrando 1998, p. 4)

35 See Ferrando 1998, pp. 4–5.
36 Gunning and English 1993, p. 157.
37 See Schenker 1997, p. 174.
38 See Health Council of the Netherlands 1997, especially p. 1 and p. 71.
39 See Health Council of the Netherlands 1997, p. 14; and Schenker 1997, p. 174.
40 See Health Council of the Netherlands 1997, p. 14 and p. 71.
41 However, Decree-Law No. 319/86 of 25 September 1986, covers the
    collection, manipulation, and preservation of sperm. (See Oliveira 1996,
    p. 68.)
42 See National Council of Ethics for the Life Sciences 1997c.
43 Information provided Joâo Carlos Loureiro.
44 It was challenged by the Popular party on enactment.

      It was contested that the law was unconstitutional because although it
      addressed matters of human rights it had not been made an organic law
      but had been enacted as ordinary law. (Gunning and English 1993, p. 164)

    See also, Gunning 1998, p. 100; and Nielsen 1996a, p. 309. It now appears
    that implementation of the Act has begun. (Information provided by Jennifer
    Gunning.)
45 See Gunning 1998, p. 101.

[46] See Sutton 1996, pp. 44–45; Nielsen 1997, p. 130; MacKellar 1997, p. 27; Schenker 1997, p. 176; and Gunning and English 1993, p. 164.

[47] See MacKellar 1997, p. 27.

[48] The Human Fertilisation and Embryology Act 1990 extends to Northern Ireland (except s. 37 amending the Abortion Act 1967): s. 48.

[49] See Latham 1998a, p. 94.

[50] The financial burdens placed on those seeking access should also be noted. In the UK, provision of assisted reproductive services by health authorities is given a low priority, so that only two clinics are wholly funded by the NHS. It has been suggested that, as a result,

> Many couples are having to remortgage their homes to pay for treatment. (Latham 1998a, p. 94)

Clearly, this means that financial means act as *de facto* eligibility criteria for many couples. This is to be contrasted with the situation in France, where couples who fulfil the legislative eligibility criteria 'will be able to be treated regardless of income for in France treatment for "sterility" is fully reimbursed by the State' (Latham 1998a p. 96). Similarly, in Germany, social security covers IVF for up to three attempts for married couples (Nielsen 1996a, p. 311).

[51] The French legislation also prevents post-mortem insemination.

[52] Part 3 of the HFEA's Code of Practice provides detailed guidance for centres on this requirement to consider the welfare of the child.

[53] There are two sections of Law No. 460 dealing with information and consent in relation to assisted reproduction generally. However, these provisions are not concerned with eligibility as such. (Information provided by Nina Schultz-Lorentzen.)

[54] See Ferrando 1998. In fact

> [d]uring the legislative period which ended in 1992, there were 100 bills concerning the regulation of Reproductive Technology, not one of which has been passed into law. (Nielsen 1996, p. 337)

[55] See Kriari-Catranis 1997, p. 58; and Gunning and English 1993, p. 147 and p. 171.

[56] See Kriari-Catranis 1997, p. 58; and Gunning and English 1993, p. 148 and p. 171.

[57] See Bernat 1993, p. 501.

[58] See, for example, Gunning and English 1993, p. 148.

[59] See Schotsmans 1998.

[60] See Gunning and English 1993, p. 148 and p. 172.

[61] See Schenker 1997, p. 181. For a wider discussion, see Gunning and English 1993, p. 148.

62 Information provided by Guido Pennings.
63 See MacKellar 1997, p. 6; EGE 1998a, p. 3; Nielsen 1996b, p. 329; and Gunning and English 1993, p. 172.
64 See MacKellar 1997, p. 6.
65 See Gunning and English 1993, p. 151; MacKellar 1997, p. 6; and Nielsen 1996a, p. 140.
66 See Kriari-Catranis 1997, p. 58; and Gunning and English 1993, p. 151.
67 See MacKellar 1997, p. 6.
68 This Act was enacted on 9 April 1999, and comes into force on 1 November 1999. (Information provided by Raimo Lahti.) It was based primarily on the report prepared by a Working Party on Medical Research on Humans, Human Embryos and Fetuses in 1994. On the wider implications of this report, see Lötjönen 1998. See also Hynninen 1998; and EGE 1998a, p. 3.
69 See Lötjönen 1999, p. 1.
70 See Lansac 1996; and EGE 1998a, p. 3.
71 See Lansac 1996, p. 1846; Nielsen 1996b, p. 329; and Latham 1998b, p. 236.
72 The Comité National d'Ethique (National Committee of Reproductive Medicine, Biology and Antenatal Diagnosis) advises the Minister of Health on which clinics to license. (See Lansac 1996, especially p. 1846.). See also, EGE 1998a, p. 3; Nielsen 1996b, p. 329; and Latham 1998b, p. 236.
73 See MacKellar 1997, p. 9.
74 See MacKellar 1997, p. 9; and EGE 1998a, p. 3.
75 See EGE 1998a, p. 3.
76 See Gunning and English 1993, p. 154; and EGE 1998a, p. 4.
77 See Gunning and English 1993, p. 154; Sutton 1996, p. 43; EGE 1998a, p. 4; Bernat 1993, p. 501; Kriari-Catranis 1997, p. 5; and Schenker 1997, p. 181.
78 See Bernat 1993, p. 501.
79 See Garanis-Papadatos 1998, p. 1; Gunning and English 1993, p. 172; and Schenker 1997, p. 180.
80 See MacKellar 1997, p. 17; and *Attorney General v X* [1992] 1. I.R 1.
81 The Eighth Amendment to the Irish Constitution is quoted in the text following table 2.1.
82 See MacKellar 1997, p. 17.
83 See MacKellar 1997, p. 17.
84 See Ferrando 1998, pp. 4–5.
85 See MacKellar 1997, p. 18.
86 See Ferrando 1998, p. 4.
87 See Gunning and English 1993, p. 172. The EGE Secretariat appears to be mis-informed as it states that the 'Dutch legislation forbids any research on embryos' (EGE 1998a, p. 5).
88 Information provided by Ghislaine van Thiel.
89 See Health Council of the Netherlands 1997.

[90] Information provided by Ghislaine van Thiel.

[91] See Oliveira 1996, p. 68.

[92] See National Council of Ethics for the Life Sciences 1995, especially p. 10.

[93] See Gunning 1998, p. 100. It now appears that implementation of the Act has begun. (Information provided by Jennifer Gunning).

[94] See MacKellar 1997, p. 25.

[95] See Sutton 1996, p. 45; and Gunning and English 1993, p. 164 and p. 173.

[96] See Sutton 1996, p. 45.

[97] See Sutton 1996, p. 45; and Gunning and English 1993, p. 164 and p. 173.

[98] See Sutton 1996, p. 45.

[99] See Gunning and English 1993, p. 164.

[100] Information provided by Hille Haker.

[101] Information provided by Hille Haker.

[102] See HGAC & HFEA 1998b, Annexe E.

[103] Information provided by Nina Schultz-Lorentzen. See also, HGAC & HFEA 1998b, Annexe E; and UNESCO 1998, p. 10.

[104] See UNESCO 1998, p. 10; and HGAC & HFEA 1998b, Annexe E.

[105] See Lötjönen 1999, p. 1.

[106] See HGAC & HFEA 1998b, Annexe E.

[107] See HGAC & HFEA 1998b, Annexe E.

[108] See UNESCO 1998, p. 10.

[109] See HGAC & HFEA 1998b, Annexe E.

[110] See HGAC & HFEA 1998b, Annexe E; and UNESCO 1998, p. 10.

> Anyone who artificially creates a human embryo with the same genetic information as another embryo, a fetus, an adult human being or a deceased person, will be punished by a term of imprisonment up to five years or by a fine. (Translated in Winter 1997, p. 191)

[111] Information provided by Hille Haker.

[112] See Dalla-Vorgia 1996, p. 281.

[113] Sheikh states that somatic cell nuclear transfer might be affected by the Control of Clinical Trials Act 1987 and the Control of Clinical Trials and Drugs Act 1990, if they are not 'too vague in their nature to include the procedure' (1997, p. 95).

[114] See UNESCO 1998, p. 10.

[115] Information provided by Roberto Mordacci.

[116] See UNESCO 1998, p. 10.

[117] See UNESCO 1998, p. 10.

[118] Information provided by Ghislaine van Thiel.

[119] Information provided by Ghislaine van Thiel.

[120] By implication, see National Council of Ethics for the Life Sciences 1997b, p. 2.

265

[121] See National Council of Ethics for the Life Sciences 1997b, p. 2.

[122] Title V of the Penal Code is translated in Lacadena 1996.

[123] See UNESCO 1998, p. 11; and HGAC & HFEA 1998b, Annexe E.

[124] See the text following Table 3.

[125] We use this definition of cloning throughout. Thus, when we claim that certain countries prohibit cloning we are claiming only that they prohibit techniques involving the deliberate creation of a human being that is genetically identical to another human being or has the same nuclear gene set as another human being.

[126] See the original 'Dolly paper': Wilmut *et al.* 1997. When this paper was published some commentators suggested that Dolly's DNA might have been derived from a 'stem cell', rather than a somatic cell as such. However, this suggestion has been dispelled by the successful cloning of two calves, and 50 mice at two different institutions.

[127] In a jointly written consultation document they state

> [t]he nuclear substitution of an embryo, or any cell whilst it forms part of the embryo is expressly prohibited by the HFE Act. Embryo splitting and nuclear replacement of eggs are not expressly prohibited, but as both involve the use or creation of embryos outside the body, they fall within the HFE Act and therefore come under the jurisdiction of the HFEA. (HGAC & HFEA 1998a, paragraph. 5.2, p. 10)

And in the final report they state

> [t]he Department of Health and the HFEA have taken Counsel's advice on this issue. As a result, both Ministers and the Authority reject this position and are content that the Act does allow the HFEA to regulate nuclear replacement into an unfertilised egg through its licensing system. (HGAC & HFEA 1998b, paragraph 3.4)

[128] Quoted in Science and Technology Committee 1997, p. xii.

[129] This has lead the House of Commons Select Committee on Science and Technology to declare

> [i]t is not satisfactory for issues as momentous as this to be left until they are decided through test cases. We recommend that the Human Fertilisation and Embryology Act should be amended to ensure that the Roslin technique [i.e., the Dolly technique] comes within its scope. (Select Committee for Science and Technology 1997, p. xii)

[130] See also, HGAC & HFEA 1998b, paragraph 3.8, and paragraph 9.2.

[131] However, the HGAC & HFEA have recommended that the UK government consider explicitly banning reproductive cloning using any technique (see HGAC & HFEA 1998b, paragraph 9.2).

[132] Jürgen Simon expands upon this point in his commentary on this report, and argues that the German EPA has at least one other flaw.

[133] The European Convention on Human Rights and Biomedicine opened for signature on 4.4.97, and its additional protocol opened for signature on 12.1.98. The ten EU countries that are signatories are Denmark, Finland, France, Greece, Italy, Luxembourg, the Netherlands, Portugal, Spain, and Sweden. Belgium has not signed it because of the dissensus within public opinion (see Schotsmans 1998, p. 2). Germany has not signed it because it considers it to be too lax, while the UK considers it to be too restrictive.

[134] Provisions implicitly prohibiting cloning include Article 1, which requires parties to the Convention to 'protect the dignity and identity of all human beings', and Article 18, which states that the creation of human embryos for research purposes is prohibited.

These provisions are important, because it is possible to sign the Convention without signing the protocol. Should a country, such as the UK, which has pre-existing laws on cloning, not wish to prohibit cloning it can make a reservation to these provisions of the Convention by invoking Article 36.

[135] Information provided by Ghislaine van Thiel.

[136] Moreover, the European Commission's former 'Group of Advisers on the Ethical Implications of Biotechnology' has condemned cloning, and so has the World Health Assembly (see HGAC & HFEA 1998b, paragraph 7.2). Jürgen Simon, in his commentary on this report, also points to the European Parliament's March 1997 resolution.

[137] This Declaration was unanimously adopted by the General Conference on 11 November 1997 (see UNESCO 1998).

[138] It might be argued that the disincentive is minimal, because the results of any investment can be protected by other intellectual property mechanisms, such as breach of confidence. However, patent protection has particular appeal to commercial organisations and the condemnatory nature of the political will behind the Directive is itself a disincentive.

[139] See Kriari-Catranis 1998, p. 53.

[140] See Rendtorff 1998, especially p. 83.

[141] See Lötjönen 1999, p. 2.

[142] See MacKellar 1997, p. 9.

[143] See Sutton 1996, p. 44.

[144] See Gunning 1998, p. 100. It now appears that implementation of the Act has begun. (Information provided by Jennifer Gunning.)

[145] See Sutton 1996, p. 45; and Gunning and English 1993, p. 164.

[146] The Declaration also declares that all procedures affecting an individual's genome should only be undertaken after 'rigorous and prior assessment of the potential risks and benefits' (Article 5(a)).

[147] See also conclusion 6 of the Bilbao declaration, which declares that,

267

Until scientific advances so allow, and as the exact functions of even one gene are not known, it is prudent to establish a moratorium on the alternation of germinal cells. (Bilbao Declaration 1994, p. 5)

[148] The term 'embryo' is not defined under the Austrian legislation. (See EGE 1998b).

[149] There is, however, a Higher Council on Human Genetics established under the Crown Order of 7 November 1973 (see Schotsmans 1998, p. 2).

[150] See Schotsmans 1998, p. 2.

[151] Information provided by Nina Schultz-Lorentzen.

[152] Information provided by Salla Lötjönen.

[153] See Schenker 1997, p. 178.

[154] See Hynninen 1998, pp. 5–6.

[155] See Viville *et al.* 1998, p. 1022. This still appears to be true. (Information provided by Jennifer Gunning.)

[156] See Viville *et al.* 1998, p. 1022.

[157] See MacKellar 1997, p. 10.

[158] See MacKellar 1997, p. 10.

[159] See Garanis-Papadatos 1998, p. 2.

[160] See Garanis-Papadatos 1998, p. 2.

[161] See Schenker 1997, p. 178.

[162] See Health Council of the Netherlands 1997, p. 31.

[163] See MacKellar 1997, p. 27.

[164] For a more detailed discussion of the German position vis-à-vis the regulation of PGD, see Jürgen Simon's commentary following this report.

[165] However, according to information provided by Hille Haker, some scientists hold that on the third day (when biopsies for PGD are usually made) no totipotent cells exist; others, such as Regine Kollek, consider the cells totipotent at the 6–10 cell stage.

[166] See also Fasouliotis 1998, p. 2242. It appears that this is still the situation in France. (Information provided by Jennifer Gunning.)

[167] S. 1 of Act 35 of November 1988. S. 12(1) explicitly authorises PGD to test for hereditary diseases in order to treat them or advise against transfer to the womb.

[168] See Mandry 1998, p. 34; and Nentwich 1997.

[169] Information provided by Hille Haker.

[170] See Moulin 1996, p. 27.

[171] See Petersen 1996, p. 79. Called the Abortion Act by Nielsen 1997, p. 132.

[172] Information provided by Nina Schultz-Lorentzen.

[173] See MacKellar 1997, p. 3.

[174] See MacKellar 1997, p. 5; Nielsen 1997, p. 132; and Moulin 1996, p. 27.

[175] Information provided by Nina Schultz-Lorentzen.

176 See Rendtorff 1998, especially p. 83.
177 See MacKellar 1997, p. 7.
178 See Lansac 1996, p. 1847. For more detailed discussion of Decree No. 97-578, see Jürgen Simon's commentary which follows this report.
179 See Sutton 1996, p. 43.
180 See MacKellar 1997, p. 8; and Lansac 1996, p. 1847.
181 See Lansac 1996, p. 1847.
182 Information provided by Sabine Michalowski.
183 Under the previous law, abortion was permitted for medical indications including hereditary diseases. This provision was removed because it was thought to have eugenic implications. (Information obtained from Schoenke and Schroeder 1997, and Sabine Michalowski.)
184 Information obtained from the same sources as above.
185 See Dalla-Vorgia 1988, p. 4; and Commission of the European Communities 1995.
186 See Dalla-Vorgia 1988, p. 4.
187 See Dalla-Vorgia 1988, p. 3.
188 See Dalla-Vorgia 1988, p. 3.
189 See Commission of the European Communities 1995; and MacKellar 1997, p. 15.
190 See Dalla-Vorgia 1988, p. 4.
191 As Finlay CJ put it,

> I . . . conclude that the proper test to be applied is that if it is established as a matter of probability that there is a real and substantial risk to the life, as distinct from the health, of the mother, which can only be avoided by the termination of her pregnancy, such termination is permissible, having regard to the true interpretation of Article 40, s. 3, sub-s. 3 of the Constitution [as inserted by the Eighth Amendment to the Constitution]. (*Attorney General v X* [1992] 1 I. R. 1, pp. 53–54)

The 'real and substantial risk to the life' of the mother was held to include the risk of suicide, so that on the facts of *AG v X* the fourteen year old girl, X, was permitted to travel to England for an abortion.

   On abortion in Ireland, see also Madden 1997, p. 103; MacKellar 1997, p. 17; and Rendtorff 1998, p. 101.
192 Information provided by Roberto Mordacci.
193 See MacKellar 1997, p. 18.
194 See MacKellar 1997, p. 19.
195 See Health Council of the Netherlands 1997, p. 50; and Van Thiel 1996, p. 103.
196 See MacKellar 1997, p. 20.
197 Information provided by João Carlos Loureiro.

198 See Gabarrón *et al.* 1997, p. 68.
199 See Gabarrón *et al.* 1997, p. 68.
200 See Loureiro 1996, p. 87; and information provided by Joâo Carlos Loureiro.
201 See MacKellar 1997, p. 23, and information provided by Joâo Carlos Loureiro.
202 See Gabarrón *et al.* 1997, p. 68; and MacKellar 1997, p. 25.
203 See Gabarrón *et al.* 1997, p. 68.
204 See MacKellar 1997, p. 27. For the position under the previous Abortion Act 1974, see Sutton 1996, p. 4.
205 See MacKellar 1997, p. 28.
206 Neither s. 37 of the Human Fertilisation and Embryology Act 1990 nor the Abortion Act 1967, extend to Northern Ireland. See s. 48 Human Fertilisation and Embryology Act 1990, and s. 7(3) Abortion Act 1967, respectively.
207 This is not to suggest that diagnosis of a serious non-genetic condition cannot legitimate abortion under the legislation of these countries.
208 In Sweden, abortion following PND is given no special status under the law.
209 See Beyleveld 'The Moral Status of the Human Embryo and Fetus', in this volume.
210 See below.
211 Vicarious moral status can also increase the protection granted to the embryo-fetus by the 'compromise' position. The effect that vicarious considerations have on the 'pro-life' position is more complex. This depends on the underpinning moral theory. If the 'pro-life' position is underpinned by a deontological moral theory, vicarious considerations can be ignored because the embryo-fetus already has the maximum moral status possible (i.e., full intrinsic moral status). However, if the 'pro-life' position is underpinned by a position which applies an aggregate calculus (such as utilitarianism), the derivative considerations can be decisive in determining our obligations towards the embryo-fetus.
212 See Beyleveld 1999 for a number of vicarious arguments that can be used to grant protection to the embryo-fetus.
213 We are, of course, aware that the possibility of a utilitarian position granting full moral status to the embryo-fetus from conception introduces a level of complexity that our line diagram largely ignores.
214 Even the title of the German Act, the 'Embryo Protection Act', suggests a 'pro-life' position.
215 One apparent problem with grounding the 'pro-life' position is that none of the possible grounds seem to appear at conception unless they are defined in an almost question-begging way.
216 The 'pro-life' position is defined as granting full moral status to the embryo-fetus from the moment of conception. Either this is to be redefined as granting full moral status from at least the moment of conception, or the ground for

such status (whether it is being human or a potential person/agent) cannot be perceived as applying to the unfertilised gamete.

[217] The National Council is a statutory body set up under Law No. 14/90 of 9 June 1990.

[218] Exclusion of GIFT using non-donated gametes in the UK Act is particularly interesting because GIFT involves more health risks to the mother than IVF (see Health Council of the Netherlands 1997, p. 30).

[219] The exclusion of non-heterosexual couples cannot be based on the moral interests of the embryo-fetus, because it is not even plausible to claim that only heterosexual couples make good parents. For example, one study found that the children of single mothers do not suffer from parental failure any more than other children; at most they suffer from the consequences of social and financial problems faced by most single mothers (see Golombok and Rust 1986, especially p. 182). Moreover,

> [t]he only British study in this area (which supports similar studies in the U.S.) [Golombok, Spencer, and Rutter 1983, 55] reports no statistically significant differences in psychiatric state between children with lesbian or heterosexual mothers and the incidence of disorder was similar to that found in heterosexual two-parent families. (Madden 1996, p. 16)

[220] As we pointed out above, the French legislation appears to be inconsistent because it prohibits non-therapeutic embryo research but permits PGD. However, unlike Austria and Germany, the French legislation has adopted an approach that is consistent between PGD and PND.

[221] Gewirth (1978) presents the argument to the *PGC,* which is defended against objections published up to 1990 in Beyleveld 1991.

[222] See also Beyleveld 'The Moral Status of the Human Embryo and Fetus' in this volume.

[223] See Beyleveld ibid. Also, on the application of the *PGC*, see Beyleveld, Quarrell, and Toddington 1997.

[224] For a discussion of this issue from a Gewirthian perspective, see Pattinson 1998.

[225] See Beyleveld, Quarrell, and Toddington 1997 for a Gewirthian perspective on some of the issues raised by this question.

References

Bacik, I. (1997), 'Abortion—Conflicting Rights, Duties and Arguments', *Medico-Legal Journal of Ireland*, pp. 82–84.

Bernat, E. (1993), 'Between Rationality and Metaphysics: The Legal Regulation of Assisted Reproduction in Germany, Austria and Switzerland—A Comparative Analysis', *Medical Law*, Vol. 12, pp. 493–505.

Beyleveld, D. (1991), *The Dialectical Necessity of Morality: An Analysis and Defense of Alan Gewirth's Argument to the Principle of Generic Consistency*, Chicago University Press: Chicago.

Beyleveld, D. (1998), 'The Moral and Legal Status of the Human Embryo', in Hildt, E. and Mieth, D. (eds), *In Vitro Fertilisation in the 1990s: Towards a Medical, Social and Ethical Evaluation*, Ashgate: Aldershot, pp. 247–260.

Beyleveld, D. (1999), 'Does Preimplantation Diagnosis Solve the Moral Problems of Prenatal Diagnosis? A Rights-Analysis', in Hildt, E. and Graumann, S. (eds), *Genetics in Human Reproduction*, Ashgate: Aldershot.

Beyleveld, D. and Pattinson, S. (1998), *Proportionality under Precaution: Justifying Duties to Apparent Non-agents*, unpublished paper. (Available from the authors.)

Beyleveld, D. and Pattinson, S. (2000), 'Precautionary Reasoning as a Link to Moral Action', forthcoming in Boylan, M. (ed.), *Medical Ethics*, Prentice-Hall: Englewood Cliffs N.J.

Beyleveld, D., Quarrell, O. and Toddington, S. (1997), 'Generic Consistency in the Reproductive Enterprise', *Medical Law International*, Vol. 3, pp. 135–158.

Bilbao Declaration (1996), 'International Workshop on the Legal Aspects of the Human Genome Project. Bilbao Declaration', *Law and the Human Genome Review*, Vol. 1 (July-December), pp. 205–209.

Commission of the European Communities (1995), *EC Working Group on Human Embryos and Research*, Office for Official Publications of the European Communities: Luxembourg.

Dalla-Vorgia, P. (1988), 'Greek Reply to the Questionnaire: Unofficial Reply', *Working Party on Genetic Screening of the Ad Hoc Committee of Experts on Progress in Biomedical Sciences (CAHBI-GS-GT)*, Council of Europe: Strasbourg.

Dalla-Vorgia, P. (1996), 'Assisted Reproduction in Greece', in Evans, D. (ed.), *Creating the Child*, Martinus Nijoff Publishers: The Hague, pp. 279–286.

EGE (European Group on Ethics in Science and New Technologies) (1998a), *Overview on Member States Legislations Concerning Human Embryo Research*, unpublished.

EGE (1998b), Opinion of the European Group on Ethics in Science and New Technologies to the European Communities: *Ethical Aspects of Research Involving the Use of Human Embryo in the Context of the 5th Framework Programme*, 23 November, Vol. 12, pp. 1–24.

Fasouliotis, S. J. and Schenker, J. G. (1998), 'Preimplantation Genetic Diagnosis Principles and Ethics', *Human Reproduction*, Vol. 13., No. 8, pp. 2238–2245.

Ferrando, G. (1998), *Assisted Reproduction in Italy: The Current Legal Situation*, unpublished Report prepared for the European Network for Biomedical Ethics.

Gabarrón, J. and Ramos, C. (1997), 'Prenatal Diagnosis in Spain', *European Journal of Human Genetics*, Vol. 5 (Supplement 1), pp. 64–69.

Garanis-Papadatos, T. and Dalla-Vorgia, P. (1998), *Greece: Some Information Regarding Regulation of Genetics in Human Reproduction*, unpublished report from Greece prepared for the European Network for Biomedical Ethics.

Golombok, S. and Rust, J. (1986), 'The Warnock Report and Single Women: What About the Children?', *Journal of Medical Ethics*, Vol. 12, pp. 182–186.

Golombok,S., Spencer, A., and Rutter, M. (1983), 'Children in Lesbian and Single Parent Households, a Psychosexual and Psychiatric Appraisal', Journal of Child Psychology and Psychiatry, Vol. 24, pp. 551–572.

Gunning, J. (1998), 'Oocyte Donation: The Legislative Framework in Western Europe', *Human Reproduction*, Vol. 13., No. 2, pp. 98–102.

Gunning, J. and English, V. (1993), *Human In Vitro Fertilization: A Case Study in the Regulation of Medical Innovation*, Dartmouth Publishing Company Limited: Aldershot.

Health Council of the Netherlands (1997), *In Vitro Fertilisation (IVF)*, Rijswijk.

HGAC & HFEA (Human Genetics Advisory Commission and Human Fertilisation and Embryology Authority) (1998a), *Cloning Issues in Reproduction, Science and Medicine: A Consultation Document*, January.

HGAC & HFEA (1998b), *Cloning Issues in Reproduction, Science, and Medicine*, December.

HFEA (Human Fertilisation and Embryology Authority) (1998), *Code of Practice*, Fourth Edition, Human Fertilisation and Embryology Authority: London.

Hynninen, A. *et al.* (1998), Unpublished Report on the Finnish legal position prepared for the European Network for Biomedical Ethics.

Kriari-Catranis, I. (1997), 'Embryo Research and Human Rights: An Overview of Developments in Europe', *European Journal of Health Law*, Vol. 4, pp. 43–67.

Lacadena, J. R. (1996), 'Genetic Manipulation Offences in Spain's New Penal Code: A Genetic Commentary', *Law and the Human Genome Review*, Vol. 5 (July-Dec), pp. 195–203.

Lansac, J. (1996), 'French Law Concerning Medically-assisted Reproduction', *Human Reproduction*, Vol. 11, No. 9, pp. 1843–1843.

Latham, M. (1998a), 'Regulating the New Reproductive Technologies: A Cross-channel Comparison', *Medical Law International*, Vol. 3, pp. 89–115.

Latham, M. (1998b), 'The French Parliamentary Guidelines of May 1997: Clarification or Fudge?', *Medical Law International*, Vol. 3, pp. 235–241.

Lötjönen, S. (1998), 'The Protection of Human Subjects in Medical Research in Finland', in Modeen, T. (eds), *Finnish National Reports to the XVth Congress of the International Academy of Comparative Law*, Finnish Lawyers' Publishing: Helsinki.

273

Lötjönen, S. (1999), Unpublished Report on the Finnish legal position prepared for the European Network for Biomedical Ethics.

Loureiro, J. C. (1996), 'Portugal II: Bioethical Legislation', *Biolaw in Europe: Basic Ethical Principles in Bioethics and Biolaw*, Centre for Ethics and Law: Copenhagen, pp. 71–90.

MacKellar, C. (1997), *Reproductive Medicine and Embryological Research: A European Handbook of Bioethical Legislation 1997–8*, European Bioethical Research: Edinburgh.

Madden, D. (1996), 'Legal Issues in Artificial Insemination', *Medico-Legal Journal of Ireland*, Vol. 12., No. 1, pp. 1–18.

Madden, D. (1997), '"Abortion and the Law"—Review and Commentary', *Medico-Legal Journal of Ireland*, pp. 103–105.

Mandry, C. (1998), 'European Legislation Concerning Reproductive Medicine and Research', *Biomedical Ethics*, Vol. 3, No. 1, pp. 33–34.

Moulin, M. (1996), 'Belgium: Federal Laws, Directives, and Regulation', *Biolaw in Europe: Basic Ethical Principles in Bioethics and Biolaw*, Centre for Ethics and Law: Copenhagen, pp. 27–29.

Mueller, S. (1997), 'Ethics and the Regulation of Preimplantation Diagnosis in Germany', *Eubios Journal of Asian and International Bioethics*, Vol. 7, pp. 5–6. (Also available at http://www.biol.tsukuba.ac.jp/~macer/EJ71/EJ7D.html.)

National Council of Ethics for the Life Sciences (Conselho Nacional de Ética Para as Cinêcia da Vida) (1995), *Report-Opinion on Experimentation on the Human Embryo* (15/CNECV/95), 4th October, Lisbon.

National Council of Ethics for the Life Sciences (1997a), *Report-Opinion on the Legislative Bills Relating to the Voluntary Interruption of Pregnancy,* (19/CNECV/97), 10th January, Lisbon.

National Council of Ethics for the Life Sciences (1997b), *Opinion on the Ethical Implications of Cloning,* (21/CNECV/97), 1st April, Lisbon.

National Council of Ethics for the Life Sciences (1997c), *Report on Draft Bill Concerning Medically-Assisted Procreation,* (23/CNEC/97), 29 July, Lisbon.

Nentwich, M. (1997), 'Flowering in the Shade', *Biolaw in Europe: Basic Ethical Principles in Bioethics and Biolaw*, Centre for Ethics and Law: Copenhagen, pp. 19–25.

Nielsen, L. (1996a), 'Legal Consensus and Divergence in Europe in the Area of Human Embryology—Room for Harmonisation?', in Evans, D. (ed.), *Creating the Child*, Martinus Nijoff Publishers: The Hague, pp. 305–324.

Nielsen, L. (1996b), 'Legal Consensus and Divergence in Europe in the Area of Human Embryology—Room for Harmonisation?', in Evans, D. (ed.), *Conceiving the Embryo*, Martinus Nijoff Publishers: The Hague, pp. 325–338.

Nielsen, L. (1997), 'Biolaw in Scandinavia: Assisted Procreation, DNA Testing, Organ Transplantation and Research on Human Beings in Denmark, Norway and Sweden', *Bioethics: From Ethics to Law, from Law to Ethics*, International

274

Colloquium, Lausanne, October 17–18, 1996, Swiss Institute of Comparative Law.

Oliveira, D. F. (1996), 'Bioethical Legislation', *Biolaw in Europe: Basic Ethical Principles in Bioethics and Biolaw*, Copenhagen: Centre for Ethics and Law, pp. 67–69.

Pattinson, S. (1998), *Access to Assisted Reproduction: Law, Morality, and Practice*, unpublished Thesis submitted for Master's Degree in Biotechnological Law and Ethics, Sheffield University.

Petersen, K. (1996), 'Abortion Laws: Comparative and Feminist Perspectives in Australia, England and the United States', *Medical Law International*, Vol. 2, pp. 22–105.

Rendtorff, J. D. (1998), *Basic Principles in European Bioethics and Biolaw: Autonomy, Dignity, Integrity, and Vulnerability*, draft report of the Biomed-II-Project, Centre for Ethics and Law in Nature and Society: Copenhagen.

Schenker, J. G. (1997), 'Assisted Reproduction in Europe: Legal and Ethical Aspects', *Human Reproduction Update*, Vol. 3, No. 2, pp. 173–184.

Schöne-Seifert, B. (1996), 'Germany: Laws, Directives, and Legal Practices', *Biolaw In Europe: Basic Ethical Principles In Bioethics and Biolaw*, Centre for Ethics and Law: Copenhagen, pp. 43–49.

Schoenke, A. and Schroeder, H. (1997), *Strafgesetzbuch*, 25th edition, C. H. Beck Verlag: Munich.

Schotsmans, P. (1998), *Medically Assisted Conception in Belgium: A Commentary on the Legal Framework*, unpublished report prepared for the European Network for Biomedical Ethics.

Science and Technology Committee (1997), *Fifth Report: The Cloning of Animals from Adult Cells*, Session 1996–1997, HC 373-I. The Stationary Office: London.

Sheikh, A. (1997), '"Time to Clone Around"—Human Cloning: A Brave New World Law, Medicine and Ethics', *Medico-Legal Journal of Ireland*, Vol. 3, No. 3, pp. 89–96.

Sutton, A. (1996), 'The British Law on Assisted Reproduction: A Liberal Law by Comparison with Many Other European Laws', *Ethics and Medicine*, Vol. 12, No. 2, pp. 41–45.

UNESCO (1998), *Reproductive Human Cloning: Ethical Questions*, (http://firewall.unesco.org/opi/eng/bio98/#legis).

Van Thiel, G. (1996) 'The Netherlands: National Laws and Directives', *Biolaw In Europe: Basic Ethical Principles In Bioethics and Biolaw*, Centre for Ethics and Law: Copenhagen, pp. 103–111.

Viville, S., Messaddeq, N., Flori, E. and Gerlinger, P. (1998), 'Preparing for Preimplantation Genetic Diagnosis in France', *Human Reproduction*, Vol. 13, No. 4, pp. 1022–1029.

Warnock, M. (1985), *A Question of Life: The Warnock Report on Human Fertilisation and Embryology*, Basil Blackwell: Oxford and New York.

(Originally published as *The Report of the Committee of Inquiry into Human Fertilisation and Embryology*, HMSO: London, 1994.)

Wilmut, I., Schnieke, A. E., McWhir, J., Kind, A. J. and Campbell, K. H. S. (1997), 'Viable Offspring Derived from Fetal and Adult Mammalian Cells', *Nature,* Vol. 385, pp. 812–813.

Winter, S. F. (1997), 'The Cornerstone for a Prohibition of Cloning Human Beings Laid Down in the European Convention on Human Rights and Biomedicine', *European Journal of Health Law,* Vol. 4, No. 2, pp. 189–193.

Comment: *The ethical and legal sense of medically assisted procreation*

Christian Byk

Procreating is not simply reproducing and ensuring the continuity of our species. Certainly, in that action of continuity there is already an anthropological sense. But beyond that, procreating is a manifestation of our culture, our identity, our individuality, relations that we establish with others, and the perception that we have of our future and the future of our descendants. As for the medical activity whose technical aspects are very much to the fore today in what is called 'artificial procreation' or 'medically assisted procreation', it has developed in a close and sometimes conflicting relationship with the society in which this practice is carried out and is acknowledged.

Medical assistance in procreation cannot, therefore, be only a medical practice that has its rules in the strict but exclusive respect for a tried technique. It has a legal and an ethical sense, because it is seen to be a medical act and is, above all, a social activity.

1 A medical act

Is what seems to be evident for practitioners and for those who consult them really evident? In what way do the 'new reproductive technologies' constitute a therapeutic act? Why should it be necessary that they be performed by a doctor? A therapeutic act? If medicine is the art of treating illness, where is the illness, where is the treatment?

Is there an illness? The doctor who receives these increasingly numerous people who suffer from disorders of the reproductive function will feel irritated, even aggressive, at this way of presenting things that seems both to denigrate his work and the reality of human suffering. And yet, shouldn't the jurist or, quite simply, anyone who is concerned that medicine—and doctors—continue to play a prominent role, and who sees this not only as a provision of services but is concerned to offer patients a minimum of fairness in access to health services, ask himself what illness and what conditions justify the implementation of these techniques?

What illness is it? Sterility or infertility is the most common justification for having recourse to medical assistance in procreation. However, some people do not hesitate to question whether the dysfunctioning of the reproductive function (always) constitutes an illness. If we accept the fact that medicine is an art that serves men living in society, we can consider that infertility might legitimately be defined as an illness.

But, once this justification has been admitted, the jurist sees other demands: there is the risk of transmitting serious and incurable genetic diseases, or even the so-called sexually transmitted diseases and in particular AIDS. Are the people concerned less worthy of consideration on the pretext that they can procreate. If they take risks: statistically, not all the children will be genetically affected nor will they be bearers of the AIDS virus. And what should we say about the people who can procreate today, but tomorrow—because they have a cancer and are undergoing chemotherapy—will no longer be able to do so? Finally, what shall we say about those who, because they are physically handicapped, have difficulty in procreating?

Often the choice is not easy: if having children constitutes an important part of our social life, to what extent should society and its health care system contribute to bringing this about when there is a problem due to illness? Under what conditions does illness (as a cause for access to medically assisted procreation) justify medical intervention?

A reminder that the diagnosis pronounced by the doctor should be real and persistent, that the prognosis should have a certain seriousness, seems to be an insult to medical practice. Yet, how often is recourse to medically assisted procreation in fact, through lack of experience or because it is fashionable, too rapid, and even unnecessary? Defining rules of conduct is the doctors' business and requires some time as these are new techniques.

This is true, but we should not open the way to abuse and thus provoke legislative intervention. Should it then be understood that, even when medically desirable, medically assisted procreation should only be an *ultima ratio* after other reasonable possibilities have been tried? No doubt, but here, too, there should be no excess and everything should be carefully considered and weighed up by the doctor in his relationship with a patient or a couple, since medically assisted procreation is not, strictly speaking, a 'treatment'.

Is there a treatment? Most often reproductive technology does not make the facts disappear that set everything in motion. This is the case with sterility caused by sexually transmitted diseases. Wouldn't it then be worthwhile to think about organising the prevention of these diseases? Moreover, in many cases, the causes of infertility remain unknown.

This is obviously also true for indications linked with the risk of transmitting an incurable genetic disorder. Not only does the cause of the disorder not disappear—except in the case of germ-line gene therapy, but the organisation of certain systematic screening programmes could even make us aware of the extent of some of these diseases. That raises, in any case, the question of the methodology with which, for certain risk groups, such screening should be carried out.

But isn't sometimes the 'treatment' worse in its consequences than the situation that it was supposed to relieve? Some people will remind us that, despite the precautions that can be taken, the risk of transmitting a serious disease to the child through a donation of sperm, even of infecting the mother if it is a viral disease, can never be totally removed. Does the desire for a child then justify the taking of a risk, even if it is calculated?

Although the percentage of genetic abnormalities in children born thanks to reproductive technology is in fact only slightly higher than for other children, the same cannot be said for the number of multiple pregnancies which, because of the practices connected with *in vitro* fertilisation, remains very high, and leads to risks or even after-effects for the mother and the children. We can add that these practices are at the root of a serious and paradoxical ethical problem: embryo reduction when the implantation of several embryos has been a success, going beyond the number of children desired.

Are these examples and observations too severe? No doubt, if one considers that each pregnancy obtained by reproductive technology will not, fortunately, give rise to all these issues and that if one of them arises, the disadvantages would, one hopes, be compensated for by the joy of the expected birth. However, the severity is not misplaced when a general analysis of practices sometimes shows a certain lack of mastery of the techniques, and even incompetence on the part of health care teams. This quite naturally leads to questions about the qualification of the practitioner: is he and should he be a doctor?

2 The act of a doctor

The medical act, even if is not therapeutic, is at least the act of a doctor. Does the procreation that is emphatically called 'medically assisted procreation' fit into this framework? And what role does its 'technicalness' leave for the doctor?

1. A technical and biological act. From the simplest (insemination) to the very complicated ICSI (Intra Cytoplasmic Sperm Injection, i.e., artificial

introduction of a spermatozoon into an ovum), assisted procreation is a technique or more precisely a group of techniques called 'new reproductive technology'. Most often it is even a technique of biologists or micromanipulators in which laboratory work plays an essential role, not only for developing the techniques but also for their applications. So, do we really need a doctor to insert the sperm or implant the embryo, just as Pasteur needed a doctor to insert his treatment into the bodies of the people who had been bitten by a rabid animal?

2. The role of the doctor. If it is not strictly justified by the 'technique', should the doctor's role be limited to legal respect for the medical monopoly? It seems to us that if there is a monopoly, it is because it gives a meaning to the relationship with the patient and it makes it possible to perceive the limits of the technique. Preserving the singular relationship between the doctor and the patient should not be something grandiloquent or paternalistic, but it should be a reminder of essential functions of the role of the doctor that medically assisted procreation greatly needs.

Listening to the patient of course means making a diagnosis and prognosis, then directing the patient according to his particular needs. But, bearing in mind the variety of the causes of infertility and the treatments that are on offer, it also means taking into account the whole body and the 'spirit', the psychology of the patient and even the couple. The doctor then is the confluence of multidisciplinary work.

Counselling the patient will first consist in informing him, clearly, loyally, and simply, so that he can make an informed decision that he will judge to be the best. That is obvious for genetic counselling for which it is well known that the doctor needs great tact and psychological skill. It is no less true for the techniques of the new reproductive technology, several of which could possibly be envisaged and all of which have advantages and disadvantages. And that is not to mention the aridity of the questions, the pressure of applications induced by publicity in the media, sometimes created by the doctors themselves and of which other doctors will be the 'victims'.

For precisely who will be better able than the doctor, i.e., the person to whom one entrusts the care of one's body, to deny, modulate, or interpret the hopes founded on a technology of which we cannot ask everything? Giving a glimpse of the limits of the technique means playing the difficult role of an intermediary between research, which is perpetually developing in the public's view, and its applications, which require time. This role has to be filled by the doctor, especially as the research biologist could be tempted—understandably—to propose to these couples who are waiting that they benefit 'immediately' from the new technologies that have never been applied to man and, it must be said, sometimes not even experimented with on animals.

This task belongs to the doctor, because he himself is subject to a rigorous deontology and acts within a legal framework that is increasingly often extremely regimented. The doctor will have the task of explaining and making the patient or the couple understand the legitimacy of the conditions that are imposed on the implementation of medically assisted procreation.

The 'commitment' that is required of the doctor cannot—this is the other facet of the key role that he plays in new reproductive technology—oblige him to implement technology that he judges to be contrary to his conscience.

So, medically assisted procreation requires medical intervention, although strictly speaking this is not a therapeutic act. Official recognition by society therefore plays an important part in medical assistance in procreation.

3 A social act

While the practice of medicine is subject to the effects of the society in which it is carried out, society too, by reacting to it is influenced by the role of medicine, in the way that some practices are socially qualified.

The 'medicalisation' of assisted procreation has contributed to the social and legal recognition of artificial insemination and *in vitro* fertilisation. As it has in this way been integrated into the 'social' realm, medically assisted procreation has, by assimilation, found its 'model', thus removing from its scope all practices that do not use the same 'referent'. However, in the eyes of some people it remains a symbolically ambiguous activity.

New reproductive technology *is* a medicalised social act. A reminder of history will allow us to grasp the capital role played by medicine in the social recognition of reproductive technology, since it has contributed to making an act that was contrary to good morals into one that is socially accepted.

Known as early as the 18th century, artificial insemination with 'donation' of sperm was developed in the second half of the 19th century by doctors. Lacking a 'laboratory technique', it had difficulty in concealing its rather doubtful nature. Or more precisely for moralists and jurists, there was no doubt that using donated sperm was doubly sinful: on the one hand, by bringing a third person into the couple to be the father of a child—wasn't this adultery?—and, on the other hand, because of the means of collecting the sperm that was morally reprehensible in the eyes of the Church.

Today, the third party is no longer a shadowy lover; he is an anonymous donor, objectively speaking, a prepared and frozen ejaculate or even, as symmetry is possible, an oocyte that has been punctured and then fused with a spermatozoon to become a frozen embryo. As for the method of collection, although for sperm it remains 'traditional', at least it takes place in the asepticised, and even distressing context of a hospital. The sin subsists, no doubt, but it is committed without pleasure. The act has thus been socialised to the point where medical assistance for procreation is the cause of 0.3 to 0.5% of births in the countries where it has become an accessible practice.

I would add that medically assisted procreation gets a lot of media attention. That covers of course the plentiful information now devoted to it by all types of media but it also means that the couples who turn to it agree to speak of their choice within the family circle, and even beyond.

What we can call rather hastily the 'evolution of morals', that is to say in this case the perception that men and women have of procreation, sexuality, family, the couple and the place of children, has no doubt facilitated the social legitimacy of new reproductive technology in leading to rapid changes in attitude, even if they correspond to a latent demand from patients. This is the case with the 'eradication' in Cyprus or Sicily of thalassaemia, which is made possible by genetic tests and antenatal diagnosis, which result in some people giving up a hoped-for marriage or others agreeing to perform a termination of pregnancy.

It can be said then that, in a way, medically assisted procreation has become an element of public health policy with regard to infertility, and even that it has been integrated into family policy. This accounts for the legal requirements that apply to its implementation.

4 The 'social model' of new reproductive technology

Once they have been 'socialised', the techniques of 'artificial procreation' lose their appearance of artificiality. More precisely, this appearance disappears thanks to the mask of a social reference, a family model that throws out of the field of reproductive technology anything that cannot be attached to that model.

The paradox—but its usefulness can be perfectly understood—is that to counterbalance this 'artificiality', the official recognition of medically assisted procreation is generally founded on reference to a family model that, sociologically, is no longer that of the family except in reproductive technology. Thus, the notion of a couple is a constant element in the activity of medically assisted procreation—or at least the access of people living alone is still under discussion—while, in France for instance, one-parent families are a reality that represents more than a million families.

Similarly, it is not rare for the legislator to introduce provisions that reserve medically assisted procreation only for married couples—in some countries like France, gamete donors also have to be married—or to limit access to non-married couples who can prove they have lived together for a certain length of time. Lastly, it must be noted that many texts expressly refer to the man and the woman who make up the couple, thus excluding homosexual couples.

5 An ambiguous act

But even in the context of the reference family model, there are taboos that the laws on reproductive technology try to clarify or shape. This is most often the case with surrogate motherhood (although it could be culturally tolerated up until now, medically assisted procreation outlaws it), *post mortem* insemination and the lucrative nature of gamete donation.

Enough is enough, some will say. In responding to the suffering of couples faced with infertility, we did not mean to build a new social framework; we asked for respect for a minimum of good practices by establishing a bureaucratic system to determine aptitude for being a parent! Isn't this 'enough' that practitioners sometimes talk about, the reflection of the fact that new reproductive technology remains, in the eyes of the public and the authorities and perhaps even certain doctors, an ambiguous act?

Medically assisted procreation highlights two of the main trends of our western industrialised society, trends that we, at one and the same time, affirm and fear: the 'cult' of the individual and the 'cult' of science. New reproductive technology seems to give the individual control over his procreation; it seems to confer on medicine exorbitant new power over man and his species. Is this so?

6 Control given to the individual over procreation

This is evident, from a legal point of view, in a double effect of the individual will: on filiation on the one hand, on the 'service' required from the doctor on the other. It is clear that medically assisted procreation reinforces the place of the will in the establishment of filiation since, despite the donation of gametes, or even embryos, the biological or genetic 'parents' disappear in favour of the authors of the 'parental project'. In particular the man who consents to the insemination of 'his' wife with the sperm of a third party donor will be considered as the father of the child or, in the case of natural filiation, his parenthood will be established by this fact. However, the jurist and also the doctor (by looking at blood groups)

283

are able to prevail over 'biological truth'. But isn't this effect of will always justified here, as in other cases, out of interest for the child rather than out of recognition of the right of the future parents?

It could be quite different if the one who wants to become a parent could force the practitioner of reproductive technology to supply his services and in this way turn the doctor, who serves an ethical code and is free in his conscience not to perform, into a provider of services.

The risk exists and is called 'medicine of desire' or 'convenience medicine'. But is the practitioner of medically assisted procreation less well armed psychologically to reply than the general practitioner who will have to refuse his patient the prescription of drugs that aim to make it possible for self-medication to be paid for by social security, or than the doctor who is asked for a medically unjustified certificate for someone to go on sick leave?

On the other hand, we have a greater worry on a legal and social level when we note that, in the case of the negative aspect of the right to a child, the right not to have a child, the Court of Justice of the European Communities has already, in 1992, qualified abortion as the provision of a service as understood by the Treaty of Rome.

7 The increased power of doctors over man and the species

Our fears, even our fantasies, lead us to want to control research but also to regulate its applications. Can one both assert the principle of the freedom of research and want to control it? It is all, no doubt, a case of balance in the choice of research and in the types of control set up.

Research on embryos is of course at the heart of the debate on medically assisted procreation and nobody is unaware of the casuistry that prevails in the search for an impossible consensus. Research: no doubt; observation: why not? Study: it is vague; experimentation: it has connotations. But aren't other kinds of research concerning the genome equally problematic? So, starting from there it is tempting to establish a more general prohibition: for eugenic practices, for example (*dixit* the French law)!

Does that then settle the issue? It does not matter if the essential issue lies in the nature of the control. Control by peers will reassure—is that so certain?—the professionals but not necessarily the public. So, the classic recourse to the administration will be accepted by everyone; doesn't this 'soft consensus' reflect the feeling of a dubious effectiveness, between finicky bureaucracy and a lack of means of control?

The sword of Damocles that is criminal law will then have its advocates, but must we wait for a major scandal before taking care of the ethics of the practices concerned? And what if, given these internal hesitations, the international community, or more simply the European authorities, could help us out of this difficulty? To some extent, they can, unless the driving force of international activity is, for its part, held back by our accumulated national slowness. Is not the solution for regulations, i. e. for doing our best to avoid abuse, to take a little, according to needs, from each of the categories enumerated?

Regulating applications consists perhaps first of all in thinking about and attending to the most simple, the most immediate problems. How can we assess the technical effectiveness of medically assisted procreation centres, how can we give correct information to couples without an obligation to establish reliable statistics? How can we meet a need for safety without setting up sanitary and biological tests and without ensuring the professional qualifications of the practitioners? How can we ensure respect for the imposed rules for access to reproductive technology and techniques for the conservation of gametes and embryos if the practitioners are not subject to certain procedures and controls?

Finally, for health care systems that attach importance to fairness, how can we monitor the cost for the health care system of medically assisted procreation? Is medically assisted procreation a technical, medical, even therapeutic activity? Certainly! But medically assisted procreation is also a social practice within a legal context, a health care policy. It gives rise to changes, takes part in evolution, but is also subject to the influence of the social project, i.e., public policies and the individual or collective actions of its actors, health care professionals, patients and citizens. Is medically assisted procreation, then, a pillar of society?

Comment on *Legal regulation of assisted procreation, genetic diagnosis and gene therapy*

Jürgen Simon

First of all I want to declare my unlimited respect for the lecture on 'Legal Regulation of Assisted Procreation, Genetic Diagnosis and Therapy' by Deryck Beyleveld and Shaun Pattinson.

If one tries from time to time to work by dint of legal comparison, it can be estimated how much work such an extensive empirical report demands. At the same time, the authors create a framework for understanding the moral and philosophical issues raised by these regulating approaches. If I make some supplementary remarks, they are not to be understood as a critique but as a supplement.

1 Part one

1.1 Comment on assisted reproduction

The work of Beyleveld and Pattinson not only takes account of the legislation in the different European countries, but furthermore the authors declare that if the procedure of assisted procreation is not regulated, the *de facto* position is shaped by non-legislative mechanisms such as professional guidelines. In those countries where statutory eligibility criteria exist, supplementary harsh *de facto* eligibility criteria are applied irrespective of the statutory position.

Furthermore, the remark of the authors is very interesting that the lack of legislation leads to the fact that assisted reproduction could be successfully regulated by non-legislative means, as is shown by the examples of Italy, Belgium and Portugal. In principle, this can be understood to mean that in nearly all European countries a kind of 'law mesh' more or less exists as a reception net for the developments of new technologies. This is amongst other things very important, because new technologies and especially their newness attract the interest of all and so their integration into the traditional legal system is greatly impeded. If, in consequence the legislators react very quickly, it can be that a regulation is created, which does not fit into this background of law very well.

That is the reason why in Germany, for example, regulation of gene tests of employees and policy holders has been demanded in decisions of the Federal Council and declarations of different commissions since the beginning of the nineties. But, to the present day, no law exists. This is very good because, on the one hand, these tests have not been made, and on the other hand, existing regulations are sufficient. Finally, a more intensive discussion with detailed risk assessment has to take place. The resulting regulation could, perhaps, lead to better integration in the legal system as it stands.

Concerning access to Assisted Procreation, the authors point to this aspect when they declare that 'ironically, as a result, both Italy and Belgium are, by default, among the most permissive countries of Europe'.

For me, it is a question whether it is really surprising and an irony of fate that Italy and Belgium are 'most permissive by default'. I have another point of view—on the basis of this report—because these countries are, because of their traditional legal background, permissive countries in other areas of biotechnology as well. It is astonishing for me, too, that Catholic countries such as Spain, Italy and Portugal are so liberal despite their faith.

1.2 Human cloning and germ-line gene therapy

Concerning human cloning and germ-line gene therapy it is impressive to read in so much detail that these techniques are prohibited in nearly all the European countries or that there exists a consensus against use.

In Germany, cloning is forbidden as the authors emphasise. But the German Embryo Protection Act has several weaknesses concerning cloning. The first is that the characteristic of 'genetically identical' is not defined. Until now, without the interpretation of the first additional protocol of the Biomedicine Convention, we do not have to follow the mathematical understanding of 'identical', but rather the juridical meaning, so that only a 99% identity of genetic material is enough to apply this rule.

The second weakness is that the Embryo Protection Act only includes offences in Germany because of its territorial principle. In consequence, Germans are allowed to go abroad for the procedure of cloning without being punished. This has to be changed by creating an international prohibition of cloning or by changing the German criminal law with respect to the punishment of acts carried out by Germans in Germany as well as in foreign countries.

Furthermore, concerning international activities, one could mention in the European area the resolution of the European Parliament of March 1997 on animal and human cloning, and the report of the European Group of Advisers about the ethical implications of Biotechnology to the European Community. This report contains a recommendation to prohibit human cloning by nuclear cell transfer, too.

The more or less unknown factor is the impact of the United States. The discussion about cloning and germ-line therapy is currently very intense in this country. And this concerns, as we all know, not only the discussion, but above all the activities of enterprises and researchers.

1.3 Pre-implantation genetic diagnosis

Concerning pre-implantation genetic diagnosis (PGD), the resolution of the European Parliament from March 1997 condemns this method, judging it to be a violation of human dignity that should not be accepted by any society.

But, as opposed to cloning and germ-line gene therapy, for example, we find PGD only prohibited in Austria, Germany and Ireland, if we focus on EU countries. In Germany, we are experiencing an intensive discussion about this method, so that I think it is only a question of time before exceptions to this prohibition are introduced. In several other countries there are legislative projects concerning PGD. For example, in Greece a law is being prepared regulating and not prohibiting IVF as well as PGD. Furthermore, a ministry prescription exists concerning PGD, which stipulates that the woman or couple must be consulted before the procedure of PGD.

In Portugal, a law about medically assisted procreation is currently being discussed. Article 7 of this draft act foresees that PGD for the child's health will be allowed.

In Italy, a draft law exists as well concerning procreation but without regulation of PGD.

1.4 Comment on prenatal diagnosis (PND) and abortion

Concerning these subjects I have only two short remarks.

In addition to the given information about France, a new decree has to be mentioned. With decree No. 97-578 of 28 May 1997, an important decision for human genetics in France has been taken to regulate the setting up of multidisciplinary centres offering prenatal diagnosis.

In Germany, abortion is basically forbidden in criminal law by paragraph 218. But, under certain circumstances, it is allowed. The described Abortion and Family Planning Act of 1995 does not exist in this form. The regulations in criminal law were changed by an act of August 1995. But this law only changed some paragraphs. It is not an act containing regulations about abortion.

These are my remarks on the first part of the 'Legal Regulation' report.

2 Part two

Concerning the second part, the authors develop a remarkable framework for analysing the regulatory structures within the EU countries. The starting point of the authors is moral positions, but at the end of the analysis we have the result that these positions often do not appear in the legal form in which they should be brought by their advocates into the political arena. The moral positions become affected and I hold the same opinion as the authors that

> looking at the regulatory structures within the EU tells us more about the compromises that have or have not been made in the legislative arena or the socio-political context of the polity, than it does about the underpinning ground for possession of intrinsic moral status. (p. 257 in this volume)

For the political area, this point of view is helpful and necessary if we want to understand the appearance of moral codes in the form of the law.

One of the basic questions concerns how far we can follow moral positions in the process of legislation. This is very difficult and one of the issues that could be addressed by future research.

These moral positions have certainly proved reliable and practicable, and these traditions have been very helpful until now, because the subject of contemplation could be considered to be relatively secure with respect to its consequences. This unity of opinion is questioned more and more by a progressive differentiation of the separate social functional systems and individuals. This concerns the religious ideas of the Europeans as well, because other religions are gaining more ground and private religions are booming. The strong increase in the number of sects may serve as an indicator for the development described above.

Additionally, there is also the fact of a general uncertainty that is fed by the realisation that the results of research and technology are not controllable anymore. Research on humans is perceived as especially worrying and risky when looked at from this point of view. Possibilities and risks resulting from modern biotechnology and methods cannot be understood and described adequately, because the positions are emotionally burdened due to the reasons mentioned above.

These are additional reasons to focus analysis on the determining aspects in the arena of legislation and at the same time on the progressive differentiation of the separate social functional systems and individuals.

Part Seven

EVALUATION AND PERSPECTIVES

Evaluation of *The European Network for Biomedical Ethics* (ENBE) (1996–1999)

Hille Haker

The task set about three years ago by the *European Network for Biomedical Ethics* (ENBE) was to gain a more up-to-date insight into the connection between infertility treatment and genetic diagnosis and therapy. Its explicit aim was to gather scientific, social, legal and ethical perspectives in both fields and to discuss their points of intersection, above all the development of pre-implantation genetic diagnosis (PGD). The results in the different fields were meant to give impetus to ethical argumentation about and evaluation of the new techniques available in assisted procreation and human genetics. It is not the place here to present a thorough evaluation of the whole project, but I will summarise at least the central issues that were discussed in this period.[1]

All of the questions that were debated during the three conferences dealt with the availability of embryos *in vitro*. In speaking of assisted procreation, we mean conception through fertilisation using the genetic make-up of the future parents or using donor eggs or sperms. At present, it is becoming possible to transfer the nucleus of one egg to another in order to avoid the transmission of mitochondrial diseases (IVONT) (See Rubenstein *et al.* 1995; Richter and Bacchetta 1999; and Bonnicksen 1998). In human genetics, the issue is now PGD, especially that involving single embryonic cells at a time when, according to most scientists and ethicists, individuation of the embryo can hardly be asserted. We are also speaking of genetic therapy at this stage (germ-line gene therapy), and we are talking about the 'therapeutic cloning' of embryos or embryonic cells for non-reproductive purposes, which was recommended at least in one European country at the end of 1998, namely in the United Kingdom.

Many different questions arise depending on the context we are concerned with: in the context of infertility treatment, the couple or future parents of a child are much more the focus of attention than in the context of embryo research for possible future therapy of common diseases. PGD appears to be somehow in the middle of both: it is meant as a help for couples, either for those who are at risk of having children with a genetic disease, or for infertile couples whose chance of having a child might be higher if the embryos to be transferred were to be examined for chromosomal or genetic disorders. However, PGD is also the central technique in the process of research on human embryos. As a technique that still is considered to be at an experimental stage, it raises many questions if offered as a kind of treatment for genetic risks or infertility problems.[2]

In the ENBE project, *clinical application* was the central focus of attention, although embryo research was not ignored as background research.[3] At present, however, new possibilities of genetic diagnosis and therapy could easily lead to a situation in which we might tend to forget about the as yet unsolved problems of clinical application, above all those of IVF and ICSI for infertility or genetic reasons. Therefore, at least those aspects concerning more or less both of these indications for IVF or the related techniques need to be kept in mind.

Ovarian stimulation

The risk of hyperstimulation and the ovarian hyperstimulation syndrome (OHSS) occurring in 2–7% of patients (Lieberman 1998), in about 1% with lethal effect (Cooke 1998), must be taken seriously in the weighing up of burdens and benefits of infertility treatment via IVF, and they must be taken even more seriously in the case of a genetic indication for IVF.

Implantation rate and overall success rate of assisted procreation techniques

Not only the physical and psychological burden for the women and/or couple must be considered in an evaluation of IVF, but also the resulting practice of transferring more than one embryo. What kind of research is needed to improve this success rate? Or is there a definite limit to assisted conception via IVF?

Two suggestions have been made. One part of the *Network* held that the only consequence can be the furthering of embryo research in order to gain more knowledge about the causes of implantation, non-implantation or early miscarriages. Scientists called for more research on the cultures used in IVF, research in cryopreservation, on metabolic needs of embryos, etc., in the hope that with better knowledge the success rate can be improved step by step.

The other part of the *Network* was more sceptical about this approach. They tended to take a more pessimistic or perhaps cautious position, saying that the cultural—and moral—costs might be too high. Ethicists called for an ethical perspective that takes human contingency and finiteness seriously. Furthermore, they were concerned to gain a more integrative perspective that considered assisted procreation at some distance to the reduced perspective of clinical practice and individual clinical cases, and at a distance to the development of a promising technology. They wanted rather to take the perspective of a social-ethical point of view that would consider the rights and interests of all members of society equally, thus taking the position of a society characterised by solidarity, which takes responsibility for providing the best possible support for those who need it, without forgetting the issue of respect for all members and a just distribution of financial resources. In a weaker version of applied ethics, this approach restricts itself to the task of proving consistencies within practices and within theories that conceptualise these practices, or of criticising inconsistencies, and making explicit important aspects that might otherwise be forgotten.

Multiple pregnancies

The transfer of two or more embryos carries the risk of twin or triplet pregnancies resulting in the side-effect of risk of prematurity, miscarriages or health risks for the women, and psycho-social risks for the future family. These risks clearly call for legal regulation that is not present in all European countries.[4] Scientific data as to how the number of transfers and the success rate are related must be evaluated on a European level, but the benefit to the child or children, the health of the mother and the social situation of the future family must also be considered.

Reasons for infertility

The reasons for infertility were another matter of interest within the *Network*. Not enough research has gone into this, especially with respect to psychological and social reasons. The psychosocial and biological factors are difficult to interpret as such, as is their interplay. This makes it difficult in individual cases to decide whether IVF is an adequate treatment or whether alternative coping strategies could be interpreted as success of treatment as well. However, there is a strong consensus that much depends on the counselling of clients or patients, and much more effort must be put into the development of adequate counselling procedures.

In recent years, ICSI has become a broadly accepted and applied method of assisted procreation. Nevertheless, at least two problems remain that need further psychological and empirical study.

First, ICSI brought to attention that in many cases men are the reason for childlessness. How do women react to the treatment of their body when male infertility is the reason for assisted conception?

Second, the risk of transferring genetic disorders by way of ICSI still cannot be excluded. Here, the problem of discrimination on the one hand and the right of the future child to be protected from calculable risks on the other must be discussed. Who should decide whether such a risk—if it exists at all—may be taken? Is there a societal responsibility to avoid these risks, under certain conditions even against the will of the couple? Or is just the opposite the case: that the right to non-discrimination leads to the conclusion that a genetic risk may not be a reason for withholding a treatment to affected persons or persons at risk? These questions point back to the general debate on the 'natural desire' to reproduce (see Lesch 1998; and Zwart 1998).[5] Most ethicists doubt, however, that this implicit presupposition of reproductive medicine is right, either factually or, even more importantly, interpreted as a normative reason for the right to be assisted in procreation. If there is some ethical progress, this would certainly also be a result of the *Network's* discussions: wherever arguments based on the (positive) right to procreation are used as a justification for certain practices of assisted conception, they will have to be stronger than those that are known at present and raise new points of consideration in order to be valid.

Restriction or promotion of access? Assisted procreation as a new form of eugenics?

Access to assisted procreation is not only dependent on indications but also on financial conditions that differ greatly in European countries. Should access be made possible to everyone, which would mean that the state would have to cover the costs? Or who has the legitimate power to determine how to set limits to publicly financed infertility treatment? These questions become even more important when couples with a genetic risk are considered. Is it in the genuine interest of a society to reduce the number of persons carrying the risk, and can it be a morally legitimate interest? Thus, eugenic thinking can easily enter the debate on different levels—one of the reasons being the financial aspect of assisted procreation (see Graumann 1999; and Sèle and Testart 1999).

One major topic at the intersection of infertility treatment, genetic diagnosis and research into genetic therapy is the treatment of supernumerary embryos. This, of course, becomes more and more important as the selection of embryos is an intended consequence of PGD, and not just a side-effect (see Haker 1999). Storage, donation or destruction are the alternatives in these cases, but there is no consensus about who should be authorised to make the decision about what to do with surplus embryos. At present, the problem has not been solved.

All these aspects need further investigation and research. In the 'Points to Consider',[6] the *Network's* co-ordinators concentrate on PGD: on the empirical level, embryology, success rate, physical and psychological well-being of the future child or children and women, public and professional attitudes, psychological and socio-cultural changes and economic aspects are mentioned. We consider these and, in a broader sense, the aspects I have mentioned above, as an overall consensus of the *Network*: research on these topics is necessary in the near future, since studies are available for only some of the issues, and a broad evaluation of those studies that have been carried out is still lacking.

A good part of the *Network's* debates concerned the social changes brought about by reproductive medicine and genetic diagnosis. We gave expression to these concerns at both of the preceding conferences, which were stressed again in this volume by Regine Kollek. In the 'Points to Consider', we address social questions of different kinds, to which all European countries will find their own or common answers. The options considered do not necessarily form a common value system. Thus, pluralism will remain as far as this level of reflection is concerned. However, in our view it is necessary to make options explicit, and to show how they stand in contrast to other options, and how dilemmas arise when it becomes possible to justify two contradicting options. Thus, we mentioned the option for individual autonomy in its relationship to the option for social responsibility. These do not contradict each other, although they can stand in sharp contrast in certain contexts. Beyond this, we talked about the option to minimise genetic risks and suffering as it relates to the option to protect vulnerable human beings; the option for scientific progress in relation to the option that recognises non-scientific options to a certain degree in specific contexts where progress appears to have a high social and moral price.

With regard to the final conference, I would like to mention two other options—one is the option for female liberation, either supported by reproductive medicine, or just the opposite, impeded by it. There might well be effects of the reproductive technologies, especially when they are applied to couples with genetic risks by screening or individual counselling, that lead to a new kind of discrimination, and a new kind of disrespect for women's autonomy. Ironically, women's autonomy was one of the central issues in promoting these techniques. Thus, societies face the question of how women's liberation and equality can be shaped in the context of reproduction and genetic medicine.

The second option was raised by Onora O'Neill. It concerns the normative concept of parenthood with its new option for acceptance of parenthood under certain conditions. Whether this change in the concept of parenthood represents progress beyond the traditional concept of unconditional acceptance and 'given', not 'chosen' parenthood, is another question modern societies will have to answer.

In the third section of the 'Points to Consider', we deal with philosophical anthropology in the sense of a basic theory that has normative implications but is not normative in itself.[7] When, for example, a concept of human rights is based on certain needs or interests necessarily accompanying human life, or even accompanying being an agent, these interests must be interpreted in the context of anthropological assumptions on which our self-understanding is based. Or, to give another example, when continuity of human life is called into question as the main concept of self-identity, then this must be brought into accordance with the still valid anthropological assumption that there is a continuity that is normatively relevant (see Wimmer 1999). As Jean-Pierre Wils showed in his paper, the possibilities for making the early embryo visual are as much a challenge to our perception—with important consequences for anthropology—as they are a challenge for a theory of recognition and respect for the other as another.

Not only with respect to PGD, as stated in the Points to Consider, but also with respect to the other fields of ENBE's work, normative questions, i.e., those dimensions of rights and duties that are categorically binding from an ethical point of view, were discussed very controversially. It is important to recognise the distinction between questions of the good life, questions of virtue, or questions of values that are meant to give some orientation in one's actions and which are formed by social options, on the one hand, and questions of overall binding imperatives for one's actions, namely those imperatives that are derived from the rights of others that every agent must respect, on the other. These imperatives, or sometimes the right application of these imperatives, are at stake when normative questions arise.[8] This may be the case when rights and duties are not well defined because the practice is singular and new, or the scope of rights is not clear, or the subject of rights or duties is unclear, and so on. Normative claims are not just to be interpreted as options that can be overruled by other options; rather, they must be justified as rules that bind every agent in the same way. Therefore, they correlate to legal regulations, although they are grounded exclusively in rational argumentation, whereas legal regulations are at least partly the result of the political process of decision-making and the result of a political consensus or compromise.

In the 'Points to Consider' we address the following quite familiar normative questions:

The status of the embryo, which has many implications
for the normative level

One of the central issues at the Maastricht conference was the ethical evaluation of PGD in relation to the status of the embryo. With PGD on totipotent embryonic cells it becomes clear that selection of at least some kinds of human being is carried out intentionally. This, at least in my opinion, is the big difference from all other practices we have come to know until now, including prenatal diagnosis with its potential to result in the abortion of a fetus, and also including the diagnosis of oocytes before fertilisation and implantation.

The difference is one of fact, but it is also a difference of the kind of action in question: in prenatal diagnosis, it is possible to describe the situation as an actual conflict between woman and fetus. This cannot be said in the same sense of pre-implantation genetic diagnosis where the argument of the woman's priority in decision-making is weak anyway. I hold that pre-implantation genetic diagnosis implicitly refuses any embryo an intrinsic moral status, because any of the fertilised embryos might be destroyed without there being a serious conflict (see Haker 1999). However, to recall just one example of a moral analysis, if Beyleveld is right, this practice and its implicit normative claim is in conflict with the claim of an intrinsic moral status that must be assumed when applying a precautionary argument.[9] Thus, the disagreement still remains, and more reflection is necessary to examine the validity of any moral argument brought up in the discussion.

The right to autonomous procreation

As has become clear during the working period of ENBE, the right to autonomous procreation is not vague as a negative right. On a regulative level, it has been expressed in the Universal and European Convention on Human Rights. However, it is not at all clear how the limit on a positive right should be set, or—as we would now say—on the strong interest in assisted procreation. Given this, the interest of couples concerned remains to be interpreted with respect to a just access to modern reproductive techniques and a general concept of justice in health care.

Public welfare

Public welfare is closely connected with the rights of individuals, and thus the normative claims on this level also have to be elaborated. However, the application and policies of public welfare are very much at stake. We did not work on this dimension thoroughly during the working period of the *Network*, but we are of the opinion that future ethical research should stress public welfare questions more than is done at present.

Justice in health care systems

The same is true of questions of justice, which can be considered as part of the public welfare project rather than as an extra point. But our intention was to stress the relationship between individual and social sphere again. We debated the right to non-discrimination of individuals, especially of those persons who have a genetic disorder or a genetic risk that will be important for their own lives as well as for their procreation. From a more social-ethical perspective, non-discrimination is one part of the theory of justice, but one is easily trapped if this means that every individual must be granted any support in procreation or genetic diagnosis because of non-discrimination. This can come into conflict not only with the status of the embryo, but also with the task of a just distribution of health goods within a society. On an ideological level, the limitation of resources, however, might be used to support eugenic arguments.

In the second part of the 'Points to Consider', we addressed the remaining controversies that I will just mention but not consider again:

- the status of the embryo;
- the controversy over procreative autonomy;
- the relationship between individual welfare or well-being and public welfare;
- questions about the right or adequate ethical theory.

Our intention, here, is not to mix up political consensus and compromise with ethical argumentation where differences sometimes cannot be overcome. We want to make explicit that the *Network* might not have covered all ethical theories equally. Furthermore, we have concentrated very much on rights-theories. Arguing from a utilitarian position, however, Birnbacher (1998) pleads for a so-called narrow term of human dignity in ethical discussions, and this can be worked on from different theories. If ethicists of different approaches could meet in this interpretation of human dignity based on just a few rights necessary to live as a human being or on being an agent, this would not be a political consensus but rather a philosophical starting point for further reflection.

Notes

1   A more detailed summary and evaluation of the whole project can be found in the Final Report of the *Network,* available at the Center for Ethics in the Sciences and Humanities, Tübingen or via the internet (http://www.uni-tuebingen.de/zew/). See also Hildt and Mieth 1998; and Hildt and Graumann 1999

2   For the scientific and ethical discussion, see Hildt and Graumann 1999.

3   An application to extend ENBE, which concentrates on research on embryos, has been made within the 5th Framework of the European Commission.

4   See Beyleveld, D. and Pattinson, S., 'Legal Regulation of Assisted Procreation, Genetic Diagnosis, and Gene Therapy', in this volume.

5   See also McLean, S., 'A Moral Right to Procreation?', in this volume.

6   See the Annexe in this volume. For a further discussion of the 'Points to Consider', see *Biomedical Ethics*, Vol. 3, No. 3, 1998.

7   The term philosophical anthropology does not refer to empirical studies in anthropology and/or ethnology. It refers to reflection on basic assumptions of human life and the meaning of humanity. These have normative implications for ideas of what it means to be a human and what it means to live the life of a human being. One part of this reflection—though perhaps not the central part of it—deals with the moral status of embryos or fetuses, and with the conceptual difference between humanity and personhood. Amongst other things, the European Convention on Human Rights and Biomedicine has been criticised for not containing this anthropological reflection, with the consequence that terms remain troublingly vague which nevertheless have far-reaching normative implications.

8   See Düwell, M., 'Moral Reasoning in Applied Ethics', in this volume.

9   See Beyleveld, D., 'The Moral Status of the Human Embryo and Fetus', in this volume.

References

Birnbacher, D. (1998), 'Do Modern Reproductive Technologies Violate Human Dignity?', in Hildt, E. and Mieth, D. (eds), *In Vitro Fertilisation in the 1990s: Towards a Medical, Social and Ethical Evaluation*, Ashgate: Aldershot, pp. 325–333.

Bonnicksen, A. L. (1998), 'Transplanting Nuclei Between Human Eggs: Implications for Germ-Line Genetics', *Politics and the Life Sciences,* Vol. 17, No. 1, pp. 3–10.

Graumann, S. (1999), 'Germ-line Gene-therapy: Public Opinions with Regard to Eugenics', in Hildt, E. and Graumann, S. (eds), *Genetics in Human Reproduction*, Ashgate: Aldershot, pp. 175–184.

Haker, H. (1999), 'Selection Through Prenatal Diagnosis and Preimplantation Diagnosis', in Hildt, E. and Graumann, S. (eds), *Genetics in Human Reproduction*, Ashgate: Aldershot, pp. 157–165.

Hildt, E., Graumann, S. (1999), (eds), *Genetics in Human Reproduction*, Ashgate: Aldershot.

Lesch, W. (1998), 'Is the Desire for a Child Too Strong? Or Is There a Right to a Child of One's Own?', in Hildt, E. and Mieth, D. (eds), *In Vitro Fertilisation in the 1990s: Towards a Medical, Social and Ethical Evaluation*, Ashgate: Aldershot, pp. 73–79.

Richter, G. and Bacchetta, D. (1999), 'Nuclear Transplantation: Medical and Ethical Aspects', in Hildt, E. and Graumann, S. (eds), *Genetics in Human Reproduction*, Ashgate: Aldershot, pp. 55–71.

Rubenstein, D. S., Thomasma, D. C., Schon, E. A. and Zinaman, M. J. (1995), 'Germ-line Therapy to Cure Mitochondrial Disease: Protocol and Ethics of In Vitro Ovum Nuclear Transplantation', *Cambridge Quarterly of Healthcare Ethics,* Vol. 4, No. 3, pp. 316–39.

Sèle, B. and Testart, J. (1999), 'Eugenics Comes Back with Medically Assisted Procreation', in Hildt, E. and Graumann, S. (eds), *Genetics in Human Reproduction*, Ashgate: Aldershot, pp. 169–174.

Wimmer, R. (1999), 'Ethics of Research on Human Embryos', in Hildt, E. and Graumann, S. (eds), *Genetics in Human Reproduction*, Ashgate: Aldershot, pp. 141–146.

Zwart, H. (1998), 'Can Nature Serve as a Criterium for the Use of Reproductive Technologies?', in Hildt, E. and Mieth, D. (eds), *In Vitro Fertilisation in the 1990s: Towards a Medical, Social and Ethical Evaluation*, Ashgate: Aldershot, pp. 349–360.

Postscript

Dietmar Mieth

1 The political controversy on embryo-perspective

In the two earlier conferences, we tried to clarify the scientific, social, legal and ethical aspects of *in vitro* fertilisation and pre-implantation genetic diagnosis. In the last EGE Opinion on Embryo Research, we find in the chapter on the legal background under 'Common Principles' (paragraph 1.21), the time limit for the use of human embryos (14 days after fertilisation), prohibition of genetic modification of normal pre-implanted embryos, prohibition of replacement *in utero* of human-animal hybrids, prohibition of replacement *in utero* of embryos that have been used in research, and the need for consent by each person whose gametes were used to bring about the creation of the embryo.

However, there is no mention of *in vitro* cloning, which is now being debated. If the genetic modification of normal embryos is prohibited, then what is '*normal*'? Is genetic modification of embryos that are not 'normal' allowed? And, what about 'replacement *in utero*'?

There is a lack of consensus concerning answers to many questions in Europe. The European Parliament and the European Commission proposed that embryo research with destruction of the embryo (which covers practically all embryo research), will not be funded by the 5th Framework Programme for Research in Biotechnology. However, the European Council of Ministers did not follow this proposal and did not include it in the 5th Framework Programme for Life Sciences. While there is a democratic consensus with a great majority on this question, it has not received the assent of biomedical experts and bioethical committees like the EGE. I think that the acceleration of the possibilities and options related to *in vitro* cloning need our special attention. But it is clear that, until now, we have only had controversial contributions on the question of embryo protection.

2 The perspective of social ethics

Even if ethical reconstructions of a just society vary, we must accept that society is changing rapidly by virtue of technological acceleration not only in biotechnology and biomedicine but also in information technologies and their application in medicine, economy, culture, and so on. What are the values that we want to stay the same, and what are the values we can accept being changed?

3 The feminist perspective

In our earlier conferences, we tried to include and to promote feminist discussion, which is in itself very rich. We learned, for example, that IVF brings some new risks of instrumentalisation and for the autonomy of women. And we learned to integrate the interests of individual women into the general situation of women. I think that this perspective merits being further developed. An example might be female 'optionalism', e.g., the choice of IVF/ET after sterilisation, recommended by physicians, or the alternation between methods *pro* and *contra* fertilisation (in extreme cases, opting for abortion or, some years later, for IVF). Even if it is clear that not all kinds of uses of a legally accepted method can be controlled and that the old scholastic principle *'abusis non tollit usum'* remains, there are a lot of ethical questions related to life planning and to moral identity.

4 The perspective of European biomedical politics

Article F of the Treaty of Amsterdam, recognises fundamental rights at Union level based on 'constitutional traditions common to the Member states'. What are these rights? What is their connection with ethically significant problems of biomedicine? If European integration is to remain at the level of 'respect for national identity' mentioned in the same treaty, it needs some ethical reflection and concerted action. Even if there are some common principles based on the 'common constitutional traditions', like the non-instrumentalisation of human beings as a whole or the non-commercialisation of the human body, as with autonomy and informed consent, there remains a need to clarify the extension, hierarchy and conflict of such principles. The option for a 'Charter of Fundamental Rights' in the European Union, discussed in 1999 by the European Parliament and the Council of Ministers, may be a motivation to intensify efforts in this field.

ANNEXE

Discussion of *The moral status of the human embryo and fetus*

*summarised by Ulrich Dettweiler
and Annika Thiem*

The discussion of Deryck Beyleveld's paper can, for the most part, be considered under three headings. First, there were questions on the definition of specific terms used in Beyleveld's paper, and second there were questions about the formal soundness of the arguments. Finally, the proportionality of the age of the embryo-fetus and its moral status with respect to an anthropological point of view was discussed.

However, before discussion commenced, *Deryck Beyleveld* made a brief response to the Comments of Nikolaus Knoeppfler and Micheline Husson. In response to Nikolaus Knoeppfler, he wished to emphasise that his intention had not been to justify the *PGC* in his presentation, but merely to indicate features of the argument that are crucial for the application of the *PGC*. Had he been attempting to justify the *PGC,* rather than to apply it, he would have considered objections to it in some depth. In response to Micheline Husson, he commented that he had no intention to dismiss the importance of the politics of consensus; but it is a different issue from the rational justification of morality. Furthermore, he objected to the suggestion that he simply rejected other positions as a starting presumption. His intention was to spell out the position of Gewirthian theory, and he did not *assume* that Gewirth is right. His conviction that Gewirth is right (and contradicting positions wrong) was based on a very elaborate and concerted argument. It was unfair to suggest that his rejection of other positions was arbitrary.

In response to *Farhan Yazdani's* request for a clear-cut definition of the word 'moral', *Deryck Beyleveld* suggested that 'morality sets categorically binding other-regarding requirements on action. Moral rules differ from non-moral norms or rules in that they set categorically binding requirements that ask us to take account of the interests of persons other than or in addition to ourselves.' However, if the argument for the *PGC* is formally sound on its premises, then how we choose to use the term 'morality' hardly matters. What matters is whether or not agents are rationally compelled to act in accordance with the *PGC,* not whether or not we call the *PGC* a 'moral' principle.

Robert Edwards contended that the term 'embryo-fetus' in Beyleveld's paper is unclear. One could also speak of a 'day-14-child' or 'embryo' or 'fetus'. He wanted to know what exactly was meant by this term. *Deryck Beyleveld* replied that use of generic terminology to cover all stages of the unborn is appropriate given that the question of rational criteria for judging on the moral status of a growing being is what is at issue. More differentiated terminology implies substantial metaphysical assumptions. The use of the term 'embryo-fetus' aims to avoid any such judgments. While Gewirth's argument does not require answers to such questions, in the practical application of the argument, whether the unborn are agents or at what stage they become agents is a relevant question that has to be addressed carefully, which is—from a philosophical perspective—a huge step. At the moment, this question cannot be answered. Therefore, the term 'embryo-fetus' should be considered a working neutral designation that does not require the status of the embryo to be differentiated from that of the fetus.

Regarding the formal soundness of the precautionary argument *Hille Haker* asked why, if the generic features of an agent are the reasons for its (intrinsic) moral status, is the precautionary argument still an argument for a direct intrinsic status. 'The moral status of an embryo is not a question of "more or less", it is a question of "whether or not".' *Deryck Beyleveld* replied that, under precaution, it is necessary to suppose that it is *possible* that the embryo possesses the features of 'agency' but is unable to express them. There is a difference between having the 'capacities' and 'being able to display them'; it is the 'possession of capacities' that is relevant for having the generic rights, but evidence of the capacities that is relevant to attribution of the generic rights. But, according to *Hille Haker*, this means that the concept of 'locked-in-agency' conflicted strongly with the theory of 'development' or with the theory of 'continuity'. Agreeing that this is the case, *Deryck Beyleveld* replied that the only point he was making was that if *(ex hypothesi)* the embryo-fetus is an agent then it has the generic rights. The point, however, is that we do not know whether or it has generic rights (and is a locked-in agent), because we do not know what capacities it has, as against is capable of exhibiting. Although the view that it develops may be more plausible than the view that the embryo-fetus is a locked-in agent, we need, under precaution (and guided by a categorical imperative), to remain sceptical about those things we cannot know for certain. Under precaution, we do not go along with what there is best evidence for, but exercise precaution in relation to the degree of evidence there is in relation to all the possibilities. Still, *Hille Haker* insisted on the formal question as to why this argument did not just give the embryo-fetus an 'indirect' status. All arguments for the moral status of the embryo are 'negative arguments', therefore no 'intrinsic' moral status can be claimed. *Deryck Beyleveld* replied that he was not sure what was meant by a 'negative argument', but he attributes direct or intrinsic moral status to a being if that status is possessed simply by virtue of the properties of that being. The embryo-fetus has direct status under precaution because the properties that the embryo-fetus has are sufficient to be a degree of evidence for being an agent, and hence sufficient for having a degree of status in proportion to the strength of that evidence under precaution.

This then lead into a more detailed discussion of the concepts of proportionality and anthropology with respect to the *PGC. Farhan Yazdani* claimed there was a problem in judging the moral status of a 'growing subject', 'un être en devenir'. The moral status of such a growing being is more a matter of recognition and acceptance by its social environment and less intrinsic. *Deryck Beyleveld* replied that, while the embryo-fetus gains status this way, that fact does not does not gainsay the argument that to be on the safe side it is important to grant the embryo the status of a possible agent, for if one disregards an actual agent as a non-agent the consequences of this failure are morally relevant. If one wrongfully recognises a non-agent as an agent, less happens or follows.

An enlightening example of this problem was given by *Alex Mauron*. A philosopher and a scientist argue about the relevance of agency in relation to a human embryo and an acorn. They consider the precautionary principle and assume the potentiality of agency under precaution. To be judged to be an agent, one needs some neuronal equipment, which neither the embryo nor the acorn have. To call an embryo then a 'locked-in-agent' one needs at least some metaphysical narratives. So, the scientist asks what is the relevant difference between considering a human embryo an 'agent' and not the acorn? What are the criteria of difference? What is the relevance of the 'potentiality'? *Deryck Beyleveld* replied that the possibility that the acorn was a locked-in-agent or the tree, itself, an agent, should by no means be altogether discounted. Nevertheless, there is a difference in species that is, from a pragmatic perspective relevant, because members of the human species are at least known to develop the capacity to display agency behaviour, whereas members of other species are not definitely known to behave in this way. This means that the same level of behaviour is better evidence when displayed by humans than when displayed by another species, which gives a human displaying the same behavioural capacities as a non-human a higher moral status.

Christiane Woopen still insisted on criteria for deciding on the different phases of human development. The question is how the ability to display the features of agency counts in this evaluation of moral status. *Deryck Beyleveld* conceded that criteria good enough to answer this question had not yet been found. Indeed, from a rationalist foundationalist point of view it might be impossible for a definitive answer to be given to it at all. Ultimately, we might have to make do at this level with an indirect societal argument: society does care a lot for the unborn, etc. However, as he had explained in his paper, such indirect considerations would be of less worth without the direct status given by precaution, which reinforces them.

Dietmar Mieth stressed the relevant connection of anthropology and ethics. The term 'agent' is a *pars pro toto* for 'human being'. One has to keep in mind that anthropological terms are reduced to form an ethical theory. However, because the rights claimed in the Gewirthian theory were explicitly not 'human rights' but 'agent rights', *Deryck Beyleveld* maintained that substantial anthropology was not to the point here. As 'agency' is defined, human beings just happen to be the beings that we have most evidence to consider agents. Nevertheless, *Dietmar Mieth* insisted that the inference between agents and human beings remained. One could not escape the questions of anthropology.

Finally, in response to the suggestion that Gewirthian theory is too rationalistic and ignores human characteristics, such as the emotions, *Deryck Beyleveld* stressed that emotions are highly relevant in Gewirthian theory. The argument to the *PGC* does not ignore emotions; either in its characterisation of agency or in what it regards as justified moral characteristics. However, as a rationalistic theory, it does aim to distinguish between rational emotions and irrational ones.

Discussion of *Autonomy and Recognition*

summarised by Christoph Holzem and Annika Thiem

The discussion on Jean-Pierre Wils' paper, 'Autonomy and Recognition', focused on the concept of 'unconditional' recognition, the problems of the 'new visibility' and the resulting ethical problems for human procreation.

Maureen Junker-Kenny opened the discussion by challenging the notion of 'strict mutuality' and demanded that the unconditionality of recognition be emphasised:

> 1. Is it really an 'overextension of the notion of recognition' to extend it to those who cannot requite it? Is it adequate to remain locked into Hegel's model of 'strict mutuality of recognition' of fully-fledged partners in autonomy and deny that autonomy is generated by anticipating it? Instead of focusing on the ideal case of requited recognition, is not the much more basic case for our genesis as subjects the situation of advocatory, vicarious, asymmetric, anticipatory and therefore innovative recognition? Adorno captures the anticipatory structure of recognition in his formulation of the pedagogical paradox: 'In order to educate towards autonomy (Mündigkeit), one has to presuppose it.' A model of strict mutuality excludes this. Rather than classify children as manifestations of 'Life', as Hegel does, it would be much more adequate to spell out this logic of anticipating their autonomy. Apart from the interaction with children, the lack of 'strict mutuality' as autonomous subjects applies also to the critical cases in medical ethics, PVS patients who can no longer respond to the care and initiative of the nurses and leave them without this reciprocated recognition Question Q.
> 2. Instead of resorting to 'emphatic imagination', it is sufficient to expound the unconditional character of obligation. If recognition is to be unconditional, we cannot insist on mutuality. To renounce to the equal recognition of the other for the sake of realising its unconditionality, however, lands us in the problems that Kant termed the

313

antinomy of Practical Reason, the disproportion between virtue and happiness that according to him can only be reconciled by the postulate of God. This is where the limit questions between Philosophical and Theological Ethics are reached. But would it be in keeping with morality to restrict the scope of ethics to what humans can fulfil themselves (since it is beyond human possibilities, it cannot be an ethical demand)? Does this not establish as the criterion for ethics a calculus of probable success? Are we not morally obliged to remain open to the possibility of our good intentions being fulfilled even if our own possibilities of realising them are exhausted - as in the case of caring for PVS patients? These are questions that Theological Ethics should insist on in the interest of moral agents.[1]

Jean-Pierre Wils warned against overinterpreting the term 'recognition' by introducing the predicate 'unconditional'. The semantics of the term recognition does not entail a concept that interprets recognition as an unconditional attitude, an unconditional aim that we have in common with other people.

> Therefore I do not use a very narrow concept of recognition. Rather I have tried do demonstrate that the concept has some typical problems. The process of recognition itself has to be open for reflection on the preconditions of recognition. In particular, the question for the kinds of perception of the other and for the construction of the other rise.

For this reason, he maintained that Maureen Junker Kenny overemphasises the term recognition when introducing a term like unconditional. From his point of view, emphatic terms like 'unconditional' or terms like 'life' are not useful in concrete moral conflicts, because these terms are very abstract and fail to provide orientation to solve such conflicts. The same problem occurs in Lévinas' book on anthropology, when he states that 'as much of him as escapes our understanding is himself', that what escapes our understanding is the self of the other. This is one of the examples of overinterpreting a right intention. When the identity of the other consists of his non-identity, or consists of what we do not recognise in this person, of a complete alienation of identity, then, especially concerning our moral responsibility, we cannot know who we actually are addressing. Therefore a concept of personal values and personal stories, a concept of narratives does not help with solving these questions, because there are some human beings who cannot tell any story, as they have no story. Due to the fact that they cannot tell stories about their identity, they are not able to construct an identity by narratives. Also, narratives are related to some preconditions of characteristics of human beings, of characteristics of personhood, of characteristics of identity. Finally, there is no state of a 'blank identity' as the starting point of the narratives.

The second part of Jean-Pierre Wils' statement focused on a comment made by *Eve-Marie Engels*. She argued that the new techniques might be responsible for the disappearing of moral awareness, of moral responsibility. Jean-Pierre Wils stressed that his point was rather that the new techniques confront us with different kinds of perception, with certain levels of abstraction that are new for us. These levels of abstraction render our moral awareness uncertain. There occurs a struggle for interpretation, such as the question of the embryo being a real human being or an illusion of one having rights or virtual rights. This is a good example for the uncertainty of perception that causes the struggle for interpretation of perception and leads to several possibilities. One can say that certain perceptions give rise to moral awareness. Other perceptions cause uncertainty regarding a distinction between objects and human beings, regarding their specific qualities with which we are confronted, and regarding how we are to act adequately in accordance with them as partners. Focusing on the categories of autonomy and recognition has the advantage that they are well defined in our modern tradition of philosophy as well as already by Hegel. Therefore, it is important to know what is going on when using these categories; we have to know the framework, the side-constraints of these categories. Hegel tries to demonstrate several things; first, the phenomena of self-awareness as a structure. He tries to show that this structure of self-awareness is the structure of the struggle for recognition. This means that the phenomenon of self-awareness has the same structure as a social structure for recognition. Also he tries to demonstrate that the result of the social struggle for recognition-relationship is, in a certain sense of the word, the perfect appearance of what we call 'self-awareness as a phenomenon.' So, self-awareness as a phenomenon is an implicit criterion that Hegel uses for the anticipation of autonomy. The anticipation of a perfect way of self-awareness is the result of the struggle for recognition. As self-awareness becomes a criterion for personhood, at the same time, it is a model for the social structure of recognition. Thus, the interpretation applies that self-awareness is seeing oneself seeing. The crossing over of seeing perspectives is in fact self-awareness. The result of this genesis of recognition is that the perfect appearance of self-awareness is a criterion for personhood and autonomy.

Regine Kollek stated that the question of autonomy, and the notions of 'context' and 'contextualisation', show that the way we look at the embryo is very important for our perception and our construction of moral relationships and action. Jean-Pierre Wils was talking about modern means of perception that use instruments like ultrasound screen and provide us with an abstract picture of the embryo, and this leads to establishing a distance between us and the fetus and embryo. This, as she herself believes and Eve-Marie Engels had pointed out earlier, contributes to a new moral evaluation of the embryo. The results are two different developments. On the one hand, pregnancy within the realm of the new techniques has become very tentative. For many weeks the relevant question for the pregnant women is whether the embryo/fetus is healthy or not, and then, fairly suddenly, it is already visible on the ultrasound screen. In this situation, it is very difficult to say which moral decision has to be made. The other development concerns pre-implantation genetic diagnosis (PGD). There, the embryo is, indeed, something like a 'heap of undifferentiated cells'. It is hard to imagine these undifferentiated cells as some moral being. Also, it is very different from prenatal diagnosis. In prenatal diagnosis (PND), the pictures we now have of the embryo somehow protect the embryo from being aborted even in the case of diagnosis of a genetic defect.

Hille Haker wanted to draw a connection between Deryck Beyleveld's paper and the paper of Jean-Pierre Wils. Perhaps the recognition theory of Hegel, or at least the way Jean-Pierre Wils interpreted it, could be one way of overcoming the weakness of Gewirthian theory in starting with the individual agent. This impression arises when taking into account that nothing but knowledge about myself being an agent follows from the precautionary principle. With the 'recognition model,' which is completely different from the 'respect model' focusing on *just the* individual, we have the turning of the self to the other. The self is a self only through the other and depending on the other. Then we have a dialogue model or a dialectic of an intersubjectivity model. There might not have been a dialogue between theories in the Kantian and Hegelian traditions to data, but attempts should be made to achieve that. This mediation can be extended a bit further, since the perception theory introduced by Deryck Beyleveld is also important for the precautionary principle because some evidence is obtained by perception.

Regarding the second point made by Hille Haker, *Deryck Beyleveld* agreed that the description of the phenomenology of recognition is one way of talking about evidence for the possibility that there is a locked-in agent. The phenomenology of recognition sets standards for how elaborate the metaphysical stories needed for the idea that the fetus is a locked-in agent have to be for the stories to be plausible. The fact that people often react to the image of a fetus on an ultrasound screen by saying 'It looks like a little person, doesn't it?' makes such stories more plausible and renders 'far-fetched' metaphysical tales more believable. Phenomenology operates at both a rational level and a purely emotional one here. However, Deryck Beyleveld was more sceptical about Hille Haker's second argument, on the ground that he did not consider that it is possible to understand and know oneself through others in the relevant way. Any theory that requires one to believe this is highly problematic.

Hub Zwart detected a certain ambiguity in the paper of Jean-Pierre Wils. On the one hand, there seems to be a kind of nostalgia of the visible in view of the loss of visibility, the emancipation of the abstract. If that is an adequate account, then Kantian ethics has addressed the question of how human beings who are not physically here can be respected. On the other side, it was indicated that science might also increase visibility. The question then is what the ethical meaning of this would be. Responding to Eve-Marie Engels, Jean-Pierre Wils had mentioned that this could lead to moral confusion and uncertainty. However, it seems more plausible to expect that the new kinds of perception introduced by science will make us more aware, more certain and allow us to react more precisely. It is not altogether clear why the increase of perception should lead to moral confusion or hesitation.

In his brief response to these statements, *Jean-Pierre Wils* stressed that he did not interpret scientific progress and the new scientific knowledge as resulting in moral confusion. His purpose was solely to give a diagnosis, not an evaluation or a moral interpretation of the changing styles of perception. Nevertheless, there is, indeed, some uncertainty of the meaning of what we are seeing and of what we are not seeing. Therefore, the examples given by Regine Kollek show that there are different interpretations of what this perception means and of what the moral implications of this perception are. There is a struggle for recognition in the Hegelian model of recognition based on preconditions, which usually are not mentioned. They are judgments on the quality of the partners in the struggle for recognition. This means that we, indeed, anticipate autonomy. However, at the same time, we have to select who can be a partner and so be subject to anticipation of future qualities. This model, obviously, becomes more difficult if perception of a partner becomes more and more difficult.

Note

[1] We thank Maureen Junker-Kenny for submitting her remarks and questions in written form.

Discussion of *Technicalisation of human procreation and social living conditions*

summarised by Jens Badura, Gisela Lotter, and Annika Thiem

Regine Kollek's reply to Hub Zwart's comment focused on two aspects. First, if we perceive needs as socially constructed then a description of the social context from a sociological perspective in the bioethical debate is necessary to understand these socially constructed needs. This is then relevant for the discussion of normative implications. A change in perspective is helpful because social rather than technical solutions should be sought. Second, the role of bioethical discourse has to be considered. Since it has become institutionalised, one can recognise that the former pluralistic and elaborated discussion (e.g., of the women's movement), where many different voices were heard, has progressively been reduced to a (philosophical) academic debate. But, since these techniques will affect all of us, we should expand the discussion again.

Hille Haker stressed the necessity of distinguishing between the biopolitical and bioethical discussion. *Regine Kollek* argued that this can be made from an analytical perspective but, in practice, a distinction can hardly be established (e.g., because of personal union). Her critique rather aims at biopolitics, although she experienced a streamlining effect of argumentation in and through the academic discourse.

Anders Nordgren wondered whether Regine Kollek had ambitions to make the debate on ART more objective by the sociological contribution or whether this account was intended to be completely critical? *Regine Kollek* claimed to aim for objectivity as far as possible, but she regarded it necessary to highlight significant points in modern technology, which cannot always be objective. Therefore, her goal was not primarily objectivity. On the question as to how the sociological account specifically differs from the bioethical debate, she answered that the question was not how we should live but how we do live and what are the motives of our actions. The social dynamics can be described better following this and rules for living together formulated more adequately, as they are characterised by contradictions and paradoxes. Therefore, as ethicists, we should refuse the image of being the ones to decide on right or wrong.

Hub Zwart argued against referring to such an image of bioethics. The role of an ethicist is not to say what is allowed or not but to show all the aspects and developments as well as contradictions and paradoxes arising in the context of moral problems. *Regine Kollek*, however, doubted this to be the dominant view of bioethics.

The question about the use of Kollek's investigations concerning practical decisions if only negative consequences are discussed and positive aspects and possibilities are not mentioned was raised by *Inga Hanschel*. *Regine Kollek* pointed out that she had mentioned the benefits (e.g., that the new techniques may, e.g., overcome infertility problems). But she was more concerned about the problems that technicalisation entails, and especially the problems that women have to face in this context. A dramatic change in our basic perception of pregnancy, etc., has occurred, and we hardly understand its dimensions yet.

Janusz Balicki pointed out that there is a difference in the debate between Europe and the USA. Women are asked for egg donation in the USA. To demonstrate this, he showed an overhead transparency of an advertisement offering $5,000 (up to $30,000 has already been offered) as compensation for the time and effort involved in donating eggs. Whether this amount compensated for the effort was questioned by *Hille Haker,* and *Ian Cooke* stated that this was difficult to assess, since there was a risk of infertility. However, this might change as technology develops. Replying to questions concerning the risks of egg donation, and whether hormone stimulation was included, he stressed that the treatment is comparable to normal IVF treatment. Nothing is definitely known about long term cancer risks. Clinical studies are not available and require at least 20 years.

As clinicians are responsible to families that ask for genetic counselling, *Karin Bengtsson* pointed out that the consequences of information about health for the social structure of these families have to be considered. She argued that the cases of families with a known disease and families newly confronted with genetic knowledge about themselves are different. Emphasising the importance of this point, *Ian Cooke* said that greater technical understanding in the public should be promoted to avoid or reduce overestimation of the technical potential of pre-implantation genetic diagnosis. *Regine Kollek* elaborated on the distinction suggested by Karin Bengtsson. If members of families with a known disease get a negative test result, this could result in some sort of 'survivor guilt'. However, if the test is positive, the affected individuals have the demanding task of imagining that they will be suffering from the disease. There are many studies of people imagining genetic knowledge about themselves. There is a need for

320

psychological counselling, so that people are supported in coping with positive test results. Stressing that she did not want to overestimate the possibilities of genetics, she tried to show what the public thinks about these possibilities (intelligence genes, etc.). The public cannot understand complex statistical results. It is hard for a 'serious' geneticist to counteract media releases from less serious scientists. Disillusioning the public would be expensive—no resources for that are available. How are we supposed to deal with misinformation? The dynamics of the scientific system also complicate matters. Scientists should be modest about what can be done (they have to state modest results) but they cannot be modest in applying for research funding.

Darren Shickle stressed the role of the commercial sector, since it raises the aspirations of the public. What expectations do people have who ask for genetic counselling? As extensive research in this area has not taken place yet, *Regine Kollek* referred to interviews with couples that showed that they were interested in specific genes when there is a known disease. In a 'no-risk-family' people would not go for genetic testing because of trivial reasons. But, with increasing knowledge (which would come from the human genome project) and available tests, it might be applied in a wider range—even on non-disease traits.

Arguing that every method has risks and benefits, *Ian Cooke* pointed out that the risk/benefit ratio is now only positive for severe diseases. But that might change if the risks become so low that it would be worth undergoing genetic testing for more trivial reasons. *Regine Kollek* argued that this applies to other techniques as well. For instance, progress in techniques like egg cell maturation *in vitro,* or storage of egg cells (e.g., from dead persons) might change this cost (or risk)/benefit ratio of IVF treatment in the future. Anticipation of future developments is important for moral reasoning in the bioethical debate. At the moment, there is no adequate freezing method for egg cells. However, Chinese scientists have found a method to grow several egg cells from one follicle. This may facilitate cloning of human embryos and generation of embryonic stem cells. There is an interesting potential in this technology. This, again, links to the debate on the moral status of embryos. To generate embryonic stem cells is not reproductive cloning, but we, nevertheless, do create embryos for tissue culture and stem cell culture (at present). *Ian Cooke* made clear that it is relevant to take into account that embryonic stem cells can be differentiated into entirely new tissues and these tissues cannot be considered human embryos. Therefore, the status of the derivatives needs to be discussed.

In the investigation of embryonic stem cells, *Farhan Yazdani* saw the possibility of scientific compliance with ethical demands resulting from the debate on the moral status of the embryo. The new techniques would not only result in reducing the risks for the mother, but also in a reduction of embryo freezing and research.

Regine Kollek, finally, said that it might become possible to create *in vitro* systems of differentiation and de-differentiation (cloning) without the need to create an embryo.

Robert Mordacci stated that the central question concerned the concept of life, since the role of health and, therefore, the ideal of perfection in our lives should not be overemphasised. Autonomy seems to be a principle in which we give up the task, as bioethicists, to try to design an image of life that is not a technological one. Autonomy in bioethics is not a Kantian autonomy. *Hub Zwart* criticised this concept of autonomy and technological control as being unrealistic: certain forms of control are introduced and increased. Also, technology increases not only control but also dependency (e.g., dependency upon experts).

This raised, according to *Christiane Woopen,* the question of how science, politics and society should discuss the problems of new genetic technologies. *Regine Kollek* suggested that it will take time to sort out the important arguments and to bring the discussion into the public arena. It is necessary to involve as many people as possible if we want knowledge and decision making to be pluralistic.

Discussion of *Moral reasoning in applied ethics*

summarised by Annika Thiem

In the discussion of *Marcus Düwell's* paper 'Moral Reasoning in Applied Ethics' and of the comments on it by *Paul van Tongeren* and *Roberto Mordacci,* the main concern was the relation between hermeneutical ethics/ethics of the good life and normative ethics, and the meaning of this relation with respect to concrete situations.

Deryck Beyleveld started by criticising Mordacci's 'thin concept of action', because in Gewirthian theory (which Marcus Düwell broadly espouses) 'one is talking not only about all of the things that are necessary for the possibility of action at all but also about those things that are necessary for the possibility of successful action.' Therefore, the Gewirthian concept of action corresponds with the structure of needs as presented in Maslow's *psychology of need*. Though the concepts of 'law', 'ethics' and 'morality' may be differentiated, Beyleveld considered this only a 'semantic' differentiation, which is not relevant for the debate. The decisive questions are: a) Are there any categorically binding obligations on us? and b) Are there any categorically binding obligations on us to respect the interests of persons other than ourselves? Transcendental arguments, of the kind presented in Kantian and Gewirthian theory, are necessary if obligations are to be justified *as* categorically binding.

Marcus Düwell contended that a distinction between law and morality is relevant in relation to enforcement of obligations. Not all moral obligations should and can be legally enforced. The importance of understanding a moral concept becomes clear when considering, for instance, the concept of shame. For someone to feel ashamed, the presupposition that one's behaviour was wrong is necessary. This means that the moral concept of shame implies the ability of self-reflection and a concept of what 'right and wrong' means, otherwise the phenomenon 'shame' would lose its meaning.

Christiane Woopen suggested that the question then concerns the relationship between rights/duties and values, and whether rights secure values. Consideration of this includes deciding whether ethics concerns the question of a successful life, or rather, under which conditions we are entitled to which rights.

Marcus Düwell, however, doubted that the alternative ethics of rights *versus* ethics of the good life really exists. Ethics of the good life is concerned with working out these conditions, while the normative level can only be reached and secured by an ethics of rights and duties.

Hille Haker identified the pivot of the discussion at this point as the relationship between something that is binding in a certain practice in a certain context and something that is universally or categorically binding on the other hand. She suggested that three different concepts had been put forward in the discussion so far. Paul van Tongeren presented the concept of a sphere of morality in which hermeneutic mediation is necessary. Within this sphere, normative force is possible, yet it is still one sphere. The notion Marcus Düwell proposed is one of a *separation* of the two spheres of the good life and of the categorically binding force of normative ethics. The third concept, which Roberto Mordacci indicated in his comment, and which she herself would support, is a distinction between two spheres that does not separate them. However, this distinction does not rule out the possibility of blendings, overlappings and oppositions of categorically normative force and morally concrete normative force in certain contexts. The problem becomes more concrete when considering, for instance, parenthood as a practice, which Onora O'Neill brought out as a highly important issue. Concerning parenthood as a practice, there are certain conditions of excellence, of virtue, which determine what it means to be a good or good-enough parent in specific traditions. As long as the tradition remains unchanged, these concepts and meanings are stable. Nowadays, however, the problem is that we perceive a radical change. In relation to their children, there might be parental duties that have never even been perceived before and which endanger unconditioned acceptance, the 'concept of the given child', as Onora O'Neill called it. This means that we are confronted with a normative problem, and in moral theory there a decision must be made between the three possible concepts.

Paul van Tongeren suggested a concept of one sphere in which different *levels* exist. The assumption of two spheres does not seem to be sensible, because if there are categorical imperatives they still need to be interpreted in order to know what they mean and with this interpretation the problems start. Therefore, if concepts in the normative sphere are meaningless until they are drawn into the hermeneutical sphere, a differentiation between two levels in one sphere is to be preferred over the two spheres model. Marcus Düwell's suggestion appears to be problematic, because, in his model, if there are no categorical imperatives, if there is no normative ethics, then there is hardly anything morally relevant left. Marcus Düwell allows all kinds of ethics of the good life, but only as a kind of an appendix to normative ethics, which has to come first. Paul van Tongeren interpreted the level of the categorical as present in the hermeneutical sphere, as a point of reference in hermeneutical dialogue. In discussions about the right interpretation of norms, values, virtues, etc., people refer to a true answer to the question. So the idea of truth, the idea of a true answer, which no-one has, but everyone is searching for, is the categorical in the hermeneutical sphere.

Roberto Mordacci perceived an agreement on the fact that there is something categorical in ethics, in moral experience. It comes from an analysis of moral experience and from trying to find out what the precondition of any moral experience is. Whatever is necessary for any moral action is categorically binding. In this way, rights might identify what is categorically binding and the hermeneutical task is to find out the concrete contextual meaning of a right. Thus, rights have the function of protecting the possibility that human life can have a meaning. Rather than protecting the agent, rights safeguard the meaning that is embedded in the agent's action.

Returning to a more concrete question regarding the relation of anthropology and ethics, *Dietmar Mieth* stressed that, at the beginning of his paper, Marcus Düwell gave an interpretation of a stage of the early embryo's development. There, he referred to the concept of identity. This, however, is already an anthropological interpretation, since anthropology involves interpreting the relevant phenomena. According to Dietmar Mieth, Marcus Düwell also necessarily evaluated the concrete meaning of words like 'acting' or 'protection' to end up with a sensible concept of moral reasoning. This evaluation then proves to be nothing other than interpretation. The problem of with Gewirthian theory is, then, that it starts with a very thin concept of action and the *PGC* ('act in accord with the generic rights of your recipients as well as of yourself') refers to freedom and well-being as necessary goods, and a hierarchy of goods is established. The questions arising at that point concern what exactly a certain good is and what acting in accord/respect means? Therefore, interpretation is essential. There seems to be no possibility of reaching the content of this principle without the work of hermeneutics. Hermeneutical reflection on the normative foundation is absolutely necessary for moral reasoning, otherwise the normative concepts cannot be controlled. The dialogue on obligations emerges whenever there are conflicting interpretations.

Marcus Düwell proposed that there are two dimensions where hermeneutics is important. The first dimension is trying to understand the world and the experiences in it. He referred to the example of giving lectures on bioethics to people outside the community of scientific discourse. The questions that are raised there concern the technologies and the respects in which they change our lives and then how this has to be interpreted. The other dimension, which is the subject of this discussion, is the one concerning the internal relation between the features of the *PGC* and its application, which is a complex process. Each concrete moral judgment also depends on some knowledge about the world, about human life and so on. However, the normative force of a moral judgment only comes from moral reasoning. In this process of moral reasoning, hermeneutics is not directly inherent.

Eve-Marie Engels re-averted to the concept of shame, since Marcus Düwell said that 'the concept of shame presupposes a normative ethics'. However, this is not the case, although 'it does presuppose some kind of cultural context where there are norms'. The concept of shame also works with a descriptive system of ethics. The norms of a society are described simply as the evaluation of the norms and the actions of persons. Therefore, a person can feel ashamed, even though, as a member of another society, he or she would not feel ashamed. A reconciliation of the dichotomies between deontological ethics and ethics of the good life has to be reached by looking for mixed strategies.

Furthermore, she suggested that the term 'applied ethics' has two meanings. First, it can denote the application of certain norms to solve specific problems in practice and to justify our actions in the concrete situation. Second, it can also mean something for which the term 'application orientated ethics' should be used, because 'applied ethics' implies that the concepts that have to be applied are already known. The situation of bioethics proves to be a situation in which we discover that, when we try to apply them, traditional concepts do not work any longer. This is equivalent to the notion of a reflective equilibrium between ethics, as normative ethics on the one hand, and concrete cases on the other (such as whether we are already dealing with an embryo in the biological sense or a pro-embryo or something else). Then there has to be a mediation between the two levels.

Marcus Düwell clarified the point he wanted to make about the phenomenon of shame. By reflecting and becoming aware that we cannot be sure about the normative quality of our cultural beliefs, we reach a level of uncertainty about whether we need to feel ashamed or not. Therefore, deeper reflection on the phenomenon of shame necessarily leads to the problem of normative ethics.

Suggesting a completely theoretical meaning for the term 'ethics', Marcus Düwell proposed not to call a concrete decision-making process 'applied ethics'. Ethics is reflection on morality and moral phenomena. Nevertheless, ethics is part of the process of decision-making. What is applied are normative frameworks and whereas, on the one hand, there has to be reasoning for the normative conditions in meta-ethics, normative concepts, which were worked out for the concrete situation, have also to be related, on the other. These are the two dimensions of applied ethics.

According to *Deryck Beyleveld,* the main concern is with this process of applying the normative concept in order to make a decision in a concrete situation. If we want to use the *PGC* to decide what we may do in some concrete situation, we first need a justification of this principle as the principle to be used. Then, if we have what we consider to a satisfactory justification for what purports to be a categorically binding principle, we will try to apply it to yield a categorically binding decision about action in a concrete situation. Understanding the *PGC* involves understanding certain inherent abstract categories, such as the concept of action, the concept of basic, non-substractive and additive needs, the various concepts of necessity and degrees of needfulness. These provide more than an abstract form for the principle, as they provide a structured set of criteria for using that particular principle, which are justified in the process of justifying the principle. However, to use the principle, *judgments* are necessary about whether objects in the real world, in the concrete situation, correspond to the abstract or the ontological concepts of the theory. Thus, application of the *PGC* requires some kind of perceptual or empirical judgment, and *interpretation* is necessarily involved in judgment connected to perception.

To further an understanding of 'interpretation', *Dietmar Mieth* provided the way we encounter an embryo as an example. At first, it is perceived as a developing human being. Then, this interpretation can be confronted with an ethical theory, from which a decision regarding acting finally emerges. An anthropological understanding has to precede the presentation of an ethical theory to be applied to it. Another example is provided by the question that Marcus Düwell also raised in his paper by stating that interpreting biological data leads us to perceive breaks in the development of the embryo. But, on the contrary, there is continuity and no break, since the break was a question of the signification coming from both sides, a biological-empirical side and a non-ethical but hermeneutical side, and it is related to a concept of identity and individuality. This means that there are two different interpretations, which have to be discussed in order to come to a decision on them. However, this conflict of interpretations cannot be solved by Gewirth.

Ruth Landau interjected that theories do not exist for their own sakes. Theories exist to solve problems, and their usefulness is to be measured by their ability to deal with all the information concerning the concrete situation in which the problem arises.

The problem, for *Darren Shickle,* was that, in certain situations, we may already have a solution in mind that we would prefer, so we are inclined to pick a particular theory because it will give us the answer we want.

However, consistency is important, which we have to be aware of in practice, due to the idea we have that morality is categorically binding.

Farhan Yazdani argued that a consensus among philosophers on issues of application, as discussed during the conference, could only be reached by also involving 'technicians' in the discourse. To technicians like himself—since he is a surgeon—ethics is a matter of practice and less of 'theoretical morality'. Ethics, in medical practice, is more concerned with concrete problem solving, and back in the 1860s the French physiologist Claude Bernard emphasised the 'sacred union' between science and philosophy. Since the dialogue between philosophers and technicians has now become vital, this exchange should take place within a multidisciplinary setting where expert considerations should be directly grounded in practical issues and the vocabulary should be adapted to the understanding of all participants.

Pre-implantation Genetic Diagnosis — Points to Consider[1]

Dietmar Mieth, in collaboration with Sigrid Graumann and Hille Haker

1 Introduction

In recent years, pre-implantation genetic diagnosis (PGD) has become an important topic in biomedical ethics.

The discussion is extremely complex and the related ethical problems are many-layered. Because the group of persons affected by PGD is quite small (e.g., in Germany about 50 couples), there has been no widespread discussion of the topic. Consequently, no public consensus has been reached on an ethical evaluation of PGD.

With this background it seems difficult to identify, co-ordinate and focus on individual problem areas. This is also evident in attempts to deal with legal and regulatory aspects of PGD on the national and European levels.

We would like, first, to present a list of points to consider, which have originated from an analysis of the PGD ethical discussion to date and the work of the *European Network for Biomedical Ethics.* Consideration of these reference points, we believe, is absolutely essential for further reflection on and evaluation of PGD. Second, the ethical controversy at different levels will be more thoroughly described and sketched in reference to ethical substantiation. Third, the consequences of European standardisation of the legal regulation of PGD will be specified. The points to consider presented here should give form to the discussion, but not prejudice it.

2 Points to consider relevant to the ethical reflection on and the evaluation of pre-implantation diagnosis

2.1 Empirical basis for evaluation

A relatively large part of clarifying questions relating to any technical evaluation are questions about facts. Accordingly, the ethical discussion of

PGD brings up a long list of scientific, medical, sociological, (health) economic and legal questions. These question must be answered empirically and must be clearly separated from normative questions. The clarification of empirical-descriptive and prognostic questions is essential as a factual basis for the ethical evaluation of PGD. The following must be clarified:

- The development of the human embryo (of upmost importance in the German discussion is how long embryonic cells are totipotent).
- Indications for PGD, including the likelihood of expected changes to, or widening of the indications for, the technique.
- Success and failure rate of PGD, including the prognosis for future improvement.
- Success rate of IVF in connection to PGD (baby take home rate).
- Effects of PGD (and IVF) on the physical and psychological well-being of the future child.
- Physical and psychological stress from PGD (and IVF) and PND on the women concerned (for the ethical discussion, a comparison of methods is eminently relevant).
- The public acceptance of PGD (and PND).
- Attitudes of those affected toward PGD (and PND), as well as attitudes of patient organisations.
- Attitudes of concerned professionals (reproduction physicians, human geneticists, possibly counsellors, psychologists, and others) toward PGD (and PND).
- Psycho-social changes due to PGD (and PND) (attitudes toward illness, the handicapped and sexuality).
- Socio-cultural changes due to PGD (and PND) (cultural values that are connected to motherhood and parenthood, cultural assertion of wishes for new possibilities and perfection).
- Cost analysis of PGD for health systems (a European and international comparison is needed).
- Economic implications of PGD.
- Current direct and indirect legal regulation of PGD (a European and international comparison is, again, needed).

Empirical and prognostic studies that would help to answer questions in the ethical discussion of PGD are available for only a few of the above mentioned points. It is, therefore, likely that these questions will either be ignored, which would lead to an impermissibly narrowed perspective, or that many aspects of the discussion will be based on speculation. Empirical studies in the above mentioned areas belong indirectly to ethical reflection, because they are essential to the ethical evaluation.

330

2.2 Social options

PGD, like biomedicine generally, must be seen in the context of modern society, which is characterised by pluralism. General value systems have lost their ability to integrate. They have been largely replaced by differing options which, however, have been only partially subjected to explicit discussion. In the PGD context, several options are open for discussion. Some of these options have been partially accepted without question, others have been favoured with reservations, and still others have led to controversy. To gain clarity by identifying points of agreement and disagreement is an important part of the ethical discussion.

- How can the relationship between the option that respects individual autonomy and the option for social solidarity be determined?
- What importance does the option have that tries to avoid genetically related suffering as well as the burdens resulting from it?
- How does that relate to the option that stands for the protection of exposed and vulnerable human beings?
- What importance does the option for progress through PGD development and application have?
- This option operates on the assumption that the potential to solve the problem is greater than the problematic implications of the solution.
- How does this relate to the option that avoids techniques that, when they spread, appear to be uncontrollable?
- What importance does the option have that tries to recognise non-technical alternatives (renunciation of reproduction, self limitation)?

Sometimes these options overlap or exclude each other. They are a mirror of a society's values, values that are effective but not necessarily grounded in reason. These, too, are an indirect part of the ethical reflection. However, the aim of an ethical evaluation must be to question the effects and implications of these options and to substantiate them.

2.3 Anthropological questions

The relationship between ethics and anthropology is important for biomedical research, although still unclear. For example, formal and weak anthropological arguments are used as presuppositions for ethical approaches that bind the respect and dignity of a person to his or her capacity to be a moral agent and/or to have interests. However, anthropological elements might have a central relevance in ethical reflection and evaluation, independent of such narrow perspectives. For instance, the search for happiness or the avoidance of suffering in the utilitarian ethical tradition is understandable only in the light of strong anthropological assumptions.

Anthropological assumptions that are used in ethical reasoning must be explained. Nevertheless, anthropology is not only to be developed from a biological description of ontogenesis, but should be understood as philosophical anthropology, which attempts to understand and interpret man independently of practical interests or ethical implications. Philosophical anthropology tries to interpret human genesis. As such, it must give a philosophical interpretation of continuity in human life. Its task is to define the concept of 'being a person' even beyond ethical relevance. Furthermore, it must explain the anthropological connotations of the concept of 'dignity.'

2.4 Normative questions

The introduction, development and use of new techniques in the medical field involve many people who have different options, or rights and responsibilities. We must differentiate among these people and judge the normative importance of their respective actions. Especially in the context of reproductive medicine, the persons affected by actions are to be specified and their rights respected. In order to judge PGD, the following points must be considered.

- The interpretation of the embryo's moral status: to protect the embryo in the various reproductive techniques in terms of urgency, efficiency and practical handling.
- The interpretation of the right to reproductive self-determination (meaning the right to reject any regimentation or secondly, to claim the best possible medical and technical support).
- The interpretation of protection and advancement of the public welfare.
- The interpretation of questions of equal opportunities (meaning equal access, avoidance of discrimination, and distributive justice in relation to the public health system and other social goods).

The rights and responsibilities are partially complementary or exclude each other, which calls for a substantiated interpretation. This discussion forces ethics back to fundamental questions, on the one hand in relation to the validity of a particular right, on the other hand in relation to the weighing of rights, which are on different levels.

332

3 Unsolved problems of evaluation that refer back to fundamental ethical questions

3.1 The embryo status controversy

The moral status of the human embryo is at the heart of ethical evaluation in biomedical research in the reproduction field. Protection of the human embryo can, therefore, be understood as the intersection point in the discussion of the social options and the specific normative questions. To reach a consensus on this question is very difficult, because many differing value backgrounds must be considered. Until now, there is no normative ethical theory that could serve as an anchor of consensus.

Therefore, it is necessary to reflect on the *special worth of protecting* the early embryo. The corporeality of the embryo is a prerequisite of continuity, which must be considered an anthropological determination of human life. Natural loss, which is often used as an argument against continuity, is not a valid argument, because the worth of protection is not affected by it. There is no normative difference in the worth of protecting the embryo whether it be inside or outside the womb.

Second, in the light of reproduction techniques, it is necessary to question the *urgency of protection* in the area of assisted reproduction. Even if each individual embryo cannot be protected, how such protection can generally be guaranteed must be specified. This is less of a problem for embryo development *in utero*. Even in the moral debate on abortion, embryo protection is considered in the situative need to balance it against the woman's rights, and therefore considered in a context of a direct moral conflict. Only since embryos *in vitro* have become available, has embryo protection become a question in itself.

Third, there must be a clarification of the *efficiency of protection*. That includes an exact investigation of the consequences of different options, as laid down in the different legal protection regulations.

Fourth, there is the question of *practical handling of the embryo* in the given context. Two inconsistencies must be avoided. First, it must be substantiated that, and how much, differing normative judgments concerning embryos (inside and outside the womb, reproductive and non-reproductive) exclude discrimination of one embryo against the other. Second, the morally relevant differences in different stages of human development must be judged according to the attribute 'dignity.' A 'tentative production' of human embryos treats them as objects, which seems incompatible with the moral injunction of dignity.

3.2 The controversy over the importance and scope of procreative self determination

The discussion about regulating abortion made the public aware of moral paternalism. Following the debate, a negative right to reproduction prevailed. This right was based on the future parents' personal values and their right to decide. Procreative self determination prohibits direct or indirect coercion in deciding or acting upon the use of medical possibilities in the area of sensitive reproductive decisions and coercion to hinder reproduction. This negative right does not, however, release future parents from their moral responsibility to make decisions on reproductive issues.

A liberal interpretation of procreative self determination endorses a positive right to institutional support of reproduction. Concretely, this endorses the claim to have one's own child, or the claim to have a child who does not have certain characteristics. But, even such a liberal interpretation of procreative self determination has limits. The well-being of the future child ('proxy consent' measured according to the best interest standard) must be taken into consideration and the use of the embryo as an object must be excluded.

3.3 The controversy over the relationship between individual welfare and public welfare

It is not possible to deal exhaustively with normative questions by only weighing individual interests and rights. The normative interpretation of public welfare, even if difficult in a pluralistic society, emphasises, in addition to the principles of distributive justice and equal treatment, the necessity of an institutional framework. Its function would be to enable the individual to act autonomously and morally justifiably. The psycho-social and socio-cultural shifts in values brought about by reproductive medicine and the engineering progress in reproduction must also be taken into account.

3.4 Fundamental ethical questions

To answer the question of how normative controversies are to be decided (such as how rights at different levels can be weighed against one another, or how a hierarchy of values can be set up) fundamental ethical theories are necessary. These theories must be founded in moral claims on the one hand, but at the same time place the ethical aspects of a particular context in the larger picture of ethical judgments. This would inevitably lead to various solutions stemming from the different ethical theories.

The ethical discussion of PGD would not take up this problem in general, but in close connection to the biomedical context. It is worth trying to characterise the points of agreement in the various theories, as well as the points of disagreement. In the ideal case, a measure of success would be achieved by formulating some binding standards that could be accepted as valid by different ethical theories.

4 Legal regulation

On the one hand, legal regulations must not contradict binding standards. On the other hand, they must be democratically authorised. The controversial ethical aspects of PGD require the setting of political and legal priorities. Such priority setting is already visible in current direct and indirect regulation of PGD in connection with different national legal traditions.

- An extensive guarantee of embryo protection in criminal law. Here, the basic prohibition of PGD is valid because of the injunction against treating human life as an object (Germany).
- Tolerant regulation. Here the individual choices, as well as scientific progress, are given special attention. Legal regulation formulates limits on the development and application of PGD by strict regulation of indications, binding to special centres or clinics, accompanying genetic counselling, and examination by a ethics commission (France).
- Liberal regulation. Here licensing for the development and application of PGD is valid. Licensing is granted on the condition of strict adherence to medical goals (prohibition of basic research), procedural standards and quality control (United Kingdom).
- Absence of any institutional regulation (Italy, Greece).

Any efforts to standardise European regulation of PGD (or more generally reproductive biomedicine) must take account of differing national legal traditions as well as binding normative standards and ethical controversy. Also in connection with this goal, laws must grant points of ethical consensus a legally binding status. Furthermore, the integration of public debate and regulation regarding new developments in biomedicine (like PGD) should be striven for on the European level. In order to name points of agreement and disagreement, the above mentioned points to consider must be thoroughly discussed throughout Europe.

Note

[1] This text was published prior to the Sheffield conference and discussed during this meeting. See *Biomedical Ethics* Vol. 3, No. 3, 1998. The original text has been subjected to very minor editing.